# Good Practices in
# Health Financing

# Good Practices in Health Financing

## Lessons from Reforms in Low- and Middle-Income Countries

*Pablo Gottret, George J. Schieber, and Hugh R. Waters*
Editors

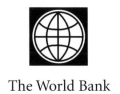

The World Bank

ISBN-13: 978-0-8213-7511-2
eISBN-13: 978-0-8213-7512-1
DOI: /10.1596/978-0-8213-7511-2

**Library of Congress Cataloging-in-Publication Data**

Good practice in health financing : lessons from reforms in low and middle-income countries / Pablo Gottret, George J. Schieber, and Hugh R. Waters, coeditors.
  p. ; cm.
  Includes bibliographical references and index.
  ISBN-13: 978-0-8213-7511-2 (alk. paper)
  ISBN-10: 0-8213-7511-3 (alk. paper)
1. Medical care—Developing countries—Finance. 2. Health care reform—Economic aspects—Developing countries 3. Medical policy—Economic aspects—Developing countries. 4. Medical care, Cost of—Developing countries. 5. Health status indicators—Developing countries. I. Gottret, Pablo E. (Pablo Enrique), 1959- II. Schieber, George. III. Waters, Hugh. IV. World Bank.
  [DNLM: 1. Health Care Reform—economics—Statistics. 2. Health Care Reform—standards—Statistics. 3. Delivery of Health Care—economics—Statistics. 4. Developing Countries—Statistics. 5. Health Care Costs—Statistics. 6. Health Expenditures—Statistics. WA 530.1 G646 2008]
  RA395.D44G66 2008
  362.1'04252091724—dc22
                    2008008389

Cover design by Rock Creek Creative.

# Contents

### Boxes

### Figures

### Tables

# Foreword

With health at the center of global development policy, the international community and developing countries are focused on scaling up health systems, in line with the Millennium Development Goals (MDGs). As a result, both global aid and individual country health reform plans are geared to improving health outcomes, securing financial protection against impoverishment, and ensuring long-term, sustainable financing to support these gains. However, with the scaling up of aid, both donors and countries have come to realize that more money alone cannot buy health improvements or prevent impoverishment due to catastrophic medical bills.

Well-targeted health spending is critical for success—including international donor aid to help in achieving sustainable results in the long term. These concerns have triggered a major debate over the need to define "results" and assemble appropriate data for decision making, monitoring, and evaluation. Central to this endeavor is the need for an analytically sound evidence base on national health financing policies that have "performed well" in terms of improving health outcomes and financial protection. Unfortunately, for want of solid evidence to inform policy makers, the policy debate is often driven by ideological, one-size-fits-all solutions.

This book attempts to partially fill the void by systematically assessing health financing reforms in nine low- and middle-income countries that have demonstrated "good performance" in expanding their populations' health insurance coverage—to both improve health status and protect against catastrophic medical expenses. Good performance also includes average or better-than-average population health outcomes relative to resources devoted to health and to national income and educational levels.

Among the low- and middle-income countries that are in the process of achieving high levels of population coverage and financial protection, nine were selected as examples of good performance by an expert steering committee representing all six World Bank Regions. They are Chile, Colombia, Costa Rica, Estonia, the Kyrgyz Republic, Sri Lanka, Thailand, Tunisia, and Vietnam. Each country case is analyzed using a standardized taxonomy that captures the key health and nonhealth sector–specific factors affecting the performance of its health financing system. Because this study relies only on post-reform information, experiments with control groups or randomization are not possible. Thus no effort is made to attribute causality. However, based on the country studies, an attempt is made to identify the common enabling factors evident in most of the cases.

The factors identified in the study make sense on conceptual grounds and would be likely hypotheses for any rigorous evaluation of the impacts of health financing changes. While these findings are interesting, their more important contribution is demonstrating that the global community must do a much better job of defining and documenting "good performance" and evaluating and disseminating the global evidence base.

To do this, at least five important actions need to be taken. First, what "good performance" means in health financing must be well defined. Second, standardized and appropriate qualitative and quantitative information must be collected. Third, health system characteristics must be described in enough detail so that the critical components and their interactions can be identified and assessed. Fourth, rigorous evaluations must be undertaken. Fifth, these evaluations—conducted in a policy-relevant and user-friendly manner—must be disseminated to all stakeholders.

In all these areas, the global community has done a rather poor job. With the growing importance of this issue, it is essential that both national and international decision makers and health policy analysts take charge and move this agenda forward. It is hoped that this volume in some small way can contribute to focusing the global health financing agenda in this direction.

Julian Schweitzer
Director, Health, Nutrition, and Population
The World Bank

# Acknowledgments

Many individuals contributed to making this report a reality. Part I was written by Lisa K. Fleisher, Pablo Gottret, Adam Leive, George J. Schieber, Ajay Tandon, and Hugh R. Waters. Part II was edited by Pablo Gottret, George J. Schieber, and Hugh R. Waters. The country case studies were prepared by country-based experts who have first-hand knowledge of the health financing and health coverage arrangements—and the history of health policy reforms—in their respective countries. The work was guided by a Steering Committee representing the World Bank's six regions. The Steering Committee in conjunction with the Health, Nutrition, and Population (HNP) unit of the Human Development Network developed criteria for the definition of a "good practice" and provided recommendations on the choice of country cases as well as appropriate experts to prepare the cases. The HNP unit, under the guidance of George Schieber, Pablo Gottret, and Hugh Waters (Johns Hopkins University), conceived and carried out this study. Ajay Tandon, Adam Leive, Lisa Fleisher, Valerie Moran, Emiliana Gunawan, Bjorn Ekman (Health Economics Program, Lund University, Sweden), and Axel Rahola (now an Adviser to the Minister of Budgeting, France) assisted in this work. The peer reviewers were Ruth Levine (Director of Programs and Senior Fellow, Center for Global Development), John Langenbrunner (Lead Health Economist, EASHD), and Christoph Kurowski (Senior Health Specialist, LCSHD). Toomas Palu provided extremely useful comments on the Estonia case study. Maureen Lewis chaired the review meeting and provided valuable comments. Kathleen A. Lynch (Editorial Consultant) provided critical editorial support.

The report was generously funded by the Swedish International Development Agency, which also provided for the technical support of Bjorn Ekman.

Other key individuals contributing to this initiative include:

*Case Study Authors*

Chile—Ricardo D. Bitrán and Urcullo C. Gonzalo, Bitrán & Asociados
Colombia—Diana Pinto, Fedesarrollo
Costa Rica—James Cercone and José Pacheco Jiménez, Sanigest Health Solutions

Estonia—Triin Habicht, Head of Health Economics Department, Estonian Health Insurance Fund; and Jarno Habicht, Head of WHO Country Office, World Health Organization Regional Office for Europe

The Kyrgyz Republic—Melitta Jakab, WHO Health Policy Advisor, the Kyrgyz Republic; and Elina Manjieva, WHO and Center for Health Systems Development, the Kyrgyz Republic

Sri Lanka—Ravi P. Rannan-Eliya and Lankani Sikurajapathy, Institute for Health Policy, Colombo, Sri Lanka

Thailand—Suwit Wibulpolprasert and Suriwan Thaiprayoon, Ministry of Health, Thailand

Tunisia—Chokri Arfa, National Institute of Labor and Social Studies, Tunisia; and Hédi Achouri, Director General of Public Health Facilities, Ministry of Public Health, Tunisia

Vietnam—Björn Ekman, Health Economics Program, Lund University, Sweden; and Sarah Bales, Health Policy Unit (HPU), Ministry of Health, Vietnam

*Steering Committee*

Paul Gertler (Former Chief Economist, Human Development Network, Professor of Economics, Haas School of Business, University of California, Berkley)

Robert Holzmann (Director, HDNSP)

Cristian Baeza (Lead Health Policy Specialist, LCSHD)

Kei Kawabata (Manager of Social Sector, IDB)

Akiko Maeda (Sector Manager, MNSHD)

Eduard Bos (Lead Population Specialist, HDNHE)

Alexander S. Preker (Lead Health Economist, AFTH2)

Peter Berman (Lead Health Economist, SASHD)

Adam Wagstaff (Lead Economist, ECSHD)

Mead Over (Lead Economist, ECSHD)

Abdo Yazbeck (Lead Health Economist, WBIHD)

Logan Brenzel (Senior Health Specialist, HDNHE)

John Langenbrunner (Lead Health Economist, EASHD)

Paolo Belli (Senior Health Economist, SASHD)

Mark Charles Dorfman (Senior Economist, HDNSP)

# Executive Summary

This volume focuses on nine countries that have completed, or are well along in the process of carrying out, major health financing reforms. These countries have significantly expanded their people's health care coverage or maintained such coverage after prolonged political or economic shocks (e.g., following the collapse of the Soviet Union). In doing so, this report seeks to expand the evidence base on "good performance" in health financing reforms in low- and middle-income countries. The countries chosen for the study were Chile, Colombia, Costa Rica, Estonia, the Kyrgyz Republic, Sri Lanka, Thailand, Tunisia, and Vietnam.

With health at the center of global development policy on humanitarian as well as economic and health security grounds, the international community and developing countries are closely focused on scaling up health systems to meet the Millennium Development Goals (MDGs), improving financial protection, and ensuring long-term financing to sustain these gains. With the scaling up of aid, both donors and countries have come to realize that money alone cannot buy health gains or prevent impoverishment due to catastrophic medical bills. This realization has sent policy makers looking for reliable evidence about what works and what does not, but they have found little to guide their search.

In 2004, the Center for Global Development published a seminal report, *Millions Saved: Proven Successes in Global Health*, which documented 17 public health interventions of "proven" effectiveness (Levine and Kinder 2004). A major contribution of the report was an explicit specification of criteria for defining "what works." The report was acclaimed as an important synthesis of the global evidence base on public health interventions.

Concomitantly, the global community and individual donors are looking closely at "results-based" aid, holistic approaches to health systems, and long-term sustainable financing. These concerns have triggered a major debate about the need to define "results" and assemble appropriate data for decision making, monitoring, and evaluation. Central to this endeavor is the need for effective, evidence-based national policies. Seminal work in areas including human resources for health, health systems, and health financing has shown that the critical evidence bases are often lacking (Joint Learning Initiative 2004; Gottret and Schieber 2006; Levine and Kinder 2004).

This study attempts to partially fill this void with assessments of reforms in low- and middle-income countries that have demonstrated good performance in expanding their people's health insurance coverage to improve their health status and protect them against catastrophic medical expenses. Coverage expansions are measured, to the extent possible, by the number of individuals covered, while financial protection is measured as the share of out-of-pocket payments in overall health spending or household consumption. Besides broadening coverage, these countries have achieved average or better-than-average population health outcomes—as measured, for example, by infant mortality rates, life expectancy, and maternal mortality rates—in relation to the resources devoted to health and their income and educational levels.

Among the few low- and middle-income countries that have almost achieved universal coverage and effective financial protection, nine—Chile, Colombia, Costa Rica, Estonia, the Kyrgyz Republic, Sri Lanka, Thailand, Tunisia, and Vietnam— were selected as examples of good performance by an expert steering committee representing all six World Bank Regions. Each country case is analyzed on a standardized taxonomy that captures most of the key health and nonhealth sector-specific factors affecting the performance of its health financing system. Because this study relies only on post-reform information, experiments with control groups or randomization are not possible. Thus, no attempt is made to attribute causality. In the discussion sections, some attempt is made to identify common enabling factors evident in most of the cases. However, as is noted subsequently, this is done more to provoke debate and generate hypotheses than to establish causality.

Of the selected cases, two countries—the Kyrgyz Republic and Vietnam—are classified by the World Bank as low income (i.e., with 2005 per capita GNI below US$875). Four countries—Costa Rica, Sri Lanka, Thailand, and Tunisia—are middle income (GNI of US$876 to US$3,465). Three countries—Chile, Colombia, and Estonia—are classified as upper middle income (GNI greater than US$3,466). All nine countries have immunization coverage rates above 88 percent. All but the Kyrgyz Republic have a life expectancy at birth above 70 years, and infant mortality rates below 25 per 1,000 live births. Most of them do well in terms of providing financial protection against high or catastrophic out-of-pocket payments. However, four of the countries—the three poorest (Kyrgyz Republic, Vietnam, Sri Lanka[1]) and Tunisia—perform less well, with out-of-pocket payments higher than 40 percent of all health spending.

Trying to generalize "enabling conditions" for good performance in health financing and coverage expansions from these nine case studies is difficult, particularly because these cases are hardly representative of all global experience and are not a random sample. To help contextualize and validate the findings, countries would have to be examined that do not have the same "conditions" and have demonstrated poor performance. Nevertheless, the cases selected do represent countries that have undertaken serious reforms and appear to have done well, based on the definitions of good performance used in this volume.

The key question is: as health reforms are very country-specific, can a common set of enabling conditions be found in these nine good performers, or is the conclusion simply that everything is so country-specific as to preclude generalizations? The paths taken by all these countries are clearly different and heavily contingent on each country's political economy and institutional arrangements. However, an analysis of expenditure, outcome, and demographic performance for these countries against global trends and the detailed case studies of each country reveals a number of general "enabling" conditions common to almost all of them.

## General "Enabling" Conditions

In most of the country cases several common institutional, societal, policy, and implementation characteristics are apparent. They are classified as follows:

- *Economic, institutional, and societal factors:* Strong and sustained economic growth; long-term political stability and sustained political commitment; a strong institutional and policy environment; and a well-educated population.
- *Policy factors:* financial resources committed to health, including private financing; commitment to equity and solidarity; health coverage and financing mandates; consolidation of risk pools; recognized limits to decentralization; and focus on primary care.
- *Implementation factors:* carefully sequenced health service delivery and provider payment reforms; good information systems and evidence-based decision making; strong stakeholder support; efficiency gains and copayments used as financing mechanisms; and flexibility and mid-course corrections.

These results, it might be argued, could have been posited without a study. However, the findings are based on a standardized definition of good performance in terms of expanded coverage and financial protection in countries that have achieved good health outcomes with average or below average spending and for most with little or no development assistance for health.

All the factors identified above make sense on conceptual grounds and would be likely hypotheses for any rigorous evaluation of the impacts of health financing changes. These findings are interesting, but their more important contribution is the evidence they present that the global community must do a much better job in defining "good performance" and evaluating and disseminating the global evidence base.

To do this, at least five important actions need to be taken. First, what good performance means in health financing must be rigorously defined. Second, standardized and appropriate qualitative and quantitative information must be collected. Third, health system characteristics must be described in enough detail so that the critical components and their interactions can be identified and assessed.

Fourth, rigorous evaluations must be undertaken. Fifth, these evaluations—conducted in a policy-relevant and user-friendly manner—must be disseminated to all stakeholders.

In all these areas, the global community has done a poor job. With the growing importance of this issue, it is incumbent on the global community to take charge and move this agenda forward. It is hoped that global stakeholders, through various aid-effectiveness forums, as well as the Group of Eight and Paris Declaration Process, will rise to the occasion and put this desperately needed work on track.

# Acronyms and Abbreviations

| | |
|---|---|
| ADB | Asian Development Bank |
| ARI | acute respiratory infection |
| BMI | body mass index |
| CCT | conditional cash transfer |
| CPI | Consumer Price Index |
| CPIA | Country Policy Institutional Assessment Index, World Bank |
| DALY | disability-adjusted life years |
| DDD | defined daily dose |
| DOTS | directly observed treatment shortcourse |
| DPT | diphtheria, pertussis, tetanus |
| DRG | diagnosis-related group |
| EAP | East Asia and Pacific Region, World Bank |
| ECA | Europe and Central Asia Region, World Bank |
| EPI | expanded program of immunization |
| EU | European Union |
| FDI | foreign direct investment |
| FSU | Former Soviet Union |
| G-8 | Group of Eight |
| GBD | global burden of disease |
| GFATM | Global Fund to Fight AIDS, Tuberculosis and Malaria |
| GHWA | Global Health Workforce Alliance |
| GNI | gross national income |
| HIPC | highly indebted poor country |
| HMN | Health Metrics Network |
| HNP | Health, Nutrition, and Population |
| HRH | human resources for health |
| IDB | Inter-American Development Bank |
| IEC | information, education, communication |
| IHP+ | Scaling up for Better Health |
| IMR | infant mortality rate |
| LAC | Latin America and Caribbean Region, World Bank |
| LIC | low-income country |

| | |
|---|---|
| MCH | Maternal and Child Health |
| MDGs | Millennium Development Goals, United Nations |
| MENA | Middle East and North Africa Region, World Bank |
| MHI | mandatory health insurance |
| MHIF | Mandatory Health Insurance Fund |
| MMR | maternal mortality rate |
| MOF | Ministry of Finance |
| MOH | Ministry of Health |
| NCD | noncommunicable disease |
| NGO | nongovernmental organization |
| NHA | National Health Accounts |
| NHS | National Health Service |
| ODA | overseas development assistance |
| OOP | out of pocket |
| PHC | primary health care |
| PPP | purchasing power parity |
| SHI | social health insurance |
| TFR | total fertility rate |
| U-5 | children under five years of age |
| UN | United Nations |
| UNDP | United Nations Development Programme |
| WDI | World Development Indicators |
| WHO | World Health Organization |
| WTO | World Trade Organization |

# Part I

# Assessing Good Practice in Health Financing Reform

*Lisa Fleisher, Pablo Gottret, Adam Leive,*
*George J. Schieber, Ajay Tandon, and Hugh R. Waters*

# 1

# Introduction

Many developing countries have recently undertaken ambitious health reforms to improve resource mobilization for health care. Their goals are universal health care coverage for their people and financial protection against impoverishment due to the costs of catastrophic illness. However, few low-income countries (LICs) or middle-income countries (MICs) have achieved universal coverage. The experiences of countries that have done so, though of great relevance to other low- and middle-income countries on the verge of similar reforms, have not been consistently evaluated and documented. To partially address this gap, the World Bank has prepared this report documenting experiences in financing significant expansions of health care coverage in low- and middle-income countries. The nine "good practice" countries selected as case studies are: Chile, Colombia, Costa Rica, Estonia, the Kyrgyz Republic, Sri Lanka, Thailand, Tunisia, and Vietnam.

Building the evidence base on health financing reforms is particularly important now, with health at the center stage of global development policy on humanitarian as well as global economic and health security grounds. The international community and developing countries themselves are increasingly focused on scaling up health systems to meet the United Nations' Millennium Development Goals (MDGs) and on providing financial protection through various risk-pooling mechanisms. Three of the MDGs directly pertain to health outcomes, but the first goal of halving extreme poverty is also relevant to this study, considering that out-of-pocket health expenditures are a major cause of impoverishment.

With the significant scaling up of aid, both donors and recipient countries have realized that money alone cannot buy results, and that development effectiveness matters. This realization has sent policy makers looking for reliable evidence about what works and what does not, but they have found little to guide them. The World Bank's new Health, Nutrition, and Population (HNP) strategy decries the lack of available evidence to assess whether billions of dollars of HNP lending over the previous decade have led to significant results (World Bank 2007b). A similar sentiment is expressed by Savedoff and Levine (2006) who argue that part of the reason for the lack of evidence is due to bureaucratic disincentives to conduct evaluations of policies and programs.

In 2004, the Center for Global Development published a seminal report on "Proven Successes in Global Health," which highlighted some 17 public health interventions of "proven" effectiveness (Levine and Kinder 2004). A major contribution of the report was an explicit specification of criteria for defining "what works," including the important element of large-scale implementation. The report was acclaimed as an important synthesis of the global evidence base on public health interventions.[1] Concomitantly, the global community and individual donors have been focusing closely on the need for results-based aid, financing, and lending.

These concerns have triggered a major debate and actions with respect to the need to define "results" and assemble appropriate data for decision making, monitoring, and evaluation. The recent creation of the Health Metrics Network (HMN) provides one example of global action to ensure availability of appropriate health information. Central to this venture is countries' need for knowledge about the global evidence base to implement effective, evidence-based policies. Seminal work in a number of areas including human resources for health, health systems, and health financing has shown that the critical evidence bases are often lacking (Joint Learning Initiative 2004; Gottret and Schieber 2006; Levine and Kinder 2004). For example, where is the comprehensive compilation of "successful" health financing reforms in developing countries?

The lack of such evidence-based policy collations reflects the complexities of the health sector, country and donor priorities, and the inherent difficulty of doing rigorous evaluations in the social sciences. Measuring health outcomes, other than sentinel events such as death, is methodologically difficult and complex, and collecting data is costly. Numerous health-related and non-health-related factors affect an individual's health status. Individual behavior is an important determinant of health outcomes—and difficult to measure and change (Schieber, Fleisher, and Gottret 2006). Figure 1.1 highlights the many different confounding factors that interact in the health-sector milieu. These complexities are exacerbated by the enormous number of interactive factors affecting most health policies.

In developing countries, lacking sufficient resources to meet many basic and often competing needs, it is not surprising that rigorous policy evaluation has not been a high priority. Similarly, in light of these needs, donors have focused their efforts on getting money out the door to assist countries dealing with catastrophic and unpredictable situations such as a tsunami or an avian flu outbreak. As a result, much of what passes for "evidence" is anecdotal and small scale: a box in a report indicating that in a particular health center or district a particular policy resulted in a particular outcome. Few rigorous evaluations are national in scope.[2]

In the health financing area, remarkably few single-country or multicountry studies have defined what is meant by a successful reform. Nor have they described the countries in question in a standardized way and with sufficient detail so that

**Figure 1.1 Determinants of Health, Nutrition, and Population Outcomes**

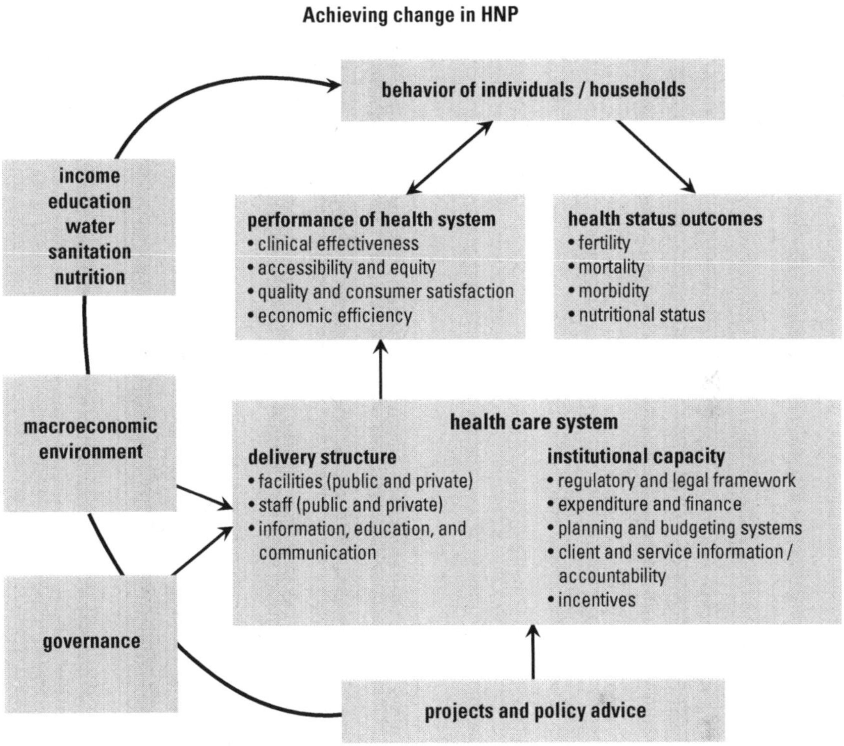

**Achieving change in HNP**

| behavior of individuals / households |

| income education water sanitation nutrition |

**performance of health system**
• clinical effectiveness
• accessibility and equity
• quality and consumer satisfaction
• economic efficiency

**health status outcomes**
• fertility
• mortality
• morbidity
• nutritional status

| macroeconomic environment |

**health care system**

**delivery structure**
• facilities (public and private)
• staff (public and private)
• information, education, and communication

**institutional capacity**
• regulatory and legal framework
• expenditure and finance
• planning and budgeting systems
• client and service information / accountability
• incentives

| governance |

**projects and policy advice**

*Source:* Wagstaff, Yazbeck, and Claeson 2004.

readers can understand the interplay of the many key factors, determine causality based on rigorous evaluation methods, and provide generalizable lessons for other countries.

The present study attempts to partially fill this void; however, it does not attempt to rigorously define "success," because failures are not defined or examined. Nor does it attempt to attribute causality in terms of what specific factors and interventions directly led to specific reform outcomes. Such comprehensive evaluations to determine successful reforms are not attempted for several reasons. The opportunity for randomized control trials to determine which policy reforms are best is rarely an option. Moreover, even good pre- and post reform evaluations are hampered by the lack of adequate baseline and follow-up data, especially since many reforms extend back for decades. The challenges involved in measuring inputs that are essential to such evaluations at the country level is underscored by the current debate over how to comprehensively institutionalize National Health Accounts (NHA) to monitor health spending patterns. In addition, measuring the breadth and depth of coverage and financial protection of the population is often difficult for lack of the necessary microdata. All of these conditions make systematic definition and evaluation of successful health reforms exceedingly problematic.

Instead, this study examines countries that have exhibited "good performance," defined in terms of coverage expansions, health outcomes, and financial protection compared with other countries with similar health spending and income levels. Financing reforms are discussed in terms of the three principal health financing functions of revenue collection, risk pooling, and purchasing, which, by assumption if effectively performed, will help achieve those objectives. The study then attempts to assess common enabling conditions for good performance. However, definitively identifying enabling conditions would require at least examining countries without such conditions, as well as those that have performed poorly with regard to the above measures, an evidence base that does not exist.

As discussed in chapter 3, nine country cases were selected by a steering committee from all six World Bank Regions. Good performers were defined as countries that have significantly increased the number of individuals covered, the depth of coverage in terms of the richness of the benefits package, and the level of financial protection. For countries that had universal coverage but have faced drastic political or economic shocks (e.g., former Soviet Union [FSU] countries), good performance is a reform that resurrects health sector revenues and expenditures and restores a benefits package to precrisis coverage and financial protection. Good performance is also implicitly based on the panel's normative judgment and on data demonstrating that these countries have attained average or better-than-average health outcomes (infant mortality, life expectancy, and maternal mortality) for their health spending and income levels. Although there are many other inputs to producing health outcomes, and health status changes cannot be attributed to health coverage expansions alone, such expansions are likely to have contributed to improvements in health status and financial protection.

Because this study relies only on existing postreform, secondary data in the nine countries, no experiments with control groups or randomization can be done. Therefore, no attempt is made to attribute causality. Moreover, due to data limitations, comparing pre- and post reform situations is limited. Each country case is described in detail, based on a standardized taxonomy that captures most key health- and non-health-sector specific factors affecting the performance of a health financing reform. Each country chapter includes a description of important background information and is organized so as to systematically address a core set of issues. However the emphasis given to the different points may vary across cases depending on the nuances of that case.

## Focal Points of the Case Studies

To facilitate understanding of the country-specific environments, detailed contextual information on underlying socioeconomic, institutional, political, and health sector characteristics are provided for each of the country cases. These include

- *The country's economic, institutional, social, and political environments. The implications of individual country's institutional structures cannot be understated and should be carefully described as part of the analysis and lessons learned.*
- *Descriptions, chronologies, assessments of reform motivations, and analysis of reforms to expand health care coverage.*
- *Overview of the health care delivery system. The breadth and depth of the benefits package.*
- *Financial protection and access to services for chronic and catastrophic conditions.*
- *Revenue sources.*
- *Health indicators, outcomes, and their distribution.*
- *Spending effectiveness.*
- *Financial sustainability of the reforms.*
- *Other key issues. These potentially include: how risk adjustment and cross-subsidization are handled; regulation of the insurance schemes; policies for opting out of insurance schemes; need for government subsidies; financing compared with depth of package (focus on "best buy"); impact on labor markets; other links between political economy and the health sector; cost-sharing mechanisms; and sustainability of financing.*
- *Scaling up the reforms.*
- *Key conditions for good performance.*
- *Lessons for other countries.*

In classifying countries by income, this study uses current World Bank definitions, based on 2005 estimates of gross national income (GNI) per capita (World Bank 2007a): low-income US$875 per capita or less; lower-middle-income, US$876 to US$3,465; upper-middle-income, US$3,466 to US$10,725; and high-income, US$10,726 or more.

The report is organized into two parts. Part I describes key issues in expanding health care coverage in low- and middle-income countries, defines what is meant by "good" performance in expansions of coverage and financial protection, discusses the criteria used to choose the country cases, and summarizes the findings from each of the nine country case studies. The concluding chapter of part I draws generalizable lessons from the country cases and provides some guidance for future efforts to enhance the global evidence base in health financing. The full set of country case studies is presented in part II.

## Audience

Governments and international policy makers, donors, staffs of stakeholder organizations, and health care analysts working in low- and middle-income countries are the target audience for this report. It is intended as a practical guide for decision makers in countries considering health financing and coverage reforms, as well as for World Bank operations teams, multilateral development organizations, bilateral aid agencies, private foundations, and other development partners. It is hoped that this modest attempt to assess good performance in major health financing changes will lead to more rigorous evaluations of such changes and important, much needed, systematic, multicountry contributions to the global evidence base.

## Endnotes

1. A recent update of the report includes three additional cases (Levine 2007).

2. Notable exceptions are the national health policy evaluations in Cambodia and Mexico. In Cambodia, different modalities of the health system reform were randomly allocated across districts and evaluated (Bhushan, Keller, and Schwartz 2002). In Mexico, the impact of conditional cash transfer programs was evaluated using a national phase-in controlled randomized design (Gertler 2004).

# 2

# Health Financing Functions

The expansion of health financing coverage is a prime focus of this report. To better understand what this entails, this chapter defines and clarifies some of the key health financing functions and concepts such as revenue generation, risk pooling, and purchasing and their importance to financial protection.

Health coverage has at least three separate and interrelated dimensions: (1) the number of people covered by organized (public and private) financing initiatives (*breadth of coverage*); (2) the extent (number and type) of services covered (*depth of coverage*); and (3) the resulting impacts on health outcomes and financial protection against high out-of-pocket expenditures. In expanding coverage to promote health outcomes and financial protection, countries need to

1. Raise *sufficient* and *sustainable* revenues *efficiently* and *equitably* to provide individuals with a basic package of essential services that both improves *health outcomes* and provides *financial protection* against unpredictable catastrophic or impoverishing financial losses caused by illness and injury.
2. Manage these revenues to *pool health risks equitably* and *efficiently* so that individuals are provided with "insurance" coverage against unpredictable catastrophic medical care costs.
3. Ensure the purchase of health services in an allocatively and technically *efficient* manner (Gottret and Schieber 2006; Mossialos et al. 2002).

The organization of the case studies in this report focuses on key health financing functions within country health care systems to meet these objectives.[1]

*Revenue collection* and *risk pooling* refer to the accumulation and management of sufficient and sustainable revenues to assure that all individuals have access to an essential package of basic services designed to improve health outcomes. These funds must be "pooled" so that the risk of large, catastrophic medical expenditures are borne collectively by all pool members and not by each member individually, thus providing all pool members with "insurance protection." Each pool member's "contribution" is prepaid through premiums, payroll taxes, and/or general tax payments.

The case studies span the range of generic health financing "models" such as national health services (NHS), mandatory health insurance (MHI) funds, and private health insurance. A simplified categorization of health insurance schemes is used here, including (1) general-tax financing, managed by an NHS or ministry of health (MOH); (2) payroll tax–financed MHI managed by a quasi-public entity; and (3) private sector–based health insurance financed by contributions to private voluntary insurers. Globally, some 100 countries have health financing systems that are predominantly financed from general taxes; another 60 have payroll tax–based MHI systems. Only a few countries have predominantly private health insurance financed systems (e.g., the United States). In practice most countries have mixed models.

Examples of high-income countries with MHI systems include Germany and Japan. Most systems based on an NHS have compulsory universal coverage financed from general government revenues, with provision also predominantly in the public sector; the United Kingdom and the Scandinavian countries are examples. In this study, Sri Lanka is the only pure NHS system. The others represent largely MHI (e.g., Estonia) or combination models (e.g., Thailand). Chile has elements of both an MHI and a private health insurance approach.

Health financing coverage is typically defined in terms of the breadth and depth of coverage as well as the resulting level of financial protection. Financial protection in health is generally taken to broadly imply that households and individuals: (1) obtain health care when needed and are not prevented from doing so by excessive costs; (2) do not incur costs when they do access health care that prevent them from obtaining other basic household necessities—including food, education, and shelter; and (3) do not fall into poverty due to excessive medical care costs and lost income resulting from illness. A plethora of empirical evidence exists concerning the economic and social impacts of adverse health shocks and the need for policies to provide everyone, but particularly the poor, with financial protection against such large and unpredictable costs (Wagstaff 2005; van Doorslaer et al. 2005; Baeza and Packard 2006).

Financial protection can be measured in a number of ways. For the health system as a whole, out-of-pocket payment as a percent of total health spending offers a rough estimate of financial protection. Evidence shows that higher levels of out-of-pocket financing in the health system are correlated with greater incidence of catastrophic payments (Xu et al. 2003; van Doorslaer et al. 2005). However, the extent of out-of-pocket financing alone does not give a complete picture because the distribution of out-of-pocket payments among population income groups or the severity of catastrophic spending or the impoverishing effect of out-of-pocket payments on households are also important to assess.

More revealing measures of financial protection therefore require individual or household-level analysis. Descriptions of such measures appear in this chapter's annex. Many of these measures are complementary and attempt to account for both the extent and the severity of out-of-pocket payments. Compared with the simple aggregate of the out-of-pocket share of total health spending, these measures highlight to various degrees the underlying notion that using health care often represents unanticipated financial shocks that may negatively impact household consumption and welfare. Given data limitations, as the case studies are all based on ex-post evaluations, information on many of these financial protection measures are unavailable for several of the countries. An example of some of these indicators for Tunisia is presented in annex 2A.

Another aspect of health financing has to do with the provision of demand-side incentives. A substantial body of evidence suggests that for governments to enhance coverage among the poor and other vulnerable populations, extensive outreach programs and/or demand-side subsidies are often required. Subsidized government health services often benefit primarily the better-off, rather than the poor for whom these services are intended. However, governments can adopt targeting measures to increase the proportion of public benefits that flow to the poor or to promote the development of separate, privately funded health care delivery mechanisms that serve the better-off (Gwatkin 2004). Demand-side approaches, such as conditional cash transfers (CCTs), have also been found to motivate the poor to seek necessary and often covered care (Rawlings 2004). CCTs provide financial support to relatively poor families contingent upon certain behaviors related to household welfare—such as sending children to school or bringing them to health centers for regular checkups.

Purchasing, the final health financing function, refers to the process by which pooled funds are paid to providers in return for delivering services. Purchasing can be broadly classified as passive—spending according to a budget, for example—or strategic—continually seeking which reimbursement schemes will maximize health system performance (WHO 2000). The types and mixes of provider payment methods constitute an important part of the purchasing arrangement. The main types of provider payment methods include capitation, fee for service; salary, global budgeting, line-item budgeting, case-based payment, and diagnosis-related groups (DRGs). Each mechanism has important incentives for providing health care, controlling costs, and improving service quality (McGuire 2000; Rice 2006; Ellis and McGuire 1996; Ellis and McGuire 1993; Jack 2005; Preker and Langenbrunner 2005).

In conclusion, health financing involves providing individuals with a basic package of benefits that is designed to improve health outcomes and ensure financial protection. Financing a basic package of health services is accomplished through revenue collection, pooling of revenue and risk, and purchasing services. Countries need to ensure that these financing mechanisms are efficient, equitable, and sustainable. In this study, a "good performance" in health financing is defined in terms of countries that have significantly increased their people's coverage for an essential package of benefits, with better-than-average health outcomes, reasonable financial protection, and better-than-average health care costs when compared with other countries with similar income.

## Annex 2A

## Definition of Financial Protection Indicators and Applications in Tunisia

The analysis in this section employs the methodology outlined in Wagstaff and van Doorslaer (2003) and van Doorslaer et al. (2007).

### Definition of Catastrophic Health Spending Indicators

The following example illustrates the catastrophic effect of out-of-pocket payments in Tunisia. The data used are from the 2003 World Health Survey, in Tunisia (WHO 2003a). However, that survey has only a limited number of questions on

---

**BOX 2A** *Measures of Financial Protection in Tunisia*

There are a number of ways to measure the incidence and the severity of out-of-pocket health payments on households, in terms of the catastrophic impact (Wagstaff and van Doorslaer 2003; van Doorslaer et al. 2007).

*Catastrophic payment headcount* is one measure often used to express the extent of out-of-pocket payments. It is the number or share of households with out-of-pocket payments exceeding some prespecified threshold of total, nonfood, or nonsubsistence consumption, expenditure, or income. Various thresholds for the budget share of out-of-pocket payments are often used (van Doorslaer et al. 2007). Some analysts consider out-of-pocket payments catastrophic when exceeding a 10 percent threshold of total expenditure (Pradhan and Prescott 2002; Wagstaff and van Doorslaer 2003; Ranson 2002). On the other hand, Xu et al. (2003) label as catastrophic spending out-of-pocket payments exceeding 40 percent of a household's non-subsistence spending, basing subsistence spending on a food-based poverty line relative to the survey.

A limitation of simply measuring the incidence of such spending is that the statistic does not reflect the severity of out-of-pocket payments (Wagstaff and van Doorslaer 2003).

*Mean positive gap* or *overshoot* is used to identify how excessive out-of-pocket payments are. It is the average amount by which the threshold is exceeded among those passing the threshold. Additionally, a normalized gap

measures the size of this gap compared with multiples of household income.

The combination of both of these measures expresses both the incidence and the intensity of out-of-pocket payments through the mean catastrophic payment gap or overshoot. This is the product of the share of the population with catastrophic spending and the mean positive gap.

To reflect normative concerns over the distribution of catastrophic payments among rich and poor households (i.e., it may be more socially acceptable for a rich household to exceed 40 percent of total spending than for a poor household to do so), both the headcount and mean positive gap can be weighted by the complement of their corresponding concentration index (Wagstaff and van Doorslaer 2003). This effectively uses a weight equal to 2 for the poorest individual and 0 for the richest, with weights declining linearly in between. By weighting based on the household's rank in income distribution, the *rank-weighted headcount* and *rank-weighted overshoot* or *gap* account for whether it is the poor or rich who generally incur catastrophic spending. Since a negative concentration index indicates a disproportionate distribution among the poor, this will increase the value of the headcount or gap. On the other hand, a positive concentration index will reduce the associated value and make the headcount or gap look less severe.

**Figure 2A.1 Payments as Share of Total and Nonfood Expenditure in Tunisia, 2003**

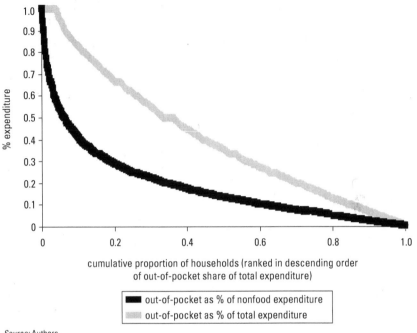

cumulative proportion of households (ranked in descending order
of out-of-pocket share of total expenditure)

■ out-of-pocket as % of nonfood expenditure
▨ out-of-pocket as % of total expenditure

*Source:* Authors.

household expenditure and does not impute the rental equivalent of housing or durable goods. Data necessary to construct a consumption aggregate, the preferred measure of living standards (Deaton and Zaidi 2002), were not available, and the use of limited expenditure data almost certainly results in measurement error. The results are therefore meant only to be illustrative and should be interpreted with caution. Data on out-of-pocket payments include expenditures on inpatient care; outpatient care; care by traditional healers or dentists; medication or drugs; health care products such as prescription glasses, hearing aids or prosthetic devices; laboratory tests; and any other health care payments. The recall period for both total expenditure and out-of-pocket health expenditure is one month.

This analysis indicates that out-of-pocket payments have catastrophic effects, at least in the short term. Figure 2A.1 graphically depicts the shares of total and nonfood expenditure per capita composed of out-of-pocket for those households having a positive expenditure (slightly less than half of all households). The incidence of these spending levels is much higher for nonfood spending and reflects that food accounts for a large share of many households' expenditure. A small but noticeable share of households appears to spend their entire monthly non-out-of-pocket consumption on food.

**Table 2A.1   Catastrophic Impact of Out-of-Pocket Payments in Threshold Expenditure Shares in Tunisia, 2003**

| Measure | Percent of total expenditure | | | Percent of nonfood expenditure | | |
|---|---|---|---|---|---|---|
| | 10 | 25 | 40 | 10 | 25 | 40 |
| Catastrophic headcount | 33.2% | 13.6% | 5.9% | 49.8% | 37.7% | 27.2% |
| Concentration index | 0.023 | −0.077 | −0.126 | 0.014 | −0.043 | −0.112 |
| Rank-weighted catastrophic headcount | 32.4% | 14.7% | 6.6% | 49.1% | 39.3% | 30.2% |
| Mean positive overshoot | 17.5% | 17.6% | 17.2% | 36.8% | 32.0% | 27.5% |
| concentration index | −0.047 | −0.091 | −0.071 | −0.072 | 0.530 | 0.060 |
| Mean catastrophic payment overshoot | 5.8% | 2.4% | 1.0% | 18.3% | 12.1% | 7.5% |
| Rank-weighted mean catastrophic payment overshoot | 6.1% | 2.6% | 1.1% | 19.7% | 5.7% | 7.0% |

*Source:* Authors.

More detailed analysis of the catastrophic impact of out-of-pocket payments appears in table 2A.1. The headcount statistics indicate a sizable number of households spending large shares of total and nonfood expenditure on out-of-pocket payments. The severity of these payments, as measured by the overshoots, is also strikingly high. Moreover, above the 25 percent and 40 percent thresholds, the poorer households incur catastrophic spending for both total and nonfood spending. The rank-weighted headcounts, which are accordingly larger than the unweighted headcounts, indicate the increasingly higher concentrations among the poor as the threshold rises. In terms of total expenditure, the severity of out-of-pocket payments is also concentrated among the poor for all thresholds; however, for the two highest thresholds of nonfood spending, the rich account for most of the excessiveness of out-of-pocket payments. In this case, more poor households surpass the thresholds, but the rich spend disproportionately more of their discretionary spending on out-of-pocket payments.

## Endnote

1. Although classifications of health systems and health financing systems performance criteria are couched differently by different organizations, all focus on the ultimate results of improvements in health outcomes and financial protection and impose efficiency, equity, and sustainable criteria as well. The World Health Organization (WHO) also included health systems' responsiveness to consumers. See for example Murray and Frenk (2000) and Gottret and Schieber (2006: chapter 2).

# 3

# Criteria for Defining "Good Practice" and Choosing Country Cases

Evaluating good performance involves a range of different components. The most important criteria for assessing good performance and selecting the country case studies can be classified in two groups, ranked by order of importance.

## First Tier Criteria

1. *Improvements in health care coverage.* The principal criterion for selection was a documented effort to increase the proportion of the population with formal health care coverage and to improve the level of financial protection.

2. *Applicability and pertinence for other low- and middle-income countries.*

3. *Large-scale initiatives.* The initiatives described and analyzed should be at a national scale, or at least involve significant national policy making. In most cases, the principal form of expansion of health care coverage is through institutional arrangements—formal sector employment, tax-based government affiliation, or market-based private insurance.[1]

4. *Availability of information and data.* Information needed to analyze the case includes the measurable key outcomes and indicators. Data availability plays a critical role in whether a "story" can be told about the performance of a country's reform efforts. Household-level data are particularly important for measuring coverage, access, and financial protection. However, this is not the most important determinant of a country's inclusion and was not a necessary precondition for selection.

## Second Tier Criteria

1. *Health indicators and outcomes.* It is extremely difficult to document a causal association between health system and financing characteristics and population-level health outcomes because many other inputs in producing health status, as well as the associated time lags, are also important. However, the ultimate goals of health coverage reforms are to improve health status and

financial protection along with responsiveness (WHO 2000). Accordingly, key population-level outcomes—including life expectancy, infant and child mortality, and immunization coverage—were used to assess the long-term success of reforms attempted in a specific country.

2. *Relation of expenditures to outcomes.* At a national level, the amount of funds devoted to health care reflects a societal commitment to promoting population health and protecting people against impoverishment from catastrophic medical care costs. However, spending levels by themselves provide little information about equity, the efficiency of spending, or the extent of financial protection for individuals. While many developing countries face severe resource constraints in mobilizing resources, and many low-income countries (LICs) cannot raise enough revenues to meet the Millennium Development Goals (MDGs), value for money in terms of health outcomes (i.e., allocative efficiency) and production costs (i.e., technical efficiency) are critical issues in all countries. Thus, it has become increasingly recognized that more money alone will not buy improved health care outcomes. Nevertheless, a direct comparison of health spending per capita across comparable income countries with health outcomes—while confounded by factors well outside the reach of the health system and often difficult to measure accurately—provides a crude comparative benchmark of how effectively a country spends its health care resources vis-à-vis its health outcomes.

One critical aspect of this study is the definition used to determine good performance in terms of coverage expansions and financial protection. Breadth of coverage is readily measured by the number of individuals formally eligible to receive benefits from a particular "insurance" (i.e., national health service [NHS], mandatory health insurance [MHI], or private health insurance [PVHI]) mechanism. Measuring the depth of coverage—the type and number of services covered—is problematic due to a lack of information on the number of users. In practice, depth of coverage is often defined and measured as the actuarial value of the benefits package per enrollee (and can be approximated by *dividing* spending *less* user fees by the number of users). Even program eligibility is not a straightforward concept to measure because individuals may be eligible for benefits in a public system but not formally enroll.[2] Even if people do enroll and become program beneficiaries, they still may not be able to access services due to both demand-side barriers (e.g., cultural or educational) and supply-side constraints (e.g., no providers in rural areas, private providers excluded from reimbursement by public programs). Moreover, putting aside the difficulty of assessing supply- and demand-side access barriers, simply measuring the number of people entitled to benefits is no easy task. Even in developed countries the number of family members eligible for coverage through the household head's eligibility may be unknown, not to mention how many actually enroll and of these how many receive covered services. All of these factors determine whether a coverage expansion achieves its health outcome and financial protection objectives.

For the purposes of this study,

- *Breadth of coverage* is measured by the number of people with formal coverage.
- *Depth of coverage* is not measured separately.
- *Financial protection* is measured in terms of out-of pocket payments as a percent of total health spending or out-of-pocket spending as a share of household consumption, when available. In principle, out-of-pocket payment shares reflect both depth and breadth of coverage and/or lack thereof.
- Infant mortality, life expectancy, and maternal mortality (health outcome measures); expenditures per capita and as a share of GDP (a crude measure of macroefficiency); and revenue to GDP and public spending on health relative to the total government budget (crude sustainability indicators) are assessed through international comparisons and relations to global averages for comparable income countries.

While good performance is measured in terms of expansions in coverage and financial protection in the context of good health outcomes and average or below overall spending levels, it was decided that, to qualify as good performers, countries did not have to attain each dimension of the first tier criteria outlined above. However, for a given country, the reforms implemented would constitute good performance overall, upon meeting the first tier criteria of achieving improvements in coverage and financial protection while also exhibiting reasonable (average or lower) overall health spending levels and average or better-than-average health outcomes for the amounts spent and/or their income levels. For countries that previously had universal coverage but encountered drastic political or economic shocks (e.g., former Soviet Union countries), good performance in a reform also resurrects health sector revenues and expenditures and restores a satisfactory benefits package of pre-economic crisis dimensions.

Based on these criteria, the study steering committee recommended the nine case study countries, a fairly heterogeneous group of low-, middle-, and upper-income countries. Tables 3.1 and 3.2 provide information for these nine countries on 15 measures of health system characteristics. Some of these statistics may differ from those provided in the individual country case studies because some of the case studies use data from different sources and years. In order to ensure comparability across countries, tables 3.1 and 3.2 provide data from the same source for the same years for all countries.

## Performance of Country Cases Globally

Many inputs go into producing health outcomes. These may include income as well as factors directly related to a health system, including health spending and the supply of doctors and hospital beds. However, many other factors, such as education, infrastructure, and geography, also play critical roles. For instance, Filmer and Pritchett (1999) find that 95 percent of the variation in child mortality across countries can be explained by just five factors: income per capita, female

**Table 3.1   Income and Health Spending, 2004**

| Country | GDP per capita (US$)[a] | Total health spending (% GDP) | Total health spending per capita (US$) | Total health spending per capita (PPP) | Government health spending (% total health spending) | Government health spending (% general government expenditures) | OOP health spending (% total health spending) | Household OOP payments (% of total household consumption) |
|---------|--------|--------|--------|--------|--------|--------|--------|--------|
| Chile | 5,894 | 6.1 | 359 | 720 | 47.0[b] | 13.1 | 24.3 | |
| Colombia | 2,155 | 7.8 | 168 | 570 | 86.0 | 20.9 | 6.9 | |
| Costa Rica | 4,349 | 6.6 | 290 | 592 | 77.0 | 21.3 | 20.4 | |
| Estonia | 8,328 | 5.3 | 463 | 752 | 76.0 | 11.5 | 21.3 | 10.6[c] |
| Kyrgyz Republic | 434 | 5.6 | 24 | 102 | 40.9 | 8.4 | 55.7 | 2.4[d] |
| Sri Lanka | 1,033 | 4.3 | 43 | 163 | 45.6 | 8.4 | 45.7 | 2.1[d] 6.3[c] |
| Thailand | 2,539 | 3.5 | 88 | 293 | 64.7 | 11.2 | 26.4 | 1.7[d] |
| Tunisia | 2,832 | 6.2 | 175 | 502 | 52.1 | 8.8 | 39.8 | 10.4[c] |
| Vietnam | 550 | 5.5 | 30 | 184 | 27.1 | 5.0 | 64.2 | 5.5[d] 6.8[c] |

*Source:* World Bank World Development Indicators; WHO 2007.

*Note:* OOP = out-of-pocket.

a. GDP per capita in current U.S. dollars.
b. A large share of health expenditure in Chile counted by the WHO as private, based on national health accounts definitions, could potentially be considered public instead since coverage of formal sector workers is mandatory although many are covered by private insurers (ISAPREs).
c. Source of household OOP payments and consumption is WHO 2003b.
d. Source of household OOP payments and consumption is van Doorslaer et al. 2007.

**Table 3.2   Health Outcome and Delivery Indicators, 2004**

| Country | Infant mortality rate (per 1,000 live births) | Life expectancy (years) | Doctors/ 1,000 | Beds/ 1,000 | Immunization, DPT (% of children ages 12–23 months) | Immunization, measles (% of children ages 12–23 months) | Self-perceived unmet need (% not receiving health care when needed)[a] |
|---|---|---|---|---|---|---|---|
| Chile | 8 | 78 | 1.09 | 2.5 | 94 | 95 | n.a. |
| Colombia | 18 | 73 | 1.35 | 1.2 | 89 | 92 | n.a. |
| Costa Rica | 11 | 79 | 1.32 | 1.4 | 90 | 88 | n.a. |
| Estonia | 6 | 73 | 4.48 | 5.8 | 94 | 96 | 2.4 |
| Kyrgyz Republic | 58 | 68 | 2.51 | 5.3 | 99 | 99 | n.a. |
| Sri Lanka | 12 | 75 | 0.55 | 2.9 | 97 | 96 | 0.4 |
| Thailand | 18 | 71 | 0.37 | 2.2 | 98 | 96 | n.a. |
| Tunisia | 21 | 73 | 1.34 | 2.1 | 97 | 95 | 1.6 |
| Vietnam | 17 | 71 | 0.53 | 2.3 | 96 | 97 | 1.0 |

*Sources:* World Bank World Development Indicators; WHO 2007.

*Note:* n.a. = not available; DPT = diptheria, pertussis, tetanus.

a. WHO 2003b.

educational attainment, extent of ethnic fractionalization, level of income inequality, and predominant religion. The importance of nonhealth systems factors for attaining health outcomes has been documented by others.[3] Nevertheless, it is instructive to situate the nine case countries by examining some of their health system indicators in a global context.

Virtually all of the countries documented in these case studies have achieved remarkable health outcomes—life expectancy, infant mortality, and access to essential services—despite low or moderate levels of income and total health spending (figure 3.1).[4] All but the Kyrgyz Republic have a life expectancy at birth above 70 years, and infant mortality rates below 25 per 1,000 live births. And, with the exception of Estonia for life expectancy and Tunisia for infant mortality, all case countries have above average outcomes for their income and health spending levels. Vietnam and Sri Lanka, in particular, are near the top of the global league.

Additionally, all nine countries perform well with respect to indicators for health services delivery (figure 3.2). Each has immunization coverage rates of at least 88 percent; most are well above 90 percent. Almost all perform better than average against comparators with regard to the percentage of births attended by skilled health personnel.

As mentioned above, all nine countries generally attain these positive health outcome and health service delivery outcomes at low levels of total health spending; in per capita terms, all countries spend about average amounts on health for their income level with the exception of Colombia, which spends slightly higher

**Figure 3.1   Population Health Indicators Relative to Income and Spending**

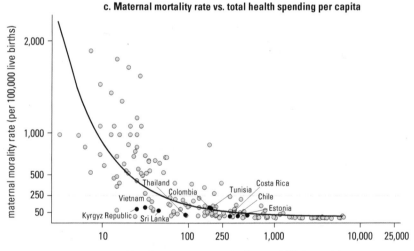

*Sources:* World Bank 2007a; WHO 2007.

than average. Thailand and Sri Lanka spend slightly below average for their income level (figure 3.3). For five of the nine case countries, health spending as a share of GDP is close to the average for their income levels; however, Estonia, Sri Lanka, and Thailand spend markedly less than their average share of GDP for their income, while Colombia spends far more (figure 3.4).

**Figure 3.2   Health Service Delivery Indicators Relative to Income and Spending**

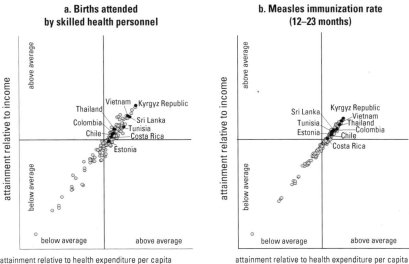

**a. Births attended
by skilled health personnel**

**b. Measles immunization rate
(12–23 months)**

attainment relative to health expenditure per capita

attainment relative to health expenditure per capita

*Sources:* World Bank 2007a; WHO 2007.

**Figure 3.3   Total Health Spending Relative to Income**

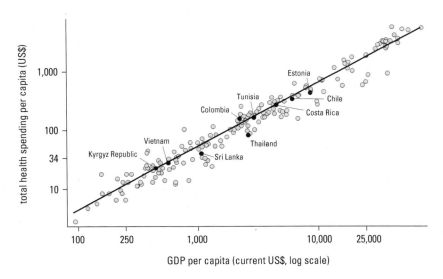

*Sources:* World Bank 2007a; WHO 2007.

**Figure 3.4   Health Spending as Share of GDP and per Capita vs. Income**

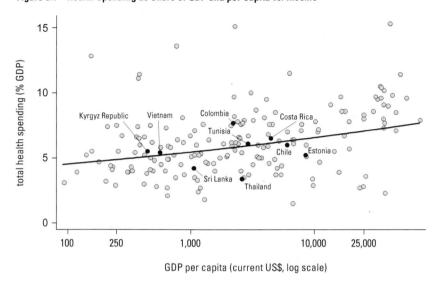

*Sources:* World Bank 2007a; WHO 2007.

Revenue-raising capacity also varies among the nine countries. Chile, Costa Rica, Sri Lanka, and Thailand raise less revenue than the average for their income level, while the remaining five countries each raises more than average (figure 3.5). Revenue-raising capacity, which tends to increase with income, is important because it provides governments with fiscal space that can be used for health spending.

Similarly, the public-private financing mix varies widely across the nine countries (figure 3.6). Colombia, Costa Rica, Estonia, and Thailand each have government shares of total health spending well above the average for their income level.[5]

Regarding financial protection, the nine countries are also mixed in terms of the shares of out-of-pocket payments comprising total health spending (figure 3.7). Five countries have average or below average levels. However, four of the countries—the three poorest, Kyrgyz Republic, Sri Lanka, Vietnam, as well as Tunisia—have relatively high out-of-pocket payments, at least 40 percent or more as a share of overall health spending.[6] This also reflects the difficulty poorer countries may have in being able to afford both a package of essential services and financial protection because some 70 percent of health spending is out of pocket in poor countries on average.

Moreover, three of the countries with high out-of-pocket levels—Kyrgyz Republic, Tunisia, and Vietnam are also countries that raise above-average revenues. These countries also show lower-than-predicted government expenditure

**Figure 3.5   Revenue to GDP Ratio vs. Income**

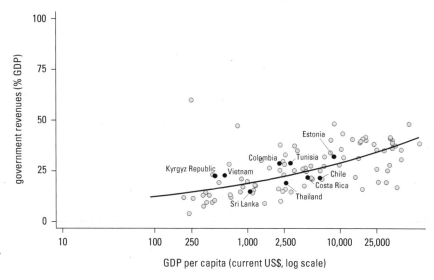

*Sources:* World Bank 2007a; WHO 2007.

**Figure 3.6   Government Share of Health vs. Income**

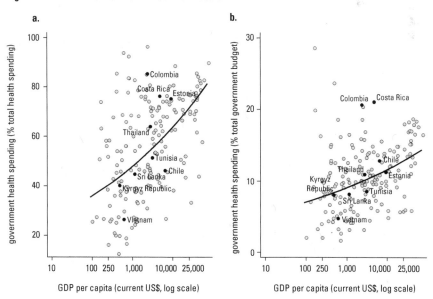

*Sources:* World Bank 2007a; WHO 2007.

**Figure 3.7   Out-of-Pocket Spending Relative to Income**

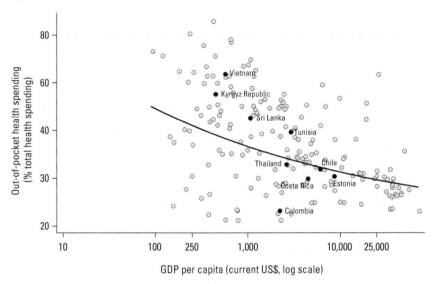

*Sources:* World Bank 2007a; WHO 2007.

shares for their income level. This may reflect the fact that health is a low priority and there are difficulties in terms of political economy in committing governments to cover an essential package of services for their population, despite good efforts in revenue collection. However, out-of-pocket levels are very low in Colombia and Costa Rica, which also have high public health spending shares of the overall government budget (annex figure 3A.3). In these countries, more than 20 percent of the government budget is spent on health.

In terms of other health service indicators, there is variation in hospital bed supply around the global average, but physician supply is above average for seven of the nine countries (figure 3.8). The former Soviet Union (FSU) countries of Estonia and the Kyrgyz Republic, despite significant reductions in recent years, still have over twice as many hospital beds and physicians compared with the other countries (table 3.2) and are far above the global averages. Sri Lanka and Vietnam also have high numbers of hospital beds, but nowhere near the levels of some of the FSU countries. Thailand is the only country among the nine cases with a significantly lower physician-to-population ratio than the global average. Perhaps a minimal physician-to-population ratio is a necessary, though not sufficient condition, for a successful expansion of health insurance coverage.

Adult literacy is another important factor that distinguishes most of these countries from others. With the exception of Tunisia, each country has above-average rates of both total adult and female adult literacy compared with countries of similar income levels (figure 3.9). This is important since the evidence of a

**Figure 3.8    Hospital Bed and Physician Capacity vs. Income**

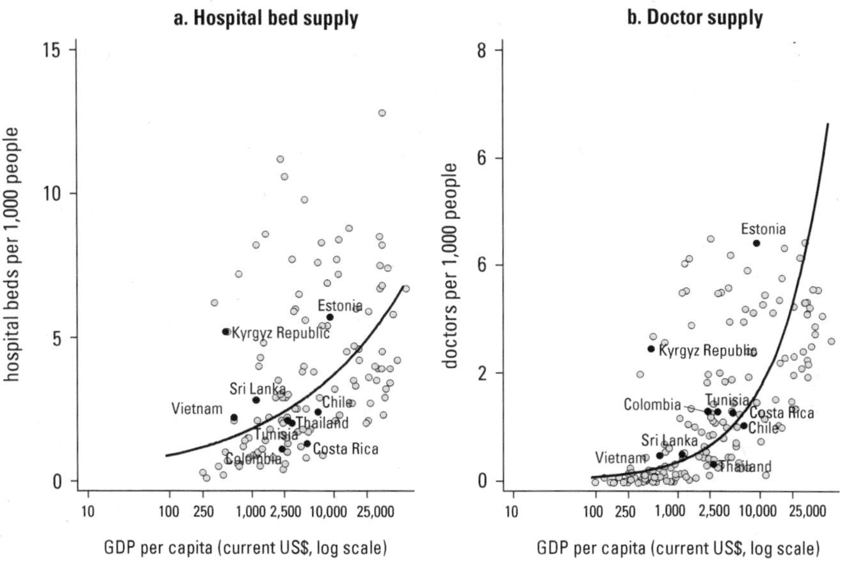

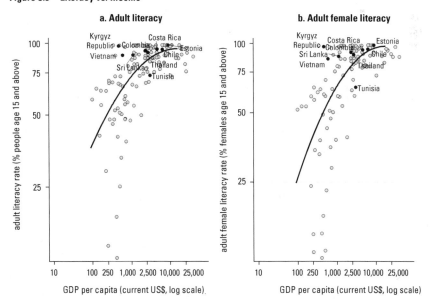

*Sources:* World Bank 2007a; WHO 2007.

**Figure 3.9    Literacy vs. Income**

*Sources:* World Bank 2007a; WHO 2007.

**Table 3.3 Correlations between Population Health Outcomes and Income, Health Spending, and Literacy Levels**

| Indicator | Life expectancy | Infant mortality | Maternal mortality |
|---|---|---|---|
| Adult female literacy rate | 0.65 | −0.75 | −0.77 |
| Adult literacy rate | 0.64 | −0.71 | −0.73 |
| GDP per capita | 0.53 | −0.50 | −0.41 |
| Health spending per capita | 0.48 | −0.45 | −0.36 |
| Public health spending per capita (US$) | 0.47 | −0.43 | −0.34 |
| Total health spending (% GDP) | 0.30 | −0.34 | −0.29 |
| Out-of-pocket/total health spending | −0.24 | 0.38 | 0.28 |

*Sources:* World Bank 2007a; WHO 2007; UNDP 2007.

strong positive link between higher education and better health outcomes is well documented (Cutler and Lleras-Muney 2006).

For the aggregate outcome and spending data used in the analysis in this chapter, the average educational attainment in the population is more highly correlated with health outcomes than other important factors, such as income and health spending.

## Endnotes

1. This focus omits countries with significant community health insurance development. However, these experiences have been well documented elsewhere (Preker and Carrin 2003; Preker et al. 2000, 2002; Gottret and Schieber 2006).

2. For example, many poor people eligible for a health card, say in Indonesia or for the Medicaid program in the United States, do not bother to register).

3. See, for instance, Cutler and Lleras-Muney (2006); Bokhari, Gai, and Gottret (2007); and Soares (2007).

4. These graphs plot the residuals for each country from two regressions: the logarithm of the health outcome is regressed first on the logarithm of GDP per capita alone and then on the logarithm of health spending per capita alone. The scatter plot of the residuals from these regressions is one concise way to assess a country's performance on the outcome compared to the global average for a given income level and total health spending per capita. See ADB (2006). The distribution of residuals lies primarily in quadrants I and III because income and health spending per capita are closely correlated (0.95) and also positively correlated with the health and delivery outcomes measured. The analysis contains observations for 178 countries for which data were available. This includes 51 low-income countries, 56 lower-middle-income countries, 36 upper-middle-income countries, and 35 high-income countries.

5. As income rises, there is a tendency for the public share of health expenditure to rise. This is often attributed to changes in relative prices and to changes in societal preferences as incomes rise.

6. In Sri Lanka out-of-pocket expenditure tends to fall on the rich, which poses less of a problem from an equity perspective.

# 4

# Summaries of Country Cases

The detailed reform experiences and lessons to be learned from each of these "good practice" cases are discussed in detail for each country in part II of this study.[1] This chapter summarizes the main reform elements and lessons from each of the countries. Chapter 5, the concluding chapter of part I of this report, attempts to assess the generalizable lessons from these country cases.

## Chile

Chile is an upper-middle-income country in the Latin America and Caribbean Region (LAC) with an average-sized population (16.3 million). Most people reside in urban settings; only 13 percent of the population lives in rural areas. In 2004, per capita GDP was US$5,894. Chile devoted some 6.1 percent of GDP (US$359 per capita) to health in 2004, a little below average for its income level. Some 53 percent of this amount is paid by private sources, including 24.3 percent paid directly by households as out-of-pocket expenditures. Health spending accounts for some 13.1 percent of the government's budget, which is above average for its income level.

In terms of health outcomes, Chile ranks among the world's highest performers. Life expectancy is 78.2 years, and infant mortality is 7.6 per 1,000 live births. In 2005, the number of physicians and hospital beds per 1,000 people were 1.09 and 2.5, respectively, slightly below average for a country of its income level.

In Chile, the expansion of a fiscally sound social security system, including health care coverage, has required considerable economic resources and was made possible by an extended period of economic growth and an efficient tax collection system. Chile is an early reformer relative to many of the countries in this study. Its reforms can be traced back over a half century, culminating in the creation of the national health system.

### Key Reform Elements and Accomplishments

The National Health Service was created in 1948 and originally provided health coverage only to public servants and private formal sector employees. In 1981,

under Pinochet's military government, reforms followed the neoliberal principles of smaller government, public subsidization of the poor, competition, and
decentralization.

The main structure of the insurance system, created in 1981, remains today. It
consists of a public insurer (Fondo Nacional de Salud, FONASA) and private
insurers (Instituciones de Salud Previsional, ISAPREs). By law, all formal sector
workers who are not self-employed, retired workers with a pension, and self-
employed workers with a retirement fund must enroll with the mandatory health
insurance (MHI) system by making a monthly contribution equal to 7 percent of
the first US$2,000 of their monthly income or pension. The required payroll con-
tribution has risen over time, from 4 percent in 1981. Other individuals may enroll
as well. They include independent workers, who can voluntarily enroll with
FONASA or an ISAPRE conditional on their 7 percent contribution, and legally
certified indigent citizens and legally unemployed workers, who are entitled to free
coverage by FONASA. ISAPRE beneficiaries may voluntarily make an extra contribution to their insurer to purchase additional coverage. However, with the return
of democracy in 1990, concerns about equity and underinvestment in government
services dominated the policy debate; the legitimacy of the existing health system
became an important and contentious issue. As a result, public health spending per
capita doubled in real terms within a few years, and efforts to regulate private
insurers were strengthened.

Today, the system covers over 86 percent of the population, close to 70 percent
through FONASA and some 16 percent through ISAPREs. Ninety-six percent of
the poorest individuals are covered by FONASA. Most of the population above 50
years of age (even within the highest income quintile) is affiliated with FONASA.
A complete subsidy (without copayments) is provided for the poorest. Financing
of these subsidies requires a solid domestic tax base for sustainability. FONASA is
also internally equitable—41 percent of its beneficiaries are indigent and make no
copayments. The share of total health expenditures paid by the public sector
through FONASA increased from 37 percent in 1998 to 49 percent in 2003. Health
services are delivered by both public and private providers. Private providers sell
their services to insurers and private consumers. The average number of services
provided per beneficiary has also increased dramatically over the years both in
FONASA and the ISAPREs. To contain public health spending, Chile has set budgetary ceilings for FONASA.

As part of the democratic reforms to improve private sector regulation, the
Superintendent of Health (Superintendencia de Salud), was created in 1991 to regulate the ISAPRES—and in 2001, the Superintendencia began regulating FONASA
as well. More recently, a minimum benefits package for all health plans was mandated in 2005. A set of new laws, collectively known as Explicit Health Guarantees
(Garantías Explícitas de Salud, GES), requires both public and private insurers to
provide coverage for 56 defined conditions—beginning with 25 conditions in July

2005 and culminating with all 56 in 2007. This effort has been the most recent concerted policy effort to improve equity in health provision and financing.

The reforms of 2005 and those over the previous half century were similarly motivated: (1) to improve the quality of public care, (2) to expand and consolidate public provision of health services, (3) to foster health insurance coverage for all citizens, (4) to promote private investment in health infrastructure, (5) to promote private-public competition in insurance, (6) to separate financing from provision in the public sector, and (7) to decentralize public health care services at all levels.

## Key Lessons

Some of the key lessons of the reforms are

- *Expansion of health care coverage requires sustained financial investments into the health sector.* In particular, expanding coverage of social insurance systems—either in terms of the population covered or the depth of benefits package—is likely to increase health care spending substantially, partly due to moral hazard and the need to subsidize the poor and the vulnerable. Therefore, it is easier to expand social security coverage when public finances are adequate to bear these costs. Such systems are usually put in place during periods of robust economic growth.

- *Increased coverage for low-income groups requires subsidies from government.* Subsidies provided to the overall population should also be progressive.

- *Cost containment measures are important.* They can prevent rampant increases in public expenditures due to moral hazard, increased population coverage with subsidies, and the introduction of new technologies. FONASA has copayments that increase with the beneficiaries' income, and the public sector has put a hard expenditure ceiling on public sector providers. The budgetary ceiling was historically based on the previous year's spending. However, an additional reform in Chile is the elimination of supply-side subsidies in the form of budget support to public sector providers.

- *Private funding support is essential for a sustainable health system.* In Chile, private financing comes mainly from two sources—copayments, which vary with the services consumed, and monthly contributions, set at 7 percent of the beneficiary's income. The average monthly salary in Chile is US$490; countries with lower income levels will likely need to charge beneficiaries higher rates to offer a comparable package of benefits. To achieve sustainability, the required contribution has risen from its starting point of 4 percent in 1981.

- *Incomplete regulation and supervision in a competitive insurance system can lead to adverse risk selection, high marketing expenses, and difficulties for beneficiaries in selection of health plans.* ISAPREs offer more than 10,000 health plans—generating asymmetries of information and making it difficult for beneficiaries to

make informed choices. The 2005 reform that mandated the same basic benefits package for both FONASA and ISAPREs sought to remedy this situation.

•  *The success of the Chilean model is highly dependent on an effective public insurance system.* If the Chilean social security system were dissolved in favor of a
completely free-market system with only private insurers, it is likely that the
process of adverse selection would leave only the lowest-risk, highest-income
individuals insured.

•  *Chile has benefited from credible, independent, and efficient institutions.* The
Superintendencia de las ISAPREs regulates the benefits packages, contribution
rates, and services provided by the ISAPREs—providing transparent rules and
fostering competition among private insurers. An efficient tax collection
mechanism and a low rate of tax evasion have also helped to ensure that the
necessary resources will be available to finance public spending.

•  *Solid political economy and consistency are important for health reform.* The initial health sector reforms in Chile were introduced during a nondemocratic
period. After 1990, successive democratic governments introduced reforms to
increase investment in the private sector, improve public sector administration, enhance coverage of the poor, tighten regulation and supervision, and
promote consumer protection. However, the current system maintains many
of the same financing, organizational, and functional characteristics of the
model initially established. Moreover, the reforms were introduced only after
attaining strong political consensus.

## Colombia

Colombia is a lower-middle-income country located in the northwestern tip of
South America. It is the continent's fourth largest country, covering 1,038,700
square kilometers. It has a population of 45.6 million and varied geography. In
2004, per capita GDP was US$2,155. In terms of health, total health expenditures
were US$168 per capita in 2004—a relatively high 7.8 percent of GDP. Only 6.9
percent of total health spending comes from out-of-pocket expenditures by
households, well below the average of countries with similar income levels.

In terms of health outcomes, with life expectancy in Colombia at 73 years and
infant mortality at 18 per 1,000 live births, Colombia performs better than other
countries of its health spending levels and income category. In terms of its delivery system, Colombia has a relatively high physician supply—1.33 doctors per
1,000 people. However, with 1.2 hospital beds per 1,000 people, Colombia ranks
somewhat below average for its income level.

Until the mid-1990s, Colombia had one of the most stable economies in Latin
America. The economy grew until 1996, when a period of economic recession
began. By 1999, unemployment had reached 20.1 percent, and 58.2 percent of the
population was below the poverty line. In recent years, the economy has been
recovering. If continued, this trend will favor the sustainability of current health
insurance expansion policies.

Prior to 1993 Colombia had a three-tiered health care system. One tier consisted of the National Health System, with a network of public facilities for health care delivery—financed from national revenues and serving roughly 50 percent of the population. A private health care delivery market grew in parallel to the public network, targeting the population with ability to pay and meeting the demand for services and quality not provided by the public sector. Private providers supplied a large part of ambulatory care services in both urban and rural areas—42 percent and 36 percent, respectively, of all visits.

A second tier was a mandated social insurance plan for workers in the public and formal private sectors, financed by employee and employer contributions and covering 20 percent of the population. The third tier consisted of private insurance or health care services paid out of pocket by higher-income groups. This market was covered by private commercial health insurers, prepaid group health organizations, and worker cooperative organizations.

Under the Colombian health system prior to 1993, access to basic health services was limited for a large proportion of the population. Health expenditures were inequitable, spending was inefficient, and there were shortcomings in the quality of the health services delivered. About 75 percent of the population was uninsured. In 1992, one out of every six individuals in the poorest income quintile who fell ill did not seek medical care because the individual could not afford to pay for it. According to national household surveys conducted in 1992, health care expenditures represented 2.4 percent of total household expenditures—but the lowest-income decile spent about 10 percent of its income on health, while the upper-income decile spent less than 0.5 percent. The cost of health care was reported by more than 55 percent of the poor as a major barrier to accessing health care services.

Public resources were poorly targeted: 40 percent of the subsidies to public hospitals benefited the wealthiest 5 percent of the population, and allocation of health care resources was biased toward more expensive, curative care, despite evidence of low productivity. Allocation of resources followed historical hospital spending trends rather than people's needs. The poor quality of health services was reflected by low use and acceptance of the network of public providers.

## Key Reform Elements and Accomplishments

The health reform proposal generated a heated debate around its goals and means between two coalitions, one supporting a promarket model (government staff in charge of economic policy) and the other favoring a welfare state (unions and bureaucracy of social security agencies and public health sector providers). The main tensions lay between the ideas of solidarity and efficiency and the roles of the public and the private sectors. To enhance the political feasibility of the reform, the government team undertook a consensus-building process before the proposal reached Congress and paired the health reform with a pension reform in a single policy-reform package. The reform was approved in 1993, with enactment of Law 100 (Gonzalez-Rossetti and Bossert 2000).

For more than a decade, Colombia's health care reform has expanded insurance coverage to 78 percent of the total population. In 1993, Colombia introduced an ambitious health care coverage reform, which created a national social health insurance (NSHI), organized as a model of "managed competition." The NSHI includes two main components. The contributory regime is the mandatory health insurance scheme for formal sector and informal (self-employed) sector workers with the ability to pay, as well as for retirees. Health insurance coverage includes immediate family members. By December 2005, 15.5 million people were enrolled in the contributory regime (37 percent of total population), including dependents.

In principle, Law 100 established universal health insurance coverage for all Colombian citizens, to be provided by the contributory regime (CR) for those with ability to pay, and by the subsidized regime (SR) for the poor. Individuals in the formal sector must contribute 12 percent of their salaries as premiums to the CR—4 percent is contributed by the employee and 8 percent by the employer. The primary sources of financing for the SR are national government transfers to *departamentos* (departments) and municipalities earmarked for health (56.3 percent of total resources); a 1 percent solidarity contribution from the CR (34.4 percent of resources); contributions from revenues of family benefits funds or Cajas de Compensación Familiar, companies that manage health and other benefits provided by employers, such as recreational services (0.5 percent of total resources); and local tax revenues earmarked for health, obtained from "sin" taxes (8.8 percent of total resources).

Solidarity is a key principle of the system—leading to subsidies from the rich to the poor and from the healthy to the sick. The subsidized regime allocates public subsidies to individual insurance premiums for the poor, following a proxy-means testing index known as Beneficiaries Identification System (Sistema de Identificación de Beneficiarios, SISBEN). SISBEN scores are calculated on the basis of a number of dimensions of poverty, including labor market participation, income, educational attainment, family structure, assets, housing material and crowding, and access to water and sanitation.

Health plans are free to establish prices for services they buy from providers, as well as the payment mechanisms. Fees for health services in the NSHI have been based on the fee schedules developed as benchmarks by public health plans prior to the reform, adjusted for inflation, but little updating for the "real cost" of services has been done. These schedules are used as ceilings for price negotiations between health plans and providers. Provider associations are currently insisting on price regulation (setting floors).

Two patterns of payment are common to all health plans: (1) preventive and primary care services are contracted mainly through capitation, and (2) most specialist and hospital care is paid on a fee-for-service basis or by service packages. The effect of these payment mechanisms on access and quality has not been evaluated.

The benefits packages— the "compulsory health plans" (Planes Obligatorios de Salud, POS)—are grouped into three levels of ascending complexity that differentiate interventions by the intensity of specialization and technology and the financial resources required for their provision. The first level of complexity includes preventive and emergency care, plus basic medical, dental, and diagnostic services. The second and third levels include specialized and rehabilitation care, hospitalizations, and the corresponding diagnostic tests.

Several key challenges remain in terms of closing some continuing health insurance gaps and ensuring the financial sustainability of the NSHI. A first and major task is finding mechanisms to enroll the informal sector, which accounted for 58 percent of the working population in 2005. About a third of this population is known as the "sandwich population," which can be sorted out in two groups. One group includes people who earn less than twice the minimum wage and who are not eligible for subsidies but for whom payment of the full contribution to the CR premium can be onerous. The second consists of workers who can contribute to the premium but who lack incentives to become affiliated. According to a household survey in 2003, the total sandwich population was about 7.3 million workers and their families, equivalent to 17 percent of the total population. Of these, 2.5 million had some capacity to pay. The administrative costs of enrolling, monitoring, and collecting contributions from this population can be substantial, and the potential for adverse selection is large. The government is currently piloting a program to provide partial subsidies to individual contributions to the premium.

A second challenge in the CR is tax evasion. To reduce evasion, Colombia has started to invest in improvements in information systems, establishing links between pension system data and health insurance contribution data. Increased enrollment of informal workers could complement these measures.

Third, in the case of the SR, not only will it be necessary to finalize the transformation of supply-side to demand-side subsidies by fully eliminating historical budgets to public providers, but it is also likely that alternative sources of financing will have to be found. Under current growth, employment, poverty, and fiscal conditions, universal health insurance is not predicted to be reached until 2010.

## Key Lessons

Some of the key lessons from the reforms are

- *The overall level of economic development is a key factor in determining the options for expanding health care coverage.* Sustained economic growth for four years before and after the implementation of the 1993 reforms was critical for popular acceptance of increases in contributions to the contributory regime, as well as for the mobilization of general revenues to finance insurance expansion.
- *Expansion of health care coverage requires substantial infusions of money into the health sector.* In particular, expanding coverage of social insurance systems—either in terms of the population covered or the depth of benefits package—is likely to lead to large increases in health care spending, partly due to moral

hazard but also due to the need to cover premiums for the poor. As Colombia's health care reforms have expanded insurance coverage from 20 percent to 78 percent of the total population, total health expenditures have grown from 6.2 percent of GDP in 1993 to 7.8 percent in 2004, mainly as a result of increases in public expenditures.

- *A clear legal and institutional framework is important in expanding formal sector insurance coverage.* The 1991 Constitution sets the legal framework and provides political legitimacy for the NSHI with the participation of the private sector.

- *In Colombia, the previous implementation of a program for the development of community-based health insurers in the rural areas allowed the NSHI to quickly enroll a large number of persons throughout the country.* The availability of SIS-BEN has given the system with an instrument for identifying its target population and for targeting subsidies to the neediest.

- *Cost containment measures are needed to limit spending increases.* These may include full separation of financing and provision by eliminating supply-side subsidies to public providers.

- *Inclusion of the informal sector is a challenge, especially people who are technically above the poverty line but for whom insurance premiums still constitute a heavy, if not impossible, expenditure.*

## Costa Rica

Costa Rica is a small (population 4.43 million) upper-middle-income country with a long tradition of political stability in the Latin America and Caribbean Region of the World Bank. It has a GDP per capita of US$4,349, about average for an upper-middle-income country. In terms of health, Costa Rica devotes some 6.6 percent of its GDP to health, which is about average for its income level, and spends about US$290 per capita on health, which is average for that income level. Some 77 percent of total health spending is public, a much larger share than in comparable countries. Only 20 percent of total health spending comes from out-of-pocket payments.

In terms of health outcomes, with life expectancy at 79 years and an infant mortality rate of 11 per 1,000 live births, Costa Rica fares better than other countries with similar income or health spending levels. In life expectancy, Costa Rica ranks with OECD countries. The country has 1.32 doctors per 1,000 people, slightly above average for its income level. However, Costa Rica is well below average in terms of hospital beds, with 1.4 per 1,000 people.

Both in terms of breadth and depth of the coverage, the health care system provides significant protection to the population. The Costa Rican Social Security Fund (Caja Costarricense de Seguro Social, CCSS) is a public entity that insures 89 percent of the population and also administers the national pension system. CCSS is also the country's principal curative health care provider. Membership and financing for the public health insurance system is based on employment;

membership is mandatory for formal sector employees. Dependents and indigent persons are provided free care under special regimes. Physical access to primary health care services in Costa Rica is universal—99 percent of the population is able to access primary health services.

The good outcomes observed in terms of coverage (both breadth and depth) are partly the result of a long history of efforts to improve the people's living conditions that date back to the 19th century. The CCSS was created in 1941. However, before health care reforms in 1994, access to primary care services was restricted to approximately 25 percent of the population.

## Key Reform Elements and Accomplishments

CCSS was set up in 1941 to oversee both the financial management and delivery of health services. The institution was originally established to protect public employees and manufacturers against the risks of illness, maternity, and work-related injuries. In 1960, the CCSS initiated efforts to achieve universal coverage by expanding the scope of benefits to farmers, independent workers, poor households, and dependants. By the mid-1970s, health insurance covered 54 percent of the population. In 1973, further vertical integration of the health system was achieved as all public hospitals were transferred from the Ministry of Health (MOH) to the CCSS. These initial reforms were further consolidated in 1993 when the health sector was reorganized. The MOH became the regulator and steward of the sector, while primary, secondary, and tertiary care was managed entirely by the CCSS.

Costa Rica's economic crisis at the beginning of the 1980s and a wide range of cumulative structural problems shook the financial situation of the CCSS and put the system at a crossroads. Coverage under primary care programs had decreased from a high of 60 percent by the end of the 1970s and further declined to 45 percent by 1994 under the traditional primary care model. Furthermore, financial problems undermined the quality of the provider network, and satisfaction with the system fell to all-time lows by the mid-1990s.

To address these issues, the government launched an ambitious reform agenda, with the financial and technical support of the World Bank and loans from the Inter-American Development Bank. These reforms aimed at correcting the structural problems and further separating financing, purchasing, and provision within the vertically integrated CCSS model. In summary, the reform process aimed to address the following objectives:

- Strengthening the primary health care network by creating new clinics and mobile teams based on a geographic model oriented to achieve full population coverage
- Introducing performance contracts with all providers in the CCSS network, to clearly establish objectives in production, quality, user satisfaction, and clinical practice
- Shifting resource allocation from historical budgeting to performance-based payments and capitation for primary health care

- Improving revenue collection through the introduction of a single, unified, Internet-based payroll collection system

The Ministry of Planning and the CCSS itself were heavily involved in the design and implementation of the reform. In addition, the two most important political parties of Costa Rica, the Partido Liberación Nacional and the Partido Unidad Social Cristiana, strongly backed the process, allowing the reform to continue despite a change of government in 1994. Opposition to the reform existed, but it was more the result of sporadic groups than it was the collective opposition of key stakeholders. Transparency and continuous communication were critical to facilitate the implementation. For instance, mixed commissions were created to involve unions and hospitals in the discussion and the understanding of the process. Hospitals also supported a pilot test of the new resource allocation model, which helped facilitate the process. In summary, one of the main advantages of the Costa Rican case was general consensus among the main stakeholders: government/ CCSS, opposition, unions, and providers.

Costa Rica represents a good example of a middle-income country with high health care coverage, considerable financial protection, and an extensive package of services. Both in terms of breadth and depth of the coverage, the health care system provides significant protection to the population.

Evidence from national surveys shows that the average Costa Rican household allocated 2.6 percent of its income to health spending in 2005. Most of households' health expenditures go for specialist and hospital services and drugs. The share of health expenditures in the richest quintile is approximately 6.6 percent of income, 3.7 times higher than the share of health expenses in the poorest quintile. In other words, most of the out-of-pocket expenditures are from wealthier families. Access to high-quality medicines is also universal and exceeds WHO basic drug list standards. The formulary includes 460 active principal drugs in 608 presentations, with products for all types of pathologies.

In Costa Rica health coverage is financed through a substantial commitment from both government and employers. Following a social insurance model, employers contribute to the CCSS 9.25 percent of the wages paid. Workers contribute an additional 5.50 percent of their wages, and the state contributes 0.25 percent of the total national wages. In sum, this amounts to 15 percent of workers' salaries. Self-employed and informal-sector workers are encouraged to join the CCSS voluntary plans where workers pay between 5.75 percent and 13.75 percent of their salaries depending on income.

The health system in Costa Rica is based on solidarity—no matter the size of a person's contribution to the system, he or she has equal access to health care services in the public delivery system. The poor are covered by the "noncontributory" and the "insured by state" regimes; an estimated 620,000 individuals belong to these two regimes, which are cross-subsidized by formal sector employees. According to CCSS actuarial studies, about 50 percent of the contributions from formal sector employees are used to cover health expenditures of pensioners, independent workers, and poorer households.

Contributions to social security are the most important source of financing, almost 60 percent of the health sector's total revenues. The second source—sales of goods and services—corresponds to out-of-pocket expenditures by households. When out-of-pocket expenditures and employee contributions to the social security are considered together, households contribute about half of the total revenues. Government contributes 7.3 percent of its total revenues (5 percent in the form of taxes and 2.3 percent in the form of contributions to the CCSS). This figure does not, however, include the government's contributions to finance health insurance for poor households. The role of external funds is minimal—less than 4 percent of total health expenditures.

These achievements are due to sustained public health expenditures and political commitment. Costa Rica has been able to apply adequate legislative and institutional arrangements to achieve high rates of health care coverage and to ensure universal provision of health services over the long term. When Costa Rica encountered difficult obstacles to achieving its coverage objectives, it was able to renew the structure by redefining the provider network and by integrating private and nongovernmental partners in the delivery of health services.

However, a number of issues pose challenges to the health system and the reform. These include (1) the monopoly of the CCSS in the administration of health insurance schemes; (2) limited choice of providers, especially of hospital services; and (3) the corruption scandal in 2004 involving the executive president and some managers of the CCSS who took advantage of the administrative restructuring, gave more power and autonomy to the latter, and severely damaged any future effort to implement further changes in the organizational, financing, and delivery structure.

## Key Lessons

Some key lessons from the reform are

- *Political commitment: both political parties agreed on the need for change.* Even though they did not agree on certain details, the common view that a health reform was required prevailed. The relatively rapid approval of the reform loans in the Congress signaled this bipartisan political support.
- *Transparency and accountability have been critical ingredients in successful expansion of health care coverage.* Political parties, the CCSS, health care providers and other workers, and MOH staff all had an important voice in shaping the reforms that have resulted in the current health coverage system. Internal institutional reforms have also played a role.
- *Wide participation of main stakeholders in the reform process extended beyond political parties.* It included CCSS workers (especially medical staff), MOH staff, medical doctors, and communities. Transparency in the flow of informa-

tion to the stakeholders was a key aspect. Several groups opposed the reforms, as expected, but continuous negotiation and a consensus building allowed the implementation of the main reform components. It is important to recognize that the original reform agenda has still not been fully implemented, and some elements are missing. For instance, allowing patients the right to choose their provider is an issue not yet resolved.

- *The creation of a dedicated purchasing unit was the most important organizational change introduced in the CCSS as part of the reforms.* It is administratively and financially independent from the CCSS hospitals. Separation of purchasing from provision functions allows one department to concentrate fully on planning, negotiating, monitoring, and evaluating the performance of health providers. It removes conflicts of interest in the purchasing relationship that might compromise the efficiency of the purchasing process.

- *Information systems have played an important role in Costa Rica.* Investments in computer systems have allowed the CCSS financial managers to monitor the flow of revenues daily, eliminating the previous 30-day delay. These systems have facilitated the implementation of new payment mechanisms between the CCSS and primary care providers to enhance provider efficiency and performance. Monitoring management agreements signed by both parties explicitly allows defining and linking coverage targets to payments.

- *These reforms take time and money to produce results.* The health reforms in Costa Rica encompassed separating purchasing from delivery functions within the CCSS, reorienting a curative-based coverage system toward preventive care, and modernizing medical technology and information. While achieving full coverage with primary care services took the country less than 15 years, universal health insurance coverage for a full benefits package will take much more time.

- *Important health outcomes were achieved by expanding primary care services as the main channel to provide universal access to the entire population.* The share of the population with access to primary services jumped from 25 percent of the population just before the reform to almost universal coverage by 2005.

- *Sustainability of the reforms depends on continuous financial support.* It is important to have a short-term budget to launch the program, such as the two reform loans approved in Congress that came from the World Bank (US$22 million) and the Inter-American Development Bank (US$42 million). A commitment to investing resources over the long run is also critical.

## Estonia

Estonia is a small upper-middle-income country in the Europe and Central Asia (ECA) Region of the World Bank, with a population of 1.3 million and GDP per capita of US$8,328. It was part of the Soviet Union, gaining independence in 1991. The economy contracted initially following separation from the Soviet

Union but recovered soon thereafter. Since then, Estonia has been one of the fastest-growing economies among formerly socialist transition economies in Eastern and Central Europe. Estonia's population, like much of Europe's, is both declining in size and aging. In 2002, more than 20 percent of the population was above 60, and the age dependency ratio is 48 percent. Almost 70 percent of the population is urban. Total health expenditure is about 5.3 percent of GDP, lower than that of other countries at similar income levels. The public share of total health expenditure is high (76 percent), with 87 percent of funds coming through the health insurance system. About 11.5 percent of the government's budget (including MHI spending) is devoted to health, about the average for Estonia's income level. In 2004, 88.3 percent of private expenditure and 21.3 percent of overall health expenditure was out-of-pocket.

Life expectancy in Estonia declined after independence, reaching a low point of 61 years for men and 73 for women in 1994. It has been on the rise ever since: in 2005, life expectancy was 66 for men and 77 for women. Average life expectancy (73 years) is still low by European Union (EU) standards, and remains lower than average for its income level. Estonia's infant mortality rate is very low: 6 per 1,000 live births in 2005. In keeping with the trend among ex-Soviet republics, the density of physicians and hospital beds per 1,000 is high at 4.48 and 5.3, respectively. Literacy rates are close to 100 percent.

Prior to reforms, Estonia's health system was that of the Soviet Union. Universal health care was centralized and provided nominally free to everybody through a state-run national health service. However, technology and clinical methods were less advanced than those in Western countries. Prereform, as was the case with other former Soviet regions, the system was characterized by input norms and targets, oversupply of hospital beds, overspecialization, and an out-migration of health personnel.

The rationale for reform was to introduce a system that would ensure secure sustainable and predictable financing for the health sector, especially given the precarious state of the economy. Following the breakup of the Soviet Union, there was a strong desire to move away from the input-based system to embrace market principles. However, it was understood that privatization and other reforms needed to be balanced by building up a sustainable health and pension system in the social sector. The first Health Insurance Act was approved by the Parliament even before political independence was achieved.

### Key Reform Elements and Accomplishments

The reform of 1991 introduced a classic Bismarkian model of coverage with MHI and decentralization. A health insurance tax of 13 percent on employee salaries was introduced, paid fully by employers. In 1994, the health insurance tax was incorporated into the social tax, with an earmarked share for the health system. Initially, funds were not pooled across the 22 noncompeting, district-based funds. As a result, some of the more deprived areas had lower resources than others.

However, this has changed. Revenue collection has been streamlined through the Government Tax Revenue Office, and since 2000, the Estonia Health Insurance Fund (EHIF), incorporated under a separate public law, has operated as a single pooled fund with selected administrative and contracting responsibilities delegated to four regional offices. The EHIF is legally obliged to balance yearly revenues and expenditures, a requirement fulfilled almost every year since the inception of the scheme.

Initially, there were no out-of-pocket payments. In 1993, however, Estonia introduced the prescription pharmaceutical reimbursement system, based on some cost sharing. Some 23 percent of out-of-pocket spending goes toward dental care. Flat copayments are charged for some types of health services such as primary care physician home visits, outpatient visits, and hospital-bed days.

The health insurance system is mandatory without an opt-out possibility. Private insurance was allowed to be taken to defray expenses not covered by mandatory health insurance. Contributions are related to being active in the workforce. Non-contributing individuals (e.g., children, pensioners) make up almost half (49 percent) of the insured population, and their expenses are implicitly subsidized by the others. The state officially contributes for only about 4 percent of the covered population.

By the end of 2003, 94 percent of the population was covered by Estonia's MHI scheme. The uninsured 6 percent are working-age individuals not employed in the formal labor market and ineligible under other criteria, such as being registered as unemployed or disabled.

The health insurance reform was accompanied by carefully phased changes in the service delivery system. Major delivery system changes included implementation of the family practice model, rationalization of the hospital sector, modernization of the pharmaceutical sector, and the adoption of incentive-based provider payment and risk-sharing mechanisms. Primary health care is now provided by private family practitioners, and hospital and specialist care predominately by autonomous public hospitals incorporated under private law as stock companies or not-for profit foundations (trusts).

However, out-of-pocket payments in Estonia have been rising. Habicht et al. (2006) found that between 1995 and 2002, the percentage of households who had out-of-pocket medical expenses exceeding 20 percent of their capacity to pay increased from 3.4 percent to 7.4 percent. Additionally, out-of-pocket payments pushed 1.3 percent of households into poverty.

## Key Lessons

Some key lessons from the reforms are

- *The reform from a Soviet NHS to a MHI model was carefully planned.* Major financing changes included a dedicated 13 percent payroll tax accompanied by carefully phased major changes in the delivery system and regulatory environment.

- *Health system revenue collection should be in line with overall fiscal policy and should take into account labor market policies, future growth and labor force projections.*
- *The reform benefited from solid economic growth*—except at the very beginning.
- *Implementing the system through the formal employment sector limited corruption and other distortions.*
- *Streamlining revenue collection through the Government Tax Revenue Office allowed the EHIF to focus on purchasing health care for its beneficiaries.*
- *A single risk pool and clear regulatory frameworks have allowed the EHIF to be an efficient administrator of MHI funds and perform as an effective purchaser of services.*
- *Annual actuarial soundness is ensured by legislatively limiting MHI spending to available revenues.*
- *The government has been adept at monitoring and undertaking mid-course corrections.* For example, risk pools and certain delivery system responsibilities initially delegated to local governments were recentralized after some instances of their capture by providers and inability to deal effectively with certain cross-regional service delivery externalities.
- *Strategically designed out-of-pocket payments—in conjunction with social insurance—can play an important role in ensuring sustainability of health care financing.* They help moderate demand and ensure that poor and other vulnerable groups receive coverage for essential health care and protection from catastrophic expenditures.
- *The reform enjoyed strong support from the medical community.*

## Kyrgyz Republic

The Kyrgyz Republic is a small (population 5.2 million), mountainous Central Asian country, with two thirds of its population rural. Beyond some gold and agriculture, it is poorly endowed with resources. In 2004, per capita GDP was US$434, about average for a low-income country. In terms of health, the country devotes some 5.6 percent of GDP, US$24 per person to health spending. Some 41 percent of total health spending is public, and health accounts for 8.4 percent of the government budget. Out-of-pocket payments account for 55.7 percent of all health spending, a high level relative to comparable income countries.

In terms of health outcomes with an infant mortality rate of 58 and life expectancy of 68, the Kyrgyz Republic compares favorably with other countries of its income or health spending levels. In terms of its delivery system, its high physician-to-population and hospital-bed-to-population ratios of 2.51 and 5.3 per 1,000, respectively, are typical of the FSU pattern. Educational levels are also high with adult literacy above 90 percent.

Before the health sector reforms of the mid-1990s, the Kyrgyz Republic had a typical Soviet norm-driven, centrally planned, general revenue–financed health system in which free health care was every citizen's right. After the breakup of the Soviet Union in 1991, the Kyrgyz economy collapsed, and between 1991 and 1996, GDP fell by more than 50 percent. The Kyrgyz Republic found itself saddled with an over-resourced, unaffordable health system in which "fixed" salary costs and infrastructure accounted for 75 percent of all health spending, private sector provision was almost nonexistent, and private payments were largely under the table "informal" payments to public providers for preferential treatment in the vast state-owned and state-managed health infrastructure.

Theoretically, the Soviet system had provided both universal and deep coverage in terms of financial protection, but in actuality supply-side rationing of technologies, diagnostic tests, and devices was rampant and manifested itself in waiting lists and informal payments. With the collapse of the Soviet Union and its drastic economic impact, the Kyrgyz Republic could no longer financially sustain this system and undertook a series of reforms to deal with both funding and delivery system improvements. Inevitably, some of the needed "financing" had to be derived from efficiency gains from streamlining the bloated health infrastructure.

## Key Reform Elements and Accomplishments

The economic decline and severe fiscal contraction of the early transition period eroded the previously high levels of financial protection and coverage. They also revealed an inequitable distribution of public resources disproportionately favoring tertiary care facilities in the capital city, an inefficiently large service delivery sector, and low health care quality. The widespread availability of data and information showed that high out-of-pocket payments (both formal and informal) were a major financial burden for many households and constituted barriers to access. With the wider economic and social reform context in the mid-1990s, emphasizing poverty reduction and expanding coverage through health reform became important instruments of the poverty reduction strategy. Strong support for health reform in its early phase from the president of the Republic played a key role in introducing coverage reforms. Additionally, Kyrgyz policy makers were willing and open to discuss the issue of high out-of-pocket payments as an irrefutable symptom of a broken system, which facilitated productive discussion of the problems and constraints besetting the health system. The huge excess capacity and limited fiscal space meant that efficiency gains had to be achieved before equity could be directly addressed. However, the objectives of increased efficiency and equity were mutually reinforcing; provider payment and service delivery reforms relaxed the need for high out-of-pocket payments and in turn improved access and financial protection.

In 1996, the Kyrgyz government undertook a two-phased health sector reform program. The first phase, from 1997 to 2001, was focused on obtaining additional revenues through the introduction of the Mandatory Health Insurance Fund (MHIF) financed by a small complimentary payroll tax. The second phase of the reform, launched in 2001, was a complete reform of the funding flows through the system and purchasing mechanisms, explicit specification of the benefits package, and a restructuring of the service delivery system.

MHIF, initiated in 1997, focused first on the economically active population who paid a 2 percent payroll tax contribution and on pensioners and the registered unemployed who were funded out of the pension and unemployment funds. Coverage, starting with 30 percent, reached 83 percent of the population in 2001 with the addition of children funded by the state and social welfare recipients funded by the social welfare funds (Meimanaliev 2003). Although the program did not significantly change the depth of coverage from Soviet times, the real benefit was to allow the step-by-step introduction of population and output-based purchasing mechanisms (Kutzin 2002). Phase 2, introduced in 2001, marked the introduction of significant provider payment and service delivery reforms, including the explicit designation of the benefits package and a subsidized outpatient drug benefit program.

The reform accomplished a number of objectives, including a focus on primary care, service delivery rationalization (reform of the bloated hospital system, improved efficiency through provider payment mechanisms, updating of treatment protocols), development of national risk pooling, diversification of health sector financing, broadening of consumer choice, encouragement of private sector provision, and the important national political benefit of clarity of entitlements to specific benefits. Although the reform has led to major improvements in efficiency and sufficient revenues to reach pre-breakup spending levels, the persistence of a high out-of-pocket share of total spending shows that the Kyrgyz Republic still faces significant financial protection and equity challenges. The average share of household consumption composed of out-of-pocket payments is 2.4 percent.

## Key Lessons

The key lessons from the reform are

- *Successes are in part due to the comprehensive approach, not a single instruments or magic bullet.*
- *Complex reforms require careful sequencing of various reform steps.*
- *Paying attention to institutional aspects was important in order to ensure sustainable benefits.* Creating the MHIF as a parastatal agency was crucial for the adoption of strategic purchasing and abandonment of inefficient input-based budgeting.
- *Phased implementation and careful sequencing were an effective implementation approach and helped build capacity and stakeholder support as well as learning by doing.*

- *Strong collaboration of the development partners facilitated harmonized support for reform design and implementation.*
- *Poor economic conditions during the implementation limited government's ability to achieve financial protection objectives.*
- *The slow pace of reforms in public financial management created a challenge for achieving health sector reforms.* Compared with other sectors in the Kyrgyz Republic, the health sector was revolutionary: it was the only one to move away from input-based line-item budgets and administrative control mechanisms toward performance-based management.
- *Elimination of copayments without commensurate increases in public funding is leading to the return of "informal" payments.*
- *For a country of its income level, the Kyrgyz Republic has a well-developed health information system that facilitated policy development, especially prospective provider reimbursement, based on enrollment at primary care facilities, hospital admissions, and outpatient utilization.*
- *The Kyrgyz reforms should be replicable in transition economies with excess capacity and reduced fiscal space.*

## Sri Lanka

With a population of 20 million and GDP per capita of just over US$1,000, Sri Lanka is a lower-middle-income country. The country is predominantly rural, with only 15 percent of the population living in urban areas. Total health spending—at US$43 per capita—is about 4.3 percent of GDP, below average for its income level. Most expenditure (54 percent) is private, 48 percent of all health spending is out of pocket. Inpatient provision is largely public (more than 95 percent). The largest part of private sector provision is ambulatory care. Government spending on health is about 8.4 percent of the overall budget.

Sri Lanka's population health indicators are better than those of comparable income countries. In 2004, life expectancy was 75 years, and the infant mortality rate was 12 per 1,000 live births. In 2005, the number of physicians and hospital beds per 1,000 was 0.55 and 2.9, respectively, higher than in comparable income countries. Government health spending is financed exclusively from general tax revenues. There is no Mandatory Health Insurance. Private insurance coverage rates are low.

Sri Lanka was an early reformer in relation to other countries included in this study. Its reforms can be traced back to 1931 and its first national elections with universal franchise. The elections resulted in the transfer of power to Sri Lankan chosen leaders while the country was still a British colony (it achieved full independence 17 years later, in 1948).

The health system prior to reforms was colonial. The emphasis was on preventive care through public health programs. The few modern urban health facilities, funded by a mixture of user fees and general revenue, catered primarily to Dutch and British residents. Most Sri Lankans depended on traditional healers. In the 1920s, the situation in the island differed little from that in most other British colonies. Government intervention in health was limited to providing health care for a small urban population that operated the colonial infrastructure and administration, for an equally small workforce involved in export agriculture, and for a sanitary regime designed to control major epidemic threats such as cholera. Motivated primarily by economic and productivity considerations, some health care was also provided for plantation workers financed by fees on exports. This group generally had better health outcomes than their rural nonplantation counterparts.

A severe malaria epidemic in 1934–35 devastated the rural population. Although by this time Sri Lanka was under elected self-rule, the new administration did little to alleviate the problems created by the epidemic. Public resentment after the inadequate response forced policy makers to reprioritize the role of the state in ensuring the people's health.

## *Key Reform Elements and Accomplishments*

Democracy has been the most important motivation for reforming health services in Sri Lanka. It was introduced expressly to empower the society's poorer groups and women to put pressure on the elites to pay attention to social and health conditions. After the 1931 elections, the political economy of the island changed irrevocably with the shift of the political power base from urban residents to the rural majority. From the perspective of the political economy of health, the impact of democracy was accentuated in Sri Lanka by the emergence of competitive politics along a left-right dimension, with two-party competition well embedded by the late 1950s; a rural bias in the delimitation of electorates; the single-member constituency system, which encouraged politicians to engage in parish-pump politics to maximize the government infrastructure built in their districts; and the smallness of the country, where each national legislator represented fewer than 10,000 voters in the 1930s.

The principal scaling up of health reforms occurred after the malaria epidemic, from the mid-1930s to the 1950s. Subsequent developments have been relatively minor and incremental to this initial fundamental shift in the structure of the health system. The introduction of democratic politics forced successive governments to continuously expand public free health services into rural areas, where the voters wanted the same standards of provision that had been established earlier for urban dwellers. Health sector managers were not averse to responding. The colonial health department was the first ministry to come under the control of local civil servants, who were imbued with a nationalist ethos of "serving the masses." A key aspect of the reform in Sri Lanka was the expansion of free health care provision to rural areas by building and staffing government hospitals and dispensaries, particularly in the 1940s. As a result of the reforms, the emphasis of the health system changed from one that was preventive and sanitation-oriented to one that emphasized universal access to curative health services through hospitals. This was driven by official recognition in the 1930s that risk protection against the impoverishing impacts of major illness was a necessary concern of public intervention.

An important government commission in 1948 later elaborated on this by finding that MHI was not necessary, because direct government provision fulfilled the same insurance function. User fees, another remnant of the colonial health system, were removed in 1951. Additionally, when resource constraints began to bite, policy makers prioritized consumer access to services over service quality. As resource limits tightened, policy makers in the health sector learned to focus on improving productivity, rather than expanding budgets. The health system changed from one in which only the urban rich had access to modern medicine—while the rural population relied primary on traditional healers—to one in which effectively the entire population has access to modern care. The density of coverage is very high: most Sri Lankans live within 2 to 3 kilometers of a public health facility.

Once democracy had served to establish a widely dispersed government health infrastructure, accessible by all, it then acted to ensure its survival under often difficult fiscal conditions. Subsequently, successful market-oriented and reform-minded governments in Sri Lanka have generally understood that the cost of adequate public health services accessible to the poor was a small fiscal price to pay for the political support that they engender to enable other more important economic reforms.

Other aspects of the Sri Lankan reform are noteworthy. The incidence of public health expenditure has been pro-poor, and the system of health financing is progressive (Rannan-Eliya, 2001). Catastrophic health spending is low (van Doorslaer et al. 2007). Out-of-pocket health expenditure is incurred primarily by the rich who are more likely to seek private care due to its (modestly) higher quality and responsiveness. Efficiency has been an important and critical element in Sri Lanka's success: it enabled it to use a limited budget to reach the poor. Sri Lankan public hospitals deliver inpatient admissions and outpatient visits at a far lower cost per capita and health-to-GDP ratio than comparable income developing countries. This has been achieved by high bed turnover rates and short average lengths of stay. Labor productivity is also high: government doctors and nurses see, on average, more inpatients and outpatients than is the norm for developing countries. As part of the reforms, public sector doctors have also been allowed to practice privately after-hours, thereby increasing their income-generation abilities and providing an incentive for relocation to rural areas (Rannan-Eliya 2001).

## Key Lessons

Some of the key lessons of the reforms are

- *Democratic accountability is important to ensure that the health system is responsive to the needs of the poor.* A key enabling factor for Sri Lanka is democracy, which has given the rural poor a voice. Anti-incumbency in a functioning democracy made the choice to pursue universal coverage an easy one (politically).[2]

- *Countries can rely on effective (and free) public provision of health that is funded out of general taxation.* Sri Lanka has no social insurance and relatively low labor market formality, again suggesting that neither is necessary for successful health financing reforms. Therefore, pushing social insurance policies in countries that are not ready for them may not be prudent.
- *Sri Lanka is not exceptional in terms of its revenue generation but has used efficiency gains to finance increases in coverage.* (At the same time, to ease the burden on the system, it has nudged the rich toward private care.) This suggests the importance of good governance in allowing for effective implementation of such policies. Sri Lanka has a history of good public administration with little corruption, both strong preconditions for its kind of NHS system.
- *The people's high educational attainment appears to have played a facilitative role in Sri Lanka.* In terms of influencing demand, it has enabled the high priority placed on health to be sustained through changes in government.

## Thailand

With a population of about 64 million and a GDP per capita of US$2,441, Thailand is a relatively large lower-middle-income country in the East Asia and Pacific Region of the World Bank. It stands out as one of the few countries in Asia never to have been colonized. Thailand was battered by the 1997 Asian financial crisis but has since recovered. Sixty-eight percent of its population is rural. At 3.5 percent, the proportion of spending on health relative to GDP in Thailand is low for its income level. In 2004, the government's share of health expenditure was 64.7 percent. Of private spending, 74.8 percent was out of pocket. Although overall health expenditures are low, a large part (11.2 percent) of the government's budget is devoted to health. Health provision is mixed, with both public and private providers.

Thailand has excellent population health outcomes. Life expectancy in 2005 was 71 years, and the infant mortality rate was 18 per 1,000 live births. There are 2.2 hospital beds and 0.37 doctors per 1,000, the latter somewhat low for a country at Thailand's income level. Literacy rates, both for adults in general and for adult females, are higher than 90 percent.

### Key Reform Elements and Accomplishments

Before the 2002 reforms expanding health coverage, Thailand sought universal health coverage through four different schemes. Social movements and the development of democracy were key contributing factors toward the series of health reforms in Thailand. The first was the Medical Welfare Scheme (MWS), introduced in 1975 by the first democratically elected government after the military dictatorship had been replaced in 1973. The MWS aimed to provide free medical care to low-income groups and covered about one quarter of the population. The scheme was funded by general taxation and covered the poor, the elderly, the disabled, and children younger than 12 years. Under this scheme, an estimated 11 million people were eligible for a comprehensive package of services without user charges at public facilities. There were some problems related to funding and targeting, and the quality of care provided was questionable (Pannarunothai 2002).

The second scheme, the Civil Servant Medical Benefit Scheme (CSMBS) was introduced in 1978 as a noncontributory regime to provide health benefits to civil servants and their dependents (a total of 7 million people). This scheme, too, was funded through general taxation. Beneficiaries were free to choose private or public providers, although only 50 percent of costs incurred not exceeding baht 3,000 were reimbursed at private health facilities. Compared with the other schemes, CSMBS had the highest expenditures as a result of its fee-for-service reimbursement model (Sriratanaban 2002).

Under a new military-led government, little progress was made for more than a decade. The Social Security Scheme (SSS), launched in 1990, covered about 8 million formal sector employees (but not their dependents). It followed a capitation model, but concerns persist about the quality of care provided (Tangcharoensathien, Willbulpholprasert, and Nitayaramphong 2002). The Voluntary Health Card Scheme (VHCS) was introduced in 1993 to cover those ineligible for any of the other schemes. The VHCS collected premiums from households, the Ministry of Public Health, and from an Asian Development Bank loan. However, there were concerns that the scheme was not reaching the intended target population and suffered from a classic adverse selection problem. The VHCS was not successful in expanding coverage due to financial nonviability (Donaldson, Pannarunothai, and Tangcharoensathien 1999).

By 1998, about 80 percent of Thailand's population was insured. In 2001, Thailand introduced a Universal Coverage Scheme (UCS) (Tangcharoensathien, Srithamrongsawat, and Pitayarangsarit 2002), motivated by the 1997 Constitution, which reintroduced a focus on populist policy. The rationale for introduction was to deal with some of the problems of the earlier schemes and to increase coverage among the uninsured.

The UCS began in 2001 as a mandatory scheme funded by general taxation and a baht 30 copayment. It merged the MWS and the VHCS and covered the remaining uninsured. Unlike many other countries of similar income levels seeking to expand coverage, Thailand's reform was rapidly implemented and scaled up nationwide within a year. All Thai citizens are eligible for the scheme, which provides a standard benefits package, and all contract provider networks—both public and private—are required to provide these services to registered beneficiaries. The uninsured have decreased from 20 percent of the population in 1998 to 5 percent in 2003. The UCS alone covers 74.7 percent of the population (47.7 million people) (Vasavid et al. 2004). More recently, the poor, the elderly, children, and the disabled have been granted exemption from copayments.

The results of the reform have been remarkably pro-poor. Since the implementation of the UCS, there has been a 25 percent increase in outpatient care and a 9 percent increase in hospitalizations, both concentrated among the poor. Additionally, government health subsidies now reach the poor at health centers, district hospitals, and provincial hospitals for both outpatient and inpatient care and thus reduce inequality in living standards among the population (Limwattananon, Tangcharoensathien, and Prakongsai 2007). The UCS has improved financial protection: the rates of catastrophic spending have decreased, and fewer people are impoverished due to out-of-pocket spending than before the reform (Limwattananon, Tangcharoensathien, and Prakongsai 2007). Regarding equity in the financing of health care, the better-off pay more than the worse-off in general taxes as a share of their income (O'Donnell et al. 2005). Accordingly, the UCS has achieved a strong pro-poor focus through improvements in the equity of utilization, public subsidies, and the health system's progressive financing structure.

Although the UCS scheme is widely regarded as successful, especially in increasing access and providing financial protection, concerns persist that it has encouraged an unsustainable increase in demand, resulting in a rapid increase in the workload of health personnel. In addition, there are no earmarked funds for the UCS, and every year it is vulnerable to budgetary competition.

## Key Lessons

Some of the key lessons of the reforms are

- *Sustained growth may help lay the foundation for expansions in coverage, but major health reforms can still occur shortly after a recession if fiscal space exists.* Even after GDP growth resumed in 1999 and 2000 after double-digit declines, total health spending still shrank slightly over this period. Significant reductions in defense spending created budgetary room for the health sector's expansion in 2001.
- *Strong political and social support for universal coverage provided the necessary conditions for a rapid scale-up.* The motto "30 baht treats all diseases" proved to be simple and popular, and the National Health Security Bill was the first bill sent to parliament because its proposal had been signed by more than 50,000 citizens.
- *The sustained development of primary care since 1980 and establishing its importance under the UCS has supported efficiency.* The gatekeeping role is especially salient because of concerns that the system is underfunded and capitation rates are too low.
- *Setting appropriate provider reimbursement through a combination of prospective payment methods has also improved efficiency.* Thailand's experience with a variety of payment schemes over the last three decades helped inform the reimbursement design in the UCS. However, the Civil Servant Medical Benefit

Scheme pays providers based on fee for service and has the highest per capita spending of any of the insurance schemes. The MWS had been conducting systematic monitoring and evaluation on DRGs since 1998; capitation has been successful at containing costs for the SSS. As a result of these experiences, the UCS was designed to use a mix of capitation, global budgets, and DRGs to put financial risks on providers to contain expenditures. Reform of the payment mechanism of the Civil Service Medical Benefits scheme is an ongoing political challenge.

- *General revenue financing has been pragmatic and beneficial to the equity in health care financing.* The VHCS suffered from adverse selection, did not expand coverage, and was not financially viable. By contrast, the UC system is funded by progressive general taxation and does not rely on household contributions, which were difficult to collect in the informal sector.

- *The rapid implementation of UCS and its achievement of national coverage within one year were possible partly because reforms were built on previous investments in the delivery system.* Thailand has had a sustained investment in the health system infrastructure for decades, including gradual development of facilities and human resources in rural areas. This network, coupled with some utilization of the private sector, greatly enabled the increase in access immediately after the "big-bang" reform.

- *Good governance arrangements have built stakeholder participation.* Partly due to the strong social movement, civil society has an influential position with the top decision-making authority for the UCS. The committee, comprising all key stakeholders and chaired by the deputy health minister, meets weekly to deal with policy implementation.

- *Excellent technical capacity and a strong evidence base for a country with Thailand's income level were important to inform policy making and facilitate implementation.* Health systems and health financing research has been active in Thailand since the late 1980s, especially after the enactment of the Health Systems Research Institute Act of 1992. This network built up enough capacity and a strong enough knowledge base to facilitate the formulation and implementation of reforms focusing on universal coverage.

## Tunisia

Tunisia is a small middle-income country in the Middle East North Africa region of the World Bank with a population of 9.91 million and per capita GDP of US$2,832. Total per capita health expenditures were US$175 in 2004—6.2 percent of GDP. About half of health spending comes from private sources, most of it (83 percent) from out-of-pocket expenditures by households.

In terms of health status, Tunisia is one of the best performers in the MENA region and above average compared with other countries with similar income levels. Life expectancy is 73.5 years, and infant mortality is 21.0 per 1,000 live births.

With respect to the delivery system, Tunisia has 1.34 physicians and 2.1 hospital beds per 1,000 people, which places the country slightly above and below average, respectively, compared with other countries of its income category. Disparities in health status between urban and rural areas, as well as among different socioeconomic groups persist: the population's health status is significantly better in urban areas than in rural areas. However, these disparities are less pronounced in Tunisia than in other MENA countries, especially in terms of infant mortality and life expectancy.

## Key Reform Elements and Accomplishments

Over the past three decades, Tunisia has developed a health system that covers nearly its entire population and which compares favorably with that of other middle-income countries. During this period, Tunisia's population has undergone dramatic demographic, socioeconomic, and health status changes that motivated the reforms. The demographic and epidemiological transitions have been characterized by an expansion of the proportion of the elderly population, a reduction of the incidence of communicable diseases, a growing incidence of accidents (traffic and work-related), and an increase of the prevalence of chronic diseases. The improvement of economic conditions and the increased living standards of Tunisians generated new expectations from the population. Tunisians became more demanding of their health system, seeking better service quality, new medical technologies, improved access, and financial protection against out-of-pocket health expenditures for vulnerable households.

Health care coverage has been expanded through substantial increases in health workers, health facilities, modern medical equipment, and health care coverage. Consequently, health care expenditures have surpassed 5 percent of GDP since the second half of the 1990s.

Until the 1980s, the health care system was based on the colonial tradition of a hospital-centered health infrastructure, concentrated in large urban areas. In the past three decades, Tunisia has progressively put into place a health system that covers nearly the entire population. It has implemented mandatory health insurance for large parts of the population, including government and other formal sector workers. At the same time, the health system has strongly emphasized preventive programs, financed completely by the government. As a result, some infectious diseases have been eradicated, and the incidence of others has been significantly reduced.

The Tunisian strategy for expanding coverage has emphasized the expansion of *geographic* coverage of the population—through primary health facilities that are geographically and financially accessible to most of the population. The strategy also focuses strongly on qualified human resources in the health sector. Tunisia has followed a consistent strategy in training and deploying medical personal since the 1960s—first concentrating on the capital, Tunis, and now decentralized, especially for nurses' training.

More than 80 percent of Tunisians are now covered by health insurance through either a health insurance scheme or a medical assistance program. There are two main types of social security systems, both mandatory and together covering about 7 million persons (71 percent of the population). The CNSS (Caisse Nationale de Sécurité Sociale) provides health care coverage for 1.2 million private sector enrollees and their families—including employees, independent workers, and other categories such as students, the disabled, nonsalaried agricultural workers, and Tunisians working abroad. The payroll contribution rate for this system is 4.75 percent. The CNRPS (Caisse Nationale de Retraite et de Prévoyance Sociale) covers about 0.6 million public sector employees and retirees and their families. The contribution rate for this scheme is 1 percent each from employers and employees. Relatively poor households are covered by two subsidized medical assistance programs provided to the enrollees and their families, together known as Assistance Médicale Gratuite (AMG). The poorest are exempt from all fees, while others who are eligible for a reduced fee scale contribute 10 Tunisian dinars annually.

The expansion of insurance coverage in Tunisia has featured the early introduction of an MHI for civil servants and formal sector employees and its gradual extension to additional groups. At the same time, additional reforms have placed a strong emphasis on preventive programs and the extension of coverage through primary health facilities, geographically and financially accessible for the entire population. Private providers have been increasingly incorporated in the health care delivery system. Private hospital bed capacity has doubled in the past 10 years, and the number of medical examinations provided in the private sector approaches that of public providers. However, the public sector remains the main health care service provider—supplying about 85 percent of all hospital beds and more than 55 percent of medical personnel.

Since 1990, the government has pursued a health sector strategy emphasizing: (1) the continuation and consolidation of gains in primary health care services, (2) improvements in hospital care—particularly in university hospitals—through structural and institutional reforms, and (3) legislative reforms to permit greater private investment in health service delivery.

In terms of health financing, the extension of the health care coverage has been accompanied during the last 16 years by an increase in the relative household contribution, a decrease in the government contribution, and a slight increase in the Mandatory Health Insurance contribution. Out-of-pocket payments have high catastrophic and poverty impacts, and the catastrophic headcounts are concentrated among the poor (see chapter annex 2A).

The health status of the Tunisian population continues to improve with the further development of preventive and curative health care services and a continued decrease in the birth rate.

## Key Lessons

Some key lessons from the reforms are

- *A strong initial commitment to primary health care contributed to the success of the Tunisian case.* This concentration has been associated with the gradual development of more intensive and more costly hospital care, influenced by the regulated introduction of new medical technologies.
- *The extensive growth of the private sector, associated with the quantitative and qualitative change in health care demand, has contributed to a significant growth in household health expenditures and poses a potential burden for poorer households.* Since the end of the 1980s, the private health care delivery has developed rapidly in terms of number of providers and health care categories. Private hospitalization, especially for surgery, has developed strongly.
- *The dimensions of the large-scale mandatory health insurance reform should not be underestimated when initially implemented.* Coverage expansions are complex and entail extensive financial commitments.
- *Regulatory and administrative capacity is critical to the successful expansion of health care coverage and must be backed up by a commitment to provide access to quality health care services.* The development of public hospitals' management capacity and the promotion of participatory management will lead to improvements in hospital performance.
- *The development of information systems is essential.* Despite substantial investments in information technology, Tunisia currently faces extensive demands in this area.

## Vietnam

With a population of about 84 million and a GDP per capita of US$550, Vietnam is one of the larger low-income countries in the East Asia and Pacific region of the World Bank. It is recognized as one of the most dynamic economies in the world, after a decade of economic growth averaging between 6 and 8 percent a year following economic reforms in the mid-1980s. The country is predominantly rural: only 25 percent of the population lives in urban areas, but the ratio of the rural to urban population is rapidly falling. In 2004, Vietnam spent about 5.5 percent of its GDP on health, about US$30 per capita—about the average for its income level. Most health spending is private—72.9 percent of total health spending, and 74.2 percent of that is out of pocket. The government spends a relatively low 5.0 percent of its budget on health.

Vietnam has excellent health outcomes for its income level. In 2005, life expectancy was 71 years, and infant mortality was 17 per 1,000. Hospital beds and physicians per 1,000 people are 2.1 and 1.34, respectively, somewhat higher than the average for other low-income countries. Both adult literacy and female literacy rates are high.

Prior to the reforms, Vietnam's health system was geared toward providing "health for all" via an extensive network of community health services and inter-communal polyclinics for primary care and government hospitals for higher levels of care (MOH 2001). Coverage was fairly widespread. However, the quality of care was low primarily due to a lack of resources, which resulted in shortages, especially of modern medical drugs and equipment. By some estimates only 8 percent of perceived need for medical equipment was met.

There were three main motivations for the health financing reforms of the past decades: (1) a historic emphasis on good health, (2) the ingrained acceptance of health as an important component for poverty eradication, and (3) a desire to make health care more affordable for the poor. Together with education and social development generally, health has historically been viewed as central to the well-being of the Vietnamese people and society. Writings of the founding father of modern Vietnam, Ho Chi Minh, emphasized good health among the population. Closely related is the general objective of poverty eradication, in which good health was and still is viewed as a cornerstone. Gradually, the Vietnamese government and local authorities became aware of the difficulties posed by the introduction of user fees for health services in the late 1980s in terms of access to care, particularly for the poor. Health financing, already pinched, became tighter at the end of the 1980s after the collapse of the Soviet Union, a country to which Vietnam looked for foreign aid. Alternate sources of finance had to be mobilized quickly if the health sector was to function effectively.

These factors led the government to introduce targeted health financing support. Initially, this support was part of other broader poverty eradication policies. Later, it took the shape of more stand-alone health financing programs aimed at the poor and other target groups, including students and children.

## Key Reform Elements and Accomplishments

Health system reforms were undertaken in the backdrop of broad economic and social reforms (*Doi Moi*) that began in 1986 with a gradual transition from a centrally planned, Soviet-style economy to a socialist-oriented, market-based one. In 1987, private health and pharmaceutical sectors were officially sanctioned. A small-scale private health sector burgeoned in the urban areas, often staffed by moonlighting government health workers. Recent estimates suggest that almost 30 percent of all delivery is now private, concentrated in the urban areas. Partial service fees and charges for drugs and diagnostics were introduced in 1989 in all public facilities, with the revenues utilized to improve services.

This "commercialization" of the health sector had an inimical impact on utilization rates among the poor, triggering the introduction of health insurance reforms in 1992: both as a means to reduce the burden on the government budget and to improve access among the poor. Insurance coverage rates increased among those with compulsory, employment-related coverage and voluntary student insurance.

However, extensions of coverage to the general population have not met expectations. As a result, the government has made several attempts—such as provision of subsidized health insurance cards for the poor and mandating free health care for children—in an effort to improve coverage among vulnerable groups.

The government's goal is to provide universal insurance coverage by 2010 through a mix of Mandatory Health Insurance, targeted health insurance for the poor and voluntary insurance schemes. In 2004, about 60 percent of the population was covered by health insurance. Compulsory insurance contribution rates are set at a modest level of 3 percent of contractual salary and basic allowances, pension, social insurance payments, scholarship or minimum wage depending on which entitlement group the insured individual belongs to. For the employed, workers pay 1 percent and their employers pay 2 percent of salary. For retirees and people receiving social insurance benefits, the contributions are paid by Vietnam social security. For the other groups the government budget pays the contributions. For the poor and the elderly aged 90 and older, the contribution is a fixed amount of US$3.1 per person per year with the contribution paid from the state budget.

The reforms in Vietnam have improved access to care and health outcomes. Inequalities remain an issue, and the government is making a special effort to target the poor in order to mitigate those. The catastrophic impact of out-of-pocket payments remain high across different thresholds and are often concentrated among the poor (van Doorslaer et al. 2007).

### Key Lessons

The key lessons from the reform are

- *Social insurance may not be a panacea, especially in a low-income setting.* Vietnam's experience indicates the difficulty of reaching high levels of coverage using social insurance alone. There is a large level of informality and, in order to cover informal workers and other vulnerable groups, the reforms had to be adjusted to incorporate special targeting programs to reach those not covered by social insurance.

- *Vietnam's and Sri Lanka's experiences contrast sharply, suggesting that many different paths can be followed to successful reform.* Sri Lanka is a democracy; Vietnam, a one-party state. Sri Lanka financed universal coverage using tax-revenue-funded public provision; Vietnam favored an approach that is more reliant on use of cost-sharing, user fees, and social insurance with adjustment to reach the uninsured. Initially, the poor suffered in Vietnam as a result of the reforms (high out-of-pocket payments and catastrophic expenses) and the focus on equity came later in the reform process. Sri Lanka started with an initial focus on equity.

- *Widespread literacy seems to have played an important role in Vietnam, as in Sri Lanka.* The people's long-standing awareness of the importance of health appears to have helped facilitate the choice and implementation of reforms.
- *Good governance has been an important enabling factor.* This has been true in terms of both implementation of social insurance and successful targeted programs such as the special funds for the poor. Decentralization in the implementation of the programs appears to have helped as well, especially in targeting.
- *Inheritance of a network of primary health care facilities was also an important enabler.* Initial conditions do matter—this was also true for some of the other cases (e.g., the Kyrgyz Republic).
- *The Vietnam case also highlights the importance of strong economic growth in helping sustain the reforms.*
- *The gradual implementation of reforms in Vietnam—as opposed to a "big-bang" approach—appears to have helped instill a learning-by-doing twist into policy making.* Deficiencies in the initial reforms triggered adjustments to solve the problem.

## Endnotes

1. Income levels, health spending and delivery system, and outcomes data in the background section of each summary are derived from the World Bank (2007a) and WHO (2007).

2. This is in line with other recent research that suggests that governments are more responsive in settings where the electorate is informed and politically active (see, for instance, Besley and Burgess 2002). Nobel laureate Amartya Sen has often made similar points about the importance of democracy and a free press in helping governments prioritize health and education. However, cross-country evidence of the positive impact of democracy on health is weak and inconclusive. Safaei (2006) does find a small positive effect of democracies on health outcomes in a cross-country setting, but many other studies have found no impact (ADB 2006).

# 5

# Enabling Factors for Expanding Coverage

The nine case countries described in this volume have all significantly expanded health care coverage, although each country is quite different and has a different story to tell. This chapter attempts to draw generalizable lessons across the nine countries and concludes by suggesting future directions for improving the global evidence base on health financing reforms.

All nine countries have one common experience: they recognized the considerable amount of time it takes to expand health care coverage and made a commitment to do it. Their good performance was assisted by political stability and economic growth and buttressed by sound planning, institutional strengthening, and financial investments in human resources, physical infrastructure, and information systems.

## Generalizable Conditions for Good Performance

Trying to generalize about enabling conditions for good performance in health financing reforms from these nine case studies is daunting—they are not representative of all global experience and do not constitute a random sample. Moreover, because failures are not assessed, the observations below are not based on the entire spectrum of financing reform outcomes. Nevertheless, all nine countries have undertaken serious reforms and by the study definitions of "good performance" have done well. These nine cases include two low-income countries and seven middle-income countries spanning the entire spectrum of middle-income countries.

The structures of the health systems also vary across the nine countries. Sri Lanka has the only pure model of a national health service (NHS). Chile represents a hybrid model of mandatory health insurance (MHI) and private health insurance. However, these categorizations are not straightforward. For example, Costa Rica's MHI system very much resembles an NHS with one fund, which owns its own facilities and is heavily subsidized from general revenues. The other countries represent MHI models, but with the exception of Estonia, each is heavily subsidized by general revenues. Estonia is one of the few countries in the world that funds virtually its entire MHI system exclusively from payroll taxes.

However, a SHI/MHI financed by payroll taxes may not be a panacea, especially in a low-income setting. In these settings, reaching broad and deep coverage is difficult, using social insurance alone (as illustrated by Vietnam); and providing health coverage to a broader segment of the population may be feasible using an NHS model (as in Sri Lanka). Labor market informality is pervasive. To cover informal workers and other vulnerable groups, the reforms had to be adjusted to incorporate special targeting programs and funding mechanisms to reach people not covered by social insurance.

As argued in chapter 2, the model a country chooses is not of primary importance. The design and implementation of the three key health financing functions are the likely determinants of the success or failure of a health financing system. Much of the detailed information is lacking to measure the equity, efficiency, and sustainability of revenue collection; the efficiency and equity of risk pooling; and the technical and allocative efficiency of purchasing. However, some indications have been presented about the *sustainability* of spending by looking at health shares of the national government budgets and revenue-to-GDP ratios. The extent of risk pooling has also been gauged by proxy through nonpooled out-of-pocket payments and, where possible, financial protection has been measured via the shares of household budgets absorbed by health spending. Allocative efficiency and technical efficiency have been crudely evaluated by comparing delivery system capacity, health outcomes, and overall spending levels to global trends.

Good performance has been examined in terms of *breadth of coverage*—defined as the percentage of the population with insurance coverage and financial protection—by looking at out-of-pocket spending as a share of total spending, and in some cases as a share of household income. More important, an attempt was made to see what common underlying factors appear to have enabled these results.

Motivations for reforms were different for Estonia and the Kyrgyz Republic. Both countries faced major financial crises after the breakup of the Soviet Union. Both countries revamped their Soviet-style systems with MHI systems, but more fundamentally made drastic changes in their inefficient delivery systems. Vietnam, ideologically a communist state, was affected financially in much the same way because of its heavy dependence on the Soviet Union for subsidies prior to the breakup. Other countries were motivated by humanitarian and solidarity considerations. In some cases, like Sri Lanka, important rural representation in the political process highlighted equity considerations related to both physical and financial access.

The different paths taken by these nine countries were heavily contingent on historical factors, as well as political economy and institutional arrangements in the individual countries. A key question remains: since health systems and health reforms are so country-specific, can a common set of enabling conditions be found in these nine good performers or are generalizations impossible? From the lessons and cross-country analyses summarized in chapter 4 and the detailed studies in part II of this volume, a number of commonalities across all nine countries emerge. The common factors identified across all or most of the nine countries include

- *Institutional and societal factors:* strong and sustained economic growth long-term political stability and sustained political commitment, strong institutional and policy environment, and a well-educated population.

- *Policy factors:* financial resources committed to health, including private financing; commitment to equity and solidarity; health coverage and financing mandates; consolidation of risk pools; limits to decentralization; and focus on primary care.

- *Implementation factors:* carefully sequenced health service delivery and provider payment reforms, good information systems and evidence-based decision making, strong stakeholder support, use of efficiency gains and copayments as financing mechanisms, and flexibility to make mid-course corrections.

These results, it might be argued, could have been posited without a study. While these case study-based findings are not the result of rigorous evaluations for the reasons previously stated, they are based on a standardized definition of good performance in terms of coverage expansions and financial protection in countries that have achieved good health outcomes with average or below average spending.

## Institutional and Societal Factors

This chapter discusses these "enabling" conditions as potentially necessary concomitants for good performance in health financing reforms. In this context, the unmet goals of these reforming countries are also highlighted.

### Strong and Sustained Economic Growth

Considering the length of the reform periods, the nine case countries faced varying economic circumstances. Virtually all of the countries, however, had long periods of favorable economic growth during much of their reform efforts (figure 5.1). Economic growth greatly facilitated health coverage expansion by bringing a greater share of the population into the formal employment sector, raising households' ability to pay for health care, and providing governments with tax revenues to subsidize health services.

Strong economic growth is particularly evident in the Latin American cases. Economic factors have been important in Colombia, where sustained economic growth for four years before and after the 1993 reforms was critical for popular acceptance of increases in contributions to the National Social Health Insurance, as well as the mobilization of general revenues to finance insurance expansions for the poor. The enrollment of a large fraction of the population through coverage of the families of contributing individuals allowed the public sector to free additional resources to provide health care for the poor.

The other countries documented in this volume also achieved substantial growth that facilitated reforms. Estonia's strong rebound after the breakup of the Soviet Union facilitated the creation of an MHI system that covers nearly the whole population funded from a 13 percent payroll tax.

**Figure 5.1   Real GDP Trends per Capita, 1960–2005**

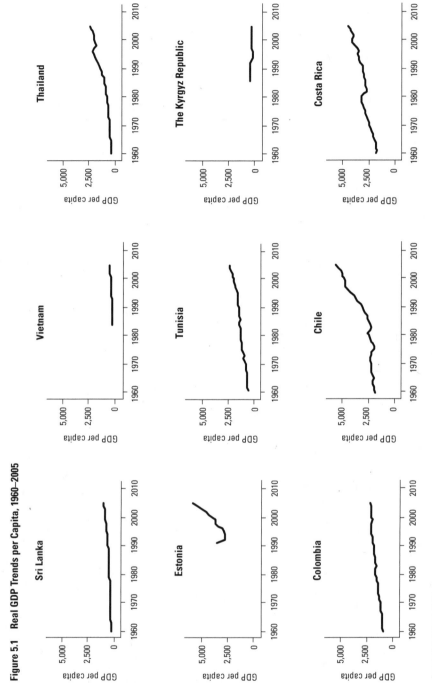

*Source:* World Bank 2007a.

Continuous and steady real growth of 5.5 percent over the past 30 years has enabled Tunisia to increase coverage and at the same time develop the delivery capacity to accommodate these expansions. It has also allowed Tunisia to reduce poverty and have a continuous improvement in its people's living conditions.

Although Thailand suffered a recession between 1996 and 1998, its economy experienced strong growth in the early 1990s. Thailand's economy also rebounded quickly from the shock and appears to have since recovered, perhaps enabling the dramatic increase in health spending after the introduction of universal coverage in 2001.

The case study of Vietnam shows that sustained economic growth over the past 15 to 20 years has enabled the government to undertake ambitious health financing reforms, currently reaching more than 60 percent of the population, with a goal of universal health insurance by 2010. In real terms, per capita spending on health has increased by two thirds during this time period. Moreover, increases in public revenues have enabled the government to significantly increase its share of health spending, creating the possibility of new programs of free health care for the poor and for children.

Similarly to Vietnam, economic liberalization has helped spur economic growth in Sri Lanka. Such growth has been an important enabling factor for the government to expand coverage and enact its propoor reforms, particularly because sustained growth can provide the basis for enhanced government revenues. It also facilitates formalization of the labor market, which can further improve the collection of revenues in MHI-based (and indeed all) financing systems. The Kyrgyz Republic is the poorest country documented in this book, but it has achieved notably improved economic circumstances since the breakup of the Soviet Union.

As these countries have experienced strong economic growth, government per capita health expenditures have also been rising. The sustainability of government spending will be a key issue as they move forward with their reforms. For example, it is not clear whether the governments of Costa Rica and Colombia can continue to devote so high a high share of their budgets to the health sector. Some countries have demonstrated fiscal discipline, such as eliminating supply-side subsidies (e.g., historical budget support to public providers) and establishing budget ceilings, as in Chile, to contain costs. Others countries will soon need to address the sustainability of government spending through supply-side controls or demand-side cost sharing.

## Long-Term Political Stability and Sustained Political Commitment

In all of the cases documented in this volume, governmental commitment to the reform has lasted for many years or decades. In no case presented here has the reform been ongoing for less than 10 years. Chile has been pursuing its reform for more than 25 years. Given the complexity of many of these reforms in terms of scope, sequencing and concomitant implementation of major delivery system changes, and the frequent development and adoption of modern health information and provider payment systems, it is not surprising that any success would require long-term government commitment. The adage that health reform is a perpetual process certainly comes to mind. Hsiao and Shaw (2007) make this same point with regard to MHI implementation experiences.

Thailand, for example, introduced its health insurance scheme for the poor in 1975. The insurance system in place today in Chile was first implemented in 1981. Both of these systems have undergone important changes over time.

The good outcomes observed in Costa Rica in terms of coverage—both breadth and depth—are the result of efforts begun in the 19th century to improve the living conditions of the population. Costa Rica has a long tradition of political stability. The Costa Rican Social Security Fund (CCSS) was created in 1941. However, before health care reforms in 1994, only 25 percent of the population had access to primary care services. At that time, the major political parties agreed on the need for change. Transparency and accountability have been critical ingredients for successful expansion of health care coverage. Political parties, the CCSS, health care providers and other workers, and MOH staff members all had an important voice in shaping the reforms that have resulted in the current health coverage system. Internal institutional reforms have also played a role.

In Sri Lanka, the principal scaling-up of health reforms stretched from the 1930s through to the 1950s, following the malaria epidemic of the mid-1930s. Subsequent developments have been relatively minor and incremental to this initial fundamental shift in the structure of the health system. One of the key aspects of the reform in Sri Lanka was the expansion of free health care provision to rural areas—through the building and staffing of government hospitals and dispensaries, particularly in the 1940s.

## Strong Institutional and Policy Environment

Institutional strength and political stability are also important enabling factors for a successful reform. Efficient tax collection and the ability to enforce mandatory membership in social insurance programs are essential functions for expanding coverage; both depend critically on institutional strength and stability. Likewise, the existence of competent, independent regulatory agencies is a prerequisite for the provision of both insurance coverage and health services.

When all nine countries started their reforms, they had—and still have—better than average institutional and policy environments, as measured by the World Bank's Country Policy Institutional Assessment Index (CPIA). The index is made up of some 16 components measuring a wide range of institutional and policy management issues including macroeconomic and trade policy, financial sectors, public sector management, social safety nets, poverty focus, environmental management, and other factors. Moreover, strong institutional environments were found for both democratic and nondemocratic countries, as shown by the polity index of democracy in figure 5.2. Higher values of the polity index signify greater degrees of democracy, and changes over time reflect changes in the nature of the polity (Marshall and Jaggers 2005).

Among the nine country cases, there are highly democratic countries like Costa Rica, Estonia, and Sri Lanka, and less democratic countries like Tunisia, the Kyrgyz Republic, and Vietnam. All the others have gone through periods of democracy and nondemocracy, although the recent trend appears to be toward democratization.

These institutional features are country-specific. An important component of the Vietnamese experience has been great economic and political stability. The one-party structure of the Vietnamese governance system has enabled the country to develop policies and implement them over an extended period of time. This is a potential advantage compared with the complexity of brokering agreements on health policy reform measures that span the political divide in many multiparty democracies. Such political stability helps obviate the risk that health reform measures may be precluded from running their course as a result of frequent changes in government.

Competent regulatory bodies are an important institutional element. This is true for both public and private health insurance. Chile in particular has benefited from credible, independent, and efficient institutions. The Superintendencia de las ISAPREs regulates the benefits packages, contribution rates, and services provided by the ISAPREs—private health insurers—providing transparent rules of the game and fostering competition among them. An efficient tax collection mechanism and a low rate of tax evasion have also helped to ensure that the necessary resources will be available to finance public spending. At the same time, the success of the Chilean model is highly dependent on an effective public insurance system.

Similarly, in Colombia a clear legal and institutional framework has proven important in expanding formal sector insurance coverage. The 1991 Constitution sets the legal framework and provides political legitimacy for the National Social Health Insurance scheme with the participation of the private sector.

In Costa Rica, transparency and accountability have likewise been critical ingredients for successful expansion of health care coverage. Political parties, the Costa Rican Social Security Fund, health care providers and other workers, and MOH staff members all had an important voice in shaping the reforms that have resulted in the current health coverage system. Internal institutional reforms have also played a role. Separation of purchasing from provision functions has allowed a single department to concentrate fully on planning, negotiating, monitoring, and evaluating the performance of health providers—and removed conflicts of interest in the purchasing relationship that might had compromised the efficiency of the purchasing process.

A strong institutional background has also marked Thailand's successful expansion of health insurance coverage. In Thailand, the proposal for universal coverage (the UCS) was the first bill sent to the national parliament because it had

**Figure 5.2   Political Freedom Trends in Case Countries, 1900–2004**

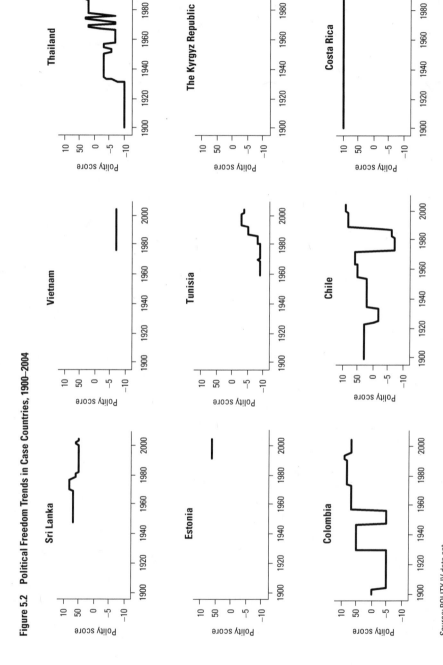

*Source:* POLITY IV data set.
*Note:* A polity score of + 10 represents a fully functional democracy and –10 represents an autocracy.

received more than 50,000 signatures from citizens. Thailand's experience with a variety of payment schemes over three decades helped inform the reimbursement system in its Universal Coverage Scheme (UCS), designed to use a mix of capitation, global budgets, and DRGs to put financial risks on providers to contain expenditures.

Some of the country studies suggest that democratic accountability can be a key facilitating factor, encouraging health systems to be responsive to the needs of the poor. Democratic accountability, achieved through free and fair elections, should not be confused with political decentralization or community participation. Sri Lanka has had little success with community participation in local government and in the running of individual facilities—but the most basic decisions about the health system are not made at the local level, but nationally, where the poor do have a voice.

## Well-Educated Population

Adult literacy is another important factor that distinguishes most of these countries from others. One can also speculate that high literacy rates made it easier to sell the reform to the population, resulted in better demand-side response to coverage expansions with respect to health seeking behaviors, and enabled individuals to be more informed consumers of both public and private care. High educational levels certainly appear to have played a facilitative role in Sri Lanka, for instance in terms of influencing demand for health by placing a high priority on this issue and sustaining it through changes in government. High literacy levels also seem to have played an important role in Vietnam. The population's awareness of the importance of health is high and that appears to have helped facilitate the choice and implementation of reforms.

## Policy Factors

In addition to strong economic growth, expansion of health care coverage requires a sustained financial commitment and continuity in other policies.

### Financial Resources Committed to Health

Sustained financial investments in the health sector are crucial. Expanding health insurance coverage—either in terms of the population covered or the depth of the benefits package—is likely to lead to substantial increases in health care spending, partly due to moral hazard and the need to subsidize the poor and the vulnerable. The insured tend to consume more physician visits, medications, and other services than the uninsured, necessitating budget ceilings for public programs. Implementing and expanding coverage is easier when public finances are adequate to bear these costs during periods of expansion and robust economic growth.

Chile devoted some 6.1 percent of GDP to health in 2004—US$359 per capita—slightly below average for its income level. Health spending accounts for some 13.1 percent of the government's budget, above average for its income level.

To contain public health spending, the Chilean reform set budgetary ceilings, based on previous year's spending.

Similarly, as health insurance coverage in Colombia has expanded from 20 percent to 78 percent of the population, total health expenditures have grown from 6.2 percent of GDP in 1993 to 7.8 percent in 2004, mainly as a result in increases in public expenditures. Costa Rica has a GDP per capita of US$4,349, about average for an upper-middle-income country. In terms of health, Costa Rica devotes some 6.6 percent of its GDP to health, above average for its income level, and spends about US$290 per capita on health, which is average. Some 77 percent of total health spending is public, well above other countries with similar income levels. Only 20 percent of total health spending comes from out-of-pocket payments.

In Estonia, 87 percent of total health expenditures come through the health insurance system, and the public share of health spending is 76 percent. Including MHI spending, 11.5 percent of the government's budget is devoted to health, about the average for Estonia's income level.

Thailand, the Kyrgyz Republic, and Sri Lanka stand out as exceptions to the general rule of substantial investment in health to achieve strong health coverage results. All three countries spend less than US$100 per person per year on health care. In Thailand and the Kyrgyz Republic, health expenditures account for just 3.5 percent and 5.6 percent of GDP, respectively. However, health expenditures account for 11.2 percent of the government budget in Thailand, and 8.4 percent in the Kyrgyz Republic.

In Sri Lanka, total health spending—at US$43 per capita—represents only 4.3 percent of GDP. Sri Lanka has been able to overcome some of the difficulties imposed by limited health financing by realizing improvements in efficiency— achieving efficiency gains in the public health system of between 1 and 4 percent a year. Sri Lanka's life expectancy of 75 years suggests that health spending alone is not the most important factor in determining health outcomes.

## Private Financing

With the exception of Sri Lanka, the cases all suggest that complementary private funding is an important factor for a sustainable health system. In Chile, the required contribution has risen over time, from 4 percent of the beneficiary's income in 1981 to 7 percent. Countries with lower income levels will likely need to charge beneficiaries higher rates to offer a comparable benefits package.

## Commitment to Equity and Solidarity

Though difficult to measure, social solidarity is also an important facilitating factor. In general, the greater the tradition of solidarity within a country—that is, the greater the number of systems and institutions working toward solidarity—the better are the chances of success for pooling arrangements, including social security and health insurance.

The governments of most of the nine countries have demonstrated strong fiscal commitment to finance coverage expansions for the poor through a combination of dedicated revenue sources and cross-subsidization through risk pooling. Many have subsidized both insurance contributions and copayment rates of the poor. For example, in Chile, the public insurer (FONASA) covers 96 percent of the poor and fully subsidizes health services for both this group and the unemployed. Colombia uses proxy-means testing to allocate subsidies to the poor in its social health insurance system. Thailand set up a new, completely revamped, general revenue funded program with no copayments for the poor, elderly, children, and disabled. Sri Lanka covers its entire population through general revenues.

The poorest are also fully exempt from copayments in the Kyrgyz Republic and Tunisia. Even in Vietnam where targeting and implementation of pro-poor policies is weaker, there remains strong government support to subsidize the poor's contributions. Additionally, creating larger risk pools to facilitate cross-subsidization from rich to poor has also demonstrated the pro-poor fiscal commitment. The transition in the Kyrgyz Republic from a system characterized by fragmented revenue collection and pooling to one with larger risk pools—first at the regional level and in 2006 at the national level—has provided the foundation for pro-poor fiscal redistribution. This move offers the prospect to improve both vertical and horizontal equity in health financing, and perhaps especially so in a country with a small population. Estonia's MHI system uses premiums from the working population to subsidize the remainder.

In Colombia, the health system is largely publicly financed—with 86 percent of total health spending coming from public sources. Only 6.9 percent of health spending comes from out-of-pocket expenditures by households, well below the average of countries with similar income levels. Solidarity is a key principle of the system where public subsidies to individual insurance premiums for the poor are allocated on the basis of a proxy-means testing index.

## Health Coverage and Financing Mandates

Solidarity—in terms of sharing both financing and risk broadly across a population requires coverage mandates. Chile and Estonia provide leading examples of mandates in the context of employment-based insurance. In Chile, health insurance is compulsory for workers in the formal sector and voluntary for those in the informal sector. Members of the health insurance system must contribute 7 percent of their earnings up to a ceiling of about US$2,000 as a premium, and may make additional voluntary contributions, in addition to copayments at the point of service.

In Estonia, the health insurance system is mandatory without an opt-out possibility. Private insurance was allowed to be taken to cover expenses not covered by the mandatory health insurance. Contributions are related to being active in the workforce. Noncontributing individuals (e.g., children, pensioners) represent almost half (49 percent) of the insured population, and their expenses are implicitly subsidized by the others. The state officially contributes for only about 4 percent of the covered population. Having a single risk pool and clear regulatory frameworks has allowed the Estonian Health Insurance Fund (EHIF) to be an efficient administrator of MHI funds and perform as an effective purchaser of services.

### Risk-Pool Consolidation

The risk-pool consolidation trend, which is increasingly apparent in both high-income and middle-income countries, is also found here in several of the case studies. Estonia and the Kyrgyz Republic have consolidated geographically defined pools into single, national-level pools. Thailand has reduced its number of major risk-pooling schemes from four to three. Sri Lanka has a single national risk pool. Among the nine cases, there are no cases of expansion in the number of risk pools, only consolidations.

### Limits to Decentralization

Estonia and the Kyrgyz Republic both established decentralized, regional risk pools then recentralized them at the national level to improve both efficiency and equity. Estonia likewise decentralized certain delivery system functions then recentralized some of them as some local governments had been captured by medical care providers and, from a provision perspective, certain economies of scale and scope required larger geographic entities to be fully exploited.

### Primary Care Focus

Every country case but Sri Lanka mentions primary care, disease prevention, or both as an important delivery system change. In some cases like Estonia and the Kyrgyz Republic, this entailed a complete reorientation of the medical system toward a family physician model. While the Sri Lanka case argues that a key success factor was a hospital-based system geographically distributed in all areas of the country, without a specific focus on cost-effectiveness, hospital outpatient units likely proved effective purveyors of primary care. In other words, the real issue may be that appropriate care can just as readily be efficiently distributed in hospital-based settings as under the more usual rural clinic and community health worker approaches. Such a focus on primary care helps explain the good health outcomes found in these countries.

## Implementation Factors

Political commitment is not a sufficient condition to ensure successful implementation of a reform. Political ability and leadership to implement the reform are equally critical. Such implementation requires a careful calibration of revenue changes with changes in the organization, composition, and management of the delivery system; dealing with the major stakeholder groups; and ensuring uptake on the demand side.

## Carefully Sequenced Health Service Delivery and Provider Payment Reforms

Perhaps it is obvious that significant coverage changes would have to be accompanied by serious delivery system reforms. This is what happened in all nine case countries. The reforms were of two types (1) enhancements in delivery capacity to accommodate the increases in coverage; and (2) significant downsizing, rationalization, and upgrading of medical practice standards in the former Soviet Union (FSU) countries.

Sequencing of delivery system changes with financing reforms has been an important element in all the reforms. Dealing with physical infrastructure and human resources for health (HRH) have gone hand in hand. Several of the countries, perhaps most notably Thailand, have implemented advanced HRH policies to staff rural areas. Implementation of modern contracting techniques, provider payment systems, and risk-sharing mechanisms has also been an important element in all the reforms. The financial resources devoted to health have increased in these countries, but most have inhibited cost escalation through prospective payment and other approaches to supply-side risk sharing. Pharmaceuticals have also been a reform target, given their high share of total and out-of-pocket health spending in terms of essential drug lists, pricing, and practice patterns (particularly in the FSU).

## Good Information Systems and Evidence-Based Decision Making

Intrinsically related to evidence-based policy, information systems were highlighted by a number of countries. Evidence-based decision making was a key enabling factor in the Thai reform. It was also important in Estonia and the Kyrgyz Republic as they adopted modern treatment protocols and, along with several other countries, modern provider payment reforms. Estonia in particular has taken a lead in terms of investments in information technology. In the mid-1990s, bills from providers were transferred to the health insurance fund on paper. All health care providers are now equipped with personal computers; electronic communication links the Estonian Health Insurance Fund with its patients, employees, and providers. In addition to facilitating efficiency in provision, electronic data transmitting has enabled the collection of high-quality data for detailed analysis such as benchmarking of providers and monitoring service utilization by specific vulnerable population groups. The Kyrgyz Republic also has a well-developed health information system that has facilitated policy development, especially the new provider payment mechanisms.

Tunisia's reforms were embodied in its investments in administrative capacity—particularly related to management and information technology in the public hospital sector. Information systems also have played an important role in Costa Rica. Investments in computer systems have allowed the financial managers of the CCSS to monitor the flow of revenues on a daily basis, instead of with the previous 30-day delay. These systems have facilitated the implementation of new payment mechanisms designed to enhance provider efficiency and performance by monitoring management agreements between the CCSS and primary care providers that explicitly define coverage targets linked to payments.

In Colombia, the previous implementation of a program for the development of community-based health insurers in the rural areas allowed the National Social Health Insurance system to quickly sign up a large number of enrollees throughout the country. The availability of SISBEN, an information system providing updated information on beneficiaries' economic status, has provided the system with an instrument for identifying its target population and directing subsidies to the neediest.

### Strong Stakeholder Support

Strong stakeholder support from the bureaucracy, consumers, medical societies, and other stakeholders were identified as important elements of the reform processes in a number of the case countries. The Estonian reform was strongly supported by the medical association, which had much to gain from the movement away from the old Soviet-style system. The support and voice of the rural poor were highlighted as important factors in the success and sustainability of the Sri Lanka reform. Strong support from the people through their political leaders has been a hallmark of the reforms in Thailand. The Costa Rican reforms have had strong support from the political parties, the CCSS itself, medical care providers, workers, and MOH staff members as they all had a voice in shaping the reform.

### Efficiency Gains and Copayments Used as Financing Mechanisms

Efficiency gains are an important means of both financing a health system and providing fiscal space for coverage expansions. Efficiency gains were a critical element in the expansions in the FSU countries and Sri Lanka. Thailand created fiscal space by reducing defense expenditures and has implemented modern provider payment systems to ensure efficiency in its new UCS program. Costa Rica has also focused on efficient purchasing arrangements to reduce outlays. Copayments have been used as both a financing mechanism and a means of containing moral hazard in Chile, Vietnam, Estonia, and to a lesser extent in Sri Lanka, the Kyrgyz Republic, and Thailand.

### Flexibility and Mid-Course Corrections

Considering the long implementation periods of the reforms in all of these countries and the careful sequencing of delivery system changes with the coverage expansions, it is not surprising that both evidence-based policies and mid-course corrections have affected implementation. Thailand prides itself on the use of evidence-based policies in all aspects of its reform efforts. It was one of the earliest developing countries to institute comprehensive national health accounts

(NHA), and it has both used and significantly contributed to the global HRH evidence base. Thailand has implemented modern provider payment and risk-sharing approaches for several of its insurance programs. It has undertaken detailed studies on equity and impoverishment due to high medical expenses. Estonia has exhibited marked flexibility in its reform and has, for example, reversed decentralization polices for risk pools and delivery system responsibilities. Colombia, Thailand, Sri Lanka, Vietnam, and the Kyrgyz Republic have made significant and explicit choices in the way that the care for the poor is subsidized through the MHI schemes.

## Next Steps for Enhancing the Global Evidence Base

This study has attempted to assess "good performance" in the context of major health financing reforms. Defining "good performance" in terms of complex financing expansions involving revenue collection, risk pooling, purchasing, and related delivery system changes is, as discussed, a complex venture. This study might be viewed as a tentative first step to provide some guidance or indeed a straw man for the global community to consider in its quest to collate the global evidence base on health financing. These concluding observations from part I of this report attempt to lay out the necessary future steps in terms of measurement, data, evaluation, and dissemination to allow needed refinements in the global evidence base on health care financing reforms.

One of the largest impediments in developing the global evidence base on health financing reforms is the difficulty of defining what is meant by "good performance" or "success." Second order questions of measurement and evaluation/attribution then arise. As discussed, all of these are problematic. Nevertheless, the global community needs to reach some consensus in these areas if it is serious about the development and dissemination of global evidence as a guide to policy making.

To do this, at least five important actions are needed:

- Define rigorously what *successes* and *good performance* mean in health financing.[1]
- Collect standardized and appropriate qualitative and quantitative information.
- Describe health systems characteristics in sufficient detail so that the critical components and their interactions can be clearly identified and assessed.
- Undertake rigorous evaluations.
- Disseminate these evaluations to all stakeholders in a policy-relevant and user-friendly manner.

## Definition of "Success" and "Good Performance"

"Good performance" with respect to health financing reforms is defined in this study in terms of countries that have expanded health coverage and financial protection in the context of reasonable and sustainable spending levels, equity, and good health outcomes relative to other comparable income countries. This definition is derived from the definitions of basic health financing function definitions and objectives outlined in chapter 2. The presumption here is that if revenue collection, risk pooling, and purchasing functions are performed effectively, the result will be better health outcomes, financial protection, equity, efficiency, and financial sustainability of the health system.

"Good practice" performers were chosen on the basis of both a priori judgments from an expert steering committee and comparative analyses of a number dimensions—including financial protection, health outcomes, equity, efficiency, and sustainability. Financial protection is explicitly defined in terms of expansions in the number of individuals who are formally covered under a publicly or privately financed health program as well as various measures of financial protection for that individual/household.[2]

The serious data gaps are openly discussed, as well as the inherent causality attribution problems. Numerous interactive factors affect health outcomes, and the multiple enabling factors are hard to attribute in so complex an area due to the difficulties of performing case control studies, including randomized trials. From the detailed case studies, the authors have attempted to highlight the critical demographic, geographic, political, socioeconomic, and health and nonhealth sector-related enabling factors. Based on the case studies and comparative data, an attempt is then made to assess whether there are common enabling factors that are likely to account for the observed performance. The factors identified make sense on conceptual grounds and are useful additions to the sparse global evidence base. The more important contribution, however, is not the findings in themselves, but rather the illustration of the need for the international community to do a better job in measurement, data development, evaluation, and dissemination of the evidence.

## Need to Collect Standardized and Appropriate Qualitative and Quantitative Information

As vividly shown in chapters 3 and 4, as well as in the case studies in part II, baseline indicators of coverage, financial protection, equity, and efficiency are generally lacking, often both pre- and postreform. Thus, first and foremost attention must be given to developing the necessary baseline and postreform information. Specifically, although most of the country cases contained information on numbers of individuals eligible for various health financing programs, there was little information on enrollment and the breadth and depth of coverage both pre- and postreform. The lack of measures of financial protection—particularly for prereform periods—is even more problematic. The postreform information came mostly from special surveys, either country-based household surveys or the "World Health Survey 2003 Results" (WHO 2003b). Definitions of total expenditure, income, and out-of-pocket spending, as well as financial protection, among these two different sources are often not equivalent and sometimes are based on different recall periods, making comparisons difficult.

Furthermore, attempts to measure changes in the aggregate spending (and revenue) accompanying these reforms (needed to assess macro efficiency and sustainability) are attenuated by the lack of reliable NHA time series information and information on revenues, particularly subnational revenues. Similarly, attempts to measure the equity aspects are limited by the lack of microdata on out-of-pocket spending, revenue incidence information, and utilization data both pre- and post-reform. Few studies bother to discuss spending efficiency in other than generic terms regarding mismatches of basic benefits packages with current and future projected disease burdens.

If individual countries—and the international community—are serious about improving the global evidence base on health financing reforms, they will need to start by ensuring the development and institutionalization of basic information such as NHA, detailed national and subnational revenue, expenditure, and utilization, output, and outcome data necessary for benefit, revenue, and net incidence assessments, and accurate counts of health program–eligible and health program–enrolled individuals. The recently established Health Metrics Network needs to give these areas appropriate focus and publicity, and countries need incentives to systematically develop and collect such information. This information will also be needed to assess aid effectiveness and the equity and efficiency of public spending. To measure health system performance fully, macrodata sets will need to be linked with microdata—not just from household surveys, but also from provider and epidemiological surveys.

## Need Health Systems Characteristics Information

Effective health coverage is important to ensure good health outcomes and financial protection. But coverage (even effective coverage in a WHO sense) is neither a necessary nor sufficient condition for reaching either of these two goals. Beyond their coverage status, numerous demographic, socioeconomic, geographic, cultural, and political factors affect individuals' behaviors, as do other complex institutional interrelations that shape health system performance in terms of health status and financial protection. Understanding these factors and, to the extent feasible, controlling and assessing their impact requires both quantitative and qualitative information on these factors themselves and on their behavioral interactions. Although the growing health policy literature (e.g., WHO Commission on Macroeconomics and Health, Millennium Project, WHO) provides important insights into the most critical factors (e.g., female education, good public sector management), detailed specification of these behavioral relationships is far from a science or complete. Nevertheless, to the extent feasible, it is important to both specify these factors upfront quantitatively and qualitatively and to control for them when attempting to draw conclusions about performance.

## Rigorous Evaluations

All new global initiatives, including the new HNP Strategy of the World Bank (World Bank 2007b), have decried the insufficient attention given to monitoring and evaluation, as well as to the previously discussed collection of critical baseline data. Studies of health financing reforms are equally implicated. Considering the complexity of evaluating such reforms and the many other factors affecting health outcomes and financial protection, the gold standard of randomized control trials or even a silver standard of case control studies with a nonrandomized control group may be less feasible as techniques for evaluating large financing changes. Although "before" and "after" evaluation techniques are more the order of the day, they too can lead to spurious conclusions, given the difficulty of teasing out the impact of secular trends that may affect health system outcomes from those that result from specific health policy interventions.

Nevertheless, it goes without saying that the global community must do a better job to develop the basic evidence and collate the existing base using the most appropriate evaluation tools. At the very least, key institutional and behavioral factors likely to affect health coverage, health status, and financial protection outcomes should be specified. The impact of these factors on the outcomes of the financing changes should then be evaluated as best as possible, qualitatively and quantitatively, through appropriate statistical and experimental methodologies.

Evaluating failures as well as success would be another needed departure from much of the present effort. Success or good performance cannot be fully evaluated without understanding what constitutes failure or poor performance—as a great deal can also be learned from failures. However, little has been written on major reforms that have not lived up to expectations such as the adoption of regionally based Mandatory Health Insurance in Russia and much of the former FSU. Although the failure of the Clinton reform in the United States has been extensively analyzed and the British attempts to introduce market incentives into the NHS have attracted great interest, their lessons for developing countries have not been well teased out.

## Dissemination of Evidence

Collation and dissemination of the global evidence is one of the key features of every new initiative—Health Metrics Network (HMN), Global Health Workforce Alliance (GHWA), Scaling Up for Better Health (IHP+), the Global Alliance for Vaccines and Immunization (GAVI), the Global Fund to Fight AIDS, Tuberculosis and Malaria (GFATM), and the Bank's new HNP Strategy. In health financing, this process is especially complex, because of the issues highlighted above, but also because of the behavior of donors and nongovernmental organizations (NGOs). Irrespective of the global evidence, donors and NGOs often push particular policy positions and/or one-size-fits-all solutions. No one is in charge of global health policy (Schieber et al. 2007), much less global health financing policy, so there is no venue for reaching agreement on appropriate indicators and responsibility for development, institutionalization, and collation of data. One ancillary outcome of the IHP+ and its focus on health systems strengthening, where the World Bank and the WHO are the secretariat for six other major development partners, might be some agreement on the needed indicators and a division of responsibility to ensure consistent development and institutionalization. This is consistent with the objectives of the IHP+ and other initiatives, including those of the G-8,[3] which has shown a strong interest in promoting risk pooling in low-income settings. The IHP+ initiative would therefore seem to present a good opportunity for collaborative development of the necessary information bases.

## Conclusions

The global community has done a poor job so far in developing, collating, and disseminating the global evidence base on what works in health financing and what does not. The G-8, as well as many individual countries, attach growing importance to health financing and risk pooling, while some organizations are pushing a single magic-bullet approach. It is incumbent on the global community to take charge and move this agenda forward in an analytically sound and policy-relevant manner. It is hoped that global stakeholders, through their aid-effectiveness forums and the G-8, IHP+, and Paris Declaration Process, will rise to the occasion and put this desperately needed effort on track.

### Endnotes

1. For purposes of this study, only good performance (not success) can be discussed, because no failures were evaluated.

2. For purposes of this financing assessment "coverage" is defined in an insurance context, not the more clinical contexts of WHO, which relate to utilization conditional on need. See Tanahashi (1978).

3. G-8 members are Germany, France, the United Kingdom, Italy, Japan, the United States, Canada (since 1976), and Russia (since 1998). The European Commission is also represented at all the meetings. German Chancellor Angela Merkel, G-8 president, invited Algeria, Brazil, China, the Arab Republic of Egypt, India, Mexico Nigeria, Senegal, and South Africa to participate in the outreach meetings in Heiligendamm, Germany, in June 2007.

## References for Part I

Abel-Smith, Brian. 1992. "Health Insurance in Developing Countries: Lessons from Experience." *Health Policy and Planning* 7 (3): 215–26.

Adams, Susan. 2005. "Vietnam's Health Care System: A Macroeconomic Perspective." Paper prepared for the International Symposium on Health Care Systems in Asia, Hanoi, Vietnam, January 21–22, 2005, Washington, DC, International Monetary Fund.

ADB (Asian Development Bank). 2006. *Measuring Policy Effectiveness in Health and Education.* Manila: ADB.

Antioch, K. M., and M. K. Walsh. 2004. "The Risk-Adjusted Vision beyond Casemix (DRG) Funding in Australia—International Lessons in High Complexity and Capitation." *European Journal of Health Economics* 5 (2): 95–109.

Aris, B. 2004. "Slovenia's Health System Out-Performs EU Neighbours. Peace and Prosperity Have Helped Slovenia Ministers Push Through Effective Reforms." *Lancet* 363 (9427): 2143–46.

Asfaw, A., and J. von Braun 2004. "Can Community Health Insurance Schemes Shield the Poor Against the Downside Health Effects of Economic Reforms? The Case of Rural Ethiopia." *Health Policy* 70 (1): 97–108.

Baeza, C., P. Crocco, M. Núñez, and M. Shaffer. 2002. *Toward Decent Work: Social Protection in Health for All Workers and Their Families.* Strategies and Tools against Social Exclusion and Poverty (STEP). Geneva: International Labour Organization.

Baeza, C., and T. Packard. 2006. *Beyond Survival: Protecting Households from Health Shocks in Latin America.* Washington, DC/Palo Alto, CA: World Bank/Stanford University Press.

Baeza, Cristian, and Fernando Montenegro Torres. 2004. "Selecting Health Care Providers." Health, Nutrition and Population (HNP) Discussion Paper. World Bank, Washington, DC.

Balabanova, D., and M. McKee. 2004. "Reforming Health Care Financing in Bulgaria: The Population Perspective." *Social Science & Medicine* 58 (4): 753–65.

Barnum, Howard, Joseph Kutzin, and Helen Saxenian. 1995. "Incentives and Provider Payment Methods." World Bank Human Resources Development and Operations Policy Working Paper No. 51, Washington, DC. http://www.worldbank.org/html/extdr/hnp/hddflash/hcwp/hrwp043.html.

Bassett, Mark. 2005. "Frameworks for Analyzing Health Systems, Health Financing and the Regulation of Health Insurance." Paper prepared for Conference on Private Health Insurance in Developing Countries cosponsored by the World Bank and the Wharton School of the University of Pennsylvania, at the Wharton School, Philadelphia, Pa., March 15–16, 2005.

Besley, T., and R. Burgess. 2002. "The Political Economy of Government Responsiveness: Theory and Evidence from India." *Quarterly Journal of Economics.* 117 (4): 1415–51.

Bhushan, I., S. Keller, and B. Schwartz. 2002. "Achieving the Twin Objectives of Efficiency and Equity: Contracting Health Services in Cambodia." *ERD Policy Brief No. 6.* Manila: Asian Development Bank.

Blau, David M. 1985. "Self-Employment and Self-Selection in Developing Country Labor Markets." *Southern Economic Journal* 51 (2): 351–63.

Bokhari, F., Y. Gai, and P. Gottret. 2007. "Government Health Expenditures and Health Outcomes. *Health Economics* 16 (3): 257–73.

Boncz, I., J. Nagy, A. Sebestyen, and L. Korosi. 2004. "Financing of Health Care Services in Hungary." *European Journal of Health Economics* 5 (3): 252–58.

Bosch, X. 2004. "French Government Approves Unpopular Health Reforms." *Lancet* 363 (9427): 2148.

Carrin, Guy, and P. Hanvoravongchai. 2003. "Provider Payments and Patient Charges as Policy Tools for Cost-Containment: How Successful Are They in High-Income Countries?" *Human Resources for Health* 1 (6): downloaded from http://www.human-resources- health.com/content/pdf/1478-4491-1-6.pdf.

Carrin, Guy, and Chris James. 2004. "Reaching Universal Coverage via Social Health Insurance: Key Design Features in the Transition Period." EIP/FER/DP.04.2, World Health Organization, Geneva.

Castañeda, Tarsicio. 2005. "Targeting Social Spending to the Poor with Proxy–Means Testing: Colombia's SISBEN System." Social Protection Discussion Paper Series, No. 0529, Social Protection Unit, Human Development Network, World Bank, Washington, DC.

Charoenparij, Sriracha, Somsak Chunharas, Dayl Donaldson, Daniel Kraushaar, Supasit Pannorunothai, Sutham Pinjaroen, Supattra Srivanichakorn, Paibul Suriyawongpaisal, Viroj Tangcharoensathien, and Aree Valyasevi. 1999. "Health Financing in Thailand: Final Integrated Report." Thailand/Boston: Health Management and Financing Study Project/ Management Sciences for Health.

Cheng, T. 2003. "Taiwan's New National Health Insurance Program: Genesis and Experience So Far." *Health Affairs* 22: 61–76.

Chollet, Deborah, and Maureen Lewis. 1997. "Private Insurance: Principles and Practice." In "Innovations in Health Care Financing," ed. George Schieber, pp. 77–103. World Bank Discussion Paper 365. World Bank, Washington, DC.

Clark, Mary. 2002. "Health Sector Reform in Costa Rica: Reinforcing a Public System." Paper prepared for Woodrow Wilson Center Workshops on the Politics of Education and Health Reforms, Washington, DC, April 2002.

Colombo, Francesca, and Nicole Tapay. 2004. "Private Health Insurance in OECD Countries: The Benefits and Costs for Individuals and Health Systems." DELSA/ELSA/WD/HEA(2004)6, Organisation for Economic Co-operation and Development, Paris.

Commission on Macroeconomics and Health. 2002. "Macroeconomics and Health: Investing in Health for Economic Development." In *Report of the Commission on Macroeconomics and Health, Commission on Macroeconomics and Health.* Geneva: World Health Organization.

Cornell, J., J. Goudge, D. McIntyre, and S. Mbatsha. 2001. "South African National Health Accounts: The Private Sector." National Health Accounts Research Team and National Department of Health, Pretoria.

Csonka, A. 2004. "Hungary Makes Slow Progress in Health-System Reform. Private Funds, Which Could Rescue Hungary's Ailing Health-Care System, Have Been Slow to Materialise." *Lancet* 363 (9425): 1957–60.

Cutler, D. M., and A. Lleras-Muney. 2006. "Education and Health: Evaluating Theories and Evidence." National Poverty Center Working Paper Series 06–19, University of Michigan, Ann Harbor.

Davoodi, H., E. Tiongson, and S. Asawanuchit. 2003. "How Useful Are Benefit Incidence Analyses of Public Education and Health Spending?" IMF Working Paper, International Monetary Fund, Washington, DC.

Deaton, A. 1997. *The Analysis of Household Surveys: A Microeconometric Approach to Development Policy.* Baltimore, MD: Johns Hopkins University Press.

Deaton, A., and S. Zaidi. 2002. "Guidelines for Constructing Consumption Aggregates for Welfare Analysis." LSMS Working Paper 135, World Bank, Washington, DC.

Docteur, E., and H. Oxley. 2003. "Health-Care Systems: Lessons from the Reform Experience." DELSA/ELSA/WD/HEA(2003)9, Organisation for Economic Co-operation and Development, Directorate for Employment, Labour and Social Affairs, Paris.

Doherty, Jane, Stephen Thomas, and Debbie Muirhead. 2002. "Health Financing and Expenditure in Post-Apartheid South Africa, 1996/97–1998/99." The National Health Accounts Project, Centre for Health Policy, University of the Witwatersrand and Health Economics Unit, University of Cape Town.

Donaldson, D., S. Pannarunothai, and V. Tangcharoensathien. 1999. *Health Financing in Thailand Summary Review and Proposed Reforms.* Nonthaburi, Thailand: Health Systems Research Institute.

Ellis, Randall P., and Thomas G. McGuire. 1993. "Supply-side Cost Sharing in Health Care." *Journal of Economic Perspectives* 7: 135–51.

———. 1996. "Hospital Response to Prospective Payment: Selection and Moral Hazard Effects." *Journal of Health Economics* 15 (3): 257–79.

El-Saharty, Sameh, Axel Róala, and Hugh Waters. 2006. "Etude du secteur de la santé en Tunisie." Human Development Department, Middle East and North Africa Region, World Bank, Washington, DC.

Ensor, Tim. 1999. "Developing Health Insurance in Transitional Asia." *Social Science & Medicine* 48 (7): 871–79.

Ensor, Tim, and Stephanie Cooper. 2004. "Overcoming Barriers to Health Service Access and Influencing the Demand Side through Purchasing." Health, Nutrition and Population (HNP) Discussion Paper 31598, World Bank, Washington, DC.

Ensor, Tim, and Robin Thompson. 1998. "Health Insurance as a Catalyst to Change in Former Communist Countries." *Social Science & Medicine* 43 (3): 203–18.

Figueras, Joseph, Ray Robinson, and Elke Jakubowski, eds. 2005. "Purchasing to Improve Health Systems Performance." European Observatory on Health Systems and Policies Series. England: Open University Press.

Filmer, D., and L. Pritchett. 1999. "The Impact of Public Spending on Health: Does Money Matter." *Social Science & Medicine* 49 (10): 1309–23.

Frenk, Julio, Jaime Sepúlveda, Octavio Gómez-Dantés, and Felicia Knaul. 2003. "Evidence-Based Health Policy: Three Generations of Reform in Mexico." *Lancet* 362 (9396): 1667–71.

Gertler, P. 2004. "Do Conditional Cash Transfers Improve Child Health? Evidence from PROGRESA's Controlled Randomized Experiment." *Health, Health Care, and Economic Development* 94 (2): 336–41.

Gertler, P., and J. van der Gaag. 1988. "Willingness to Pay for Social Services in Developing Countries." Measurement Study (LSMS) Working Paper 45, World Bank, Washington, DC.

Gertler, Paul, and Jonathan Gruber. 2002. "Insuring Consumption against Illness." *American Economic Review* 92 (1): 51–76.

Gill, I., and N. Ilahi. 2000. "Economic Insecurity, Individual Behavior, and Social Policy." Background Paper for the Regional Study on Economic Insecurity, Office of the Chief Economist, Latin America and the Caribbean, World Bank, Washington, DC.

Gill, I., T. Packard, and J. Yermo. 2004. *Keeping the Promise of Social Security in Latin America.* Latin American Development Forum. Washington, DC: World Bank.

Goglio, Alessandro. 2005. "In Search of Efficiency: Improving Health Care in Hungary." Organisation for Economic Co-operation and Development, Paris.

Gomez-Dantes, O., J. Gomez-Jauregui, and C. Inclan. 2004. "La equidad y la imparcialidad en la reforma del sistema mexicano de salud." [Equity and fairness in the Mexican health system reform]. *Salud Pública de México* 46 (5): 399–416.

González-Rossetti, A., and T. Bossert. 2000. "Enhancing the Political Feasibility of Health Reform: A Comparative Analysis of Chile, Colombia and Mexico." Harvard School of Public Health, Department of Population Studies and International Health, Data for Decision Making Project and the Latin American and Caribbean Health Sector Reform Initiative, Cambridge, MA.

Gottret, Pablo, and George Schieber. 2006. *Health Financing Revisited.* Washington DC: World Bank.

Government of Taiwan. 2003. *Statistical Yearbook.* http://www.gio.gov.tw/Taiwan-website/5-gp/yearbook/chpt02.htm#1.

Gwatkin, Davidson. 2004. "Are Free Government Health Services the Best Way to Reach the Poor?" Health, Nutrition and Population (HNP) Discussion Paper 29185, World Bank, Washington, DC.

Habicht, J., K. Xu, A. Couffinhal, and J. Kutzin. 2006. "Detecting Changes in Financial Protection: Creating Evidence for Policy in Estonia." *Health Policy and Planning* 21 (6): 421–31.

Hauck, Katharina, Peter C. Smith, and Maria Goddard. 2004. "The Economics of Priority Setting for Health Care: A Literature Review." Health, Nutrition and Population (HNP) Discussion Paper 28878, World Bank, Washington, DC.

Hlavačka, S., R. Wágner, and A. Riesberg. 2004. "Health Care Systems in Transition: Slovakia." WHO Regional Office for Europe on behalf of the European Observatory on Health Systems and Policies, Copenhagen.

Hsiao, W., and P. Shaw. 2007. *Social Health Insurance for Developing Nations.* Washington, DC: World Bank.

Hsiao, William. 2000. "What Should Macroeconomists Know about Health Care Policy? A Primer." IMF Working Paper WP/00/136. International Monetary Fund, Washington, DC. http://www.imf.org/external/pubs/cat/longres.cfm?sk&sk=3701.0

Hu, T. W. 2004. "Financing and Organization of China's Health Care." *Bulletin of the World Health Organization* 82 (7): 480.

Ikegami, N., and J. C. Campbell. 2004. "Japan's Health Care System: Containing Costs and Attempting Reform." *Health Affairs* 23 (3): 26–36.

Institute of Policy Studies. 2001. "Equity in Financing and Delivery of Health Services in Bangladesh, Nepal and Sri Lanka: Results of the Tri-country Study." Colombo: Institute of Policy Studies.

Institute of Policy Studies of Sri Lanka. 2001. "Sri Lanka National Health Accounts—Sri Lanka National Health Expenditures 1990–1999." Ministry of Health. Health Policy Programme supported by the IDA/WB Health Services Project. Ministry of Health, Nutrition and Welfare and Institute of Policy Studies, Colombo.

ILO (International Labour Office). 2002. "Extending Social Protection through Community-Based Health Organizations—Evidence and Challenges." Discussion Paper. Geneva: International Labour Office.

Jack, W. 2005. "Purchasing Health Care Services from Providers with Unknown Altruism." *Journal of Health Economics* 24 (1): 73–93.

Jegers, M., K. Kesteloot, D. De Graeve, and W. Gilles. 2002. "A Typology for Provider Payment Systems in Health Care." *Health Policy* 60 (3): 255–73.

Jesse, M., J. Habicht, A. Aaviksoo, A. Koppel, A. Irs, and S. Thomson. 2004. "Health Care Systems in Transition: Estonia." WHO Regional Office for Europe on behalf of the European Observatory on Health Systems and Policies, Copenhagen.

John, T., S. Charles, R. Nathan, K. Wilczynska, L. Mgalula, C. Mbuya, R. Mswia, F. Manzi, D. de Savigny, D. Schellenberg, and C. Victora. 2004. "Effectiveness and Cost of Facility-Based Integrated Management of Childhood Illness (IMCI) in Tanzania." *Lancet* 364 (9445): 1583–94.

Joint Learning Initiative. 2004. *Human Resources for Health: Overcoming the Crisis.* Cambridge, MA: Harvard University Press.

Karashkevica, J. 2004. "Latvia's Health Care System on the Move." *Cahiers de sociologie et de demographie medicales* 44 (2): 221–42.

Kuszewski, K., and C. Gericke. 2005. *Health Systems in Transition: Poland.* WHO Regional Office for Europe on behalf of the European Observatory on Health Systems and Policies, Copenhagen.

Kutzin, Joseph. 2001. "A Descriptive Framework for Country-Level Analysis of Health Care Financing Arrangements." *Health Policy* 56: 171–204.

———. 2002. *Health Care in Central Asia.* Policy Brief. Copenhagen: European Observatory on Health Care Systems.

La Forgia, Gerard, ed. 2004. "Health System Innovations in Central America—Lessons and Impact of New Approaches." World Bank Working Paper 57, World Bank, Washington, DC.

Langenbrunner, John C., and Xingzhu Liu. 2004. "How to Pay? Understanding and Using Incentives." Health, Nutrition and Population (HNP) Discussion Paper 31633, World Bank, Washington, DC.

Levine, R. 2007. *Case Studies in Global Health: Millions Saved.* Washington, DC: Center for Global Development.

Levine, R., and M. Kinder. 2004. *Millions Saved: Proven Successes in Global Health.* Washington, DC: Center for Global Development.

Lim, M. K. 2004. "Shifting the Burden of Health Care Finance: A Case Study of Public-Private Partnership in Singapore." *Health Policy* 69 (1): 83–92.

Limwattananon, S., V. Tangcharoensathien, and P. Prakongsai. 2007. "Catastrophic and Poverty Impacts of Health Payments: Results from National Household Surveys in Thailand." *Bulletin of the World Health Organization* 85 (8): 569–48.

Liu, Xingzhu, and Sheila O'Dougherty. 2004. "Purchasing Priority Public Health Services." Health, Nutrition and Population (HNP) Discussion Paper 31593, World Bank, Washington, DC.

Londoño, J. 1996. "Estructurando pluralismo en los servicios de salud: la experiencia colombiana." *Revista de análisis económico* 11 (2): 37–60.

Londoño, J., and J. Frenk. 1997. "Structured Pluralism: Toward an Innovative Model for Health System Reform in Latin America." *Health Policy* 41 (1): 1–36.

Maceira, Daniel. 1998. "Provider Payment Mechanisms in Health Care: Incentives, Outcomes, and Organizational Impact in Developing Countries." Major Applied Research 2, Working Paper 2. Partnerships for Health Reform Project, Abt Associates Inc. Bethesda, MD. http://www.phrproject.com/publicat/arp/download/mar2/m2wp2fin.pdf.

Marek, Tonia, Rena Eichler, and Philip Schnab. 2004. "Resource Allocation and Purchasing in Africa: What Is Effective in Improving the Health of the Poor?" Africa Region Human Development Working Paper Series, World Bank, Washington, DC.

Markota, Mladen, Igor Švab, Ksenija Sarazin Klemenèiè, and Tit Albreht. 1999. "Slovenian Experience on Health Care Reform." *Croatian Medical Journal* 40 (2): 190–94.

Marshall, M. G., and K. Jaggers. 2005. "Polity IV Project: Political Regime Characteristics and Transactions, 1800–2004." University of Maryland and George Mason University, College Park, MD, and Fairfax, VA.

McGuire, T. 2000. "Physician Agency." In *Handbook of Health Economics*, ed. J. Newhouse and A. Culyer, 461–536. The Netherlands: Elsevier.

Meimanaliev, Tilek. 2003. *Kyrgyz Model of Health Care System.* Bishkek: Uchkun.

Meimanaliev, A. S., A. Ibraimova, B. Elebesov, and B. Rechel. 2005. "Health Care Systems in Transition: Kyrgyz Republic." WHO Regional Office for Europe on behalf of the European Observatory on Health Systems and Policies, Copenhagen.

Meng, Q., C. Rehnberg, N. Zhuang, Y. Bian, G. Tomson, and S. Tang. 2004. "The Impact of Urban Health Insurance Reform on Hospital Charges: A Case Study from Two Cities in China." *Health Policy* 68 (2): 197–209.

MOH (Ministry of Health, Vietnam). 2001. *55 Years of Developing Vietnam's Revolutionary Health System.* Hanoi: Medical Publishing House.

MOH (Ministry of Public Health, Thailand). 2002. *Thailand Health Profile 1999–2000.* Thailand: Bureau of Policy and Strategy.

Montenegro, F., and R. Nazareli. 2004. "Health and Household Income and Consumption: A Review of the Literature." Background Paper, World Bank, Washington, DC.

Morlock, Laura, Alan Sorkin, and Hugh Waters, eds. Forthcoming. *National Health Insurance in Taiwan: What Lessons May Be Learned?* New York: Elsevier.

Morlock, Laura, Hugh Waters, Alan Lyles, Haluk Özsari, and Göksenin Aktulay. 2004. "Health Care Reform in Turkey—Charting the Way Forward." Final report submitted to The Turkish Industrialists' and Businessmen's Association Turk Sanayici ve Isadamlari Dernegi (TÜSIAD). Baltimore, MD: Johns Hopkins University.

Mossialos, Elias, Anna Dixon, Joseph Figueras, and Joe Kutzin, eds. 2002. "Funding Health-care: Options for Europe." European Observatory on Health Care Systems Series, Open University Press, Buckingham and Philadelphia.

Murray, C., and J. Frenk. 2000. "A Framework for Assessing the Performance of Health Systems." *Bulletin of the World Health Organization* 78 (6): 717–28.

Musgrove, P. 1996. "Un fundamento conceptual para el rol público y privado en la salud." *Análisis Económico* 11 (2): 9–36.

Musgrove, Philip, Riadh Zeramdini, and Guy Carrin. 2002. "Basic Patterns of Health Expenditure." *Bulletin of the World Health Organization* 80: 134–42.

O'Donnell, O., Eddy van Doorslaer, Ravi P. Rannan-Eliya, Aparnaa Somanathan, Shiva Raj Adhikari, Deni Harbianto, Charu C. Garg, Piya Hanvoravongchai, Mohammed N. Huq, Anup Karan, Gabriel M. Leung, Chiu Wan Ng, Badri Raj Pande, Keith Tin, Kanjana Tisayaticom, Laksono Trisnantoro, Yuhui Zhang, and Yuxin Zhao 2007. "The Incidence of Public Spending on Health Care: Comparative Evidence from Asia." *World Bank Economic Review* 21: 93–123.

O'Donnell, O., Eddy van Doorslaer, Ravi P. Rannan-Eliya, Aparnaa Somanathan, Charu C. Garg, Piya Hanvoravongchai, Mohammed N. Huq, Anup Karan, Gabriel M. Leung, Keith Tin, and Chitpranee Vasavid. 2005. "Explaining the Incidence of Catastrophic Expenditures on Health Care: Comparative Evidence from Asia." EQUITAP Project, Working Paper 5. Erasmus University, Rotterdam and Institute of Policy Studies, Colombo.

OECD (Organisation for Economic Co-operation and Development). 2002. "The Reform of Health Care: A Comparative Analysis of Seven OECD Countries." Health Policy Studies, No. 2. Paris.

———. 2003. *OECD Reviews of Health Systems—Korea.* Paris: OECD.

———. 2004. *Proposal for a Taxonomy of Health Insurance.* OECD Study on Private Health Insurance. Paris: OECD.

———. 2005. *OECD Reviews of Health Systems—Mexico.* Paris: OECD.

Packard, T., and A. Barr. 2002. "Revealed Preference and Self-Insurance: Can We Learn from the Self-Employed in Chile?" Policy Research Working Paper 2754, World Bank, Washington, DC.

PAHO (Pan American Health Organization). 1999. *Cuba Profile of the Health Services System.* Program on Organization and Management of Health Systems and Services, Division of Health Systems and Services Development. Washington, DC: PAHO.

———. 2002. *Profile of the Health Services System of Costa Rica,* 2d ed. Program on Organization and Management of Health Systems and Services, Division of Health Systems and Services Development. Washington, DC: PAHO.

Pannarunothai, S. 2002. "Medical Welfare Scheme: Financing and Targeting the Poor." In *Health Insurance Systems in Thailand,* ed. P. Pramualratana and S. Wibulpolprasert, 62–78. Nonthaburi, Thailand: Health Systems Research Institute.

Pannarunothai, S., D. Patmasiriwat, and S. Srithamrongsawat. 2004. "Universal Health Coverage in Thailand: Ideas for Reform and Policy Struggling." *Health Policy* 68 (1): 17–30.

Pauly, Mark. 1986. "Taxation, Health Insurance, and Market Failure in the Medical Economy." *Journal of Economic Literature,* 24 (2): 629–75.

Phelps, C. E. 1978. "Illness Prevention and Medical Insurance." *Journal of Human Resources* 13: 183–207. Supplement. National Bureau of Economic Research Conference on the Economics of Physician and Patient Behavior.

POLITY IV dataset: http://www.cidcm.umd.edu/polity/data/.

Pradhan, M., and N. Prescott. 2002. "Social Risk Management Options for Medical Care in Indonesia." *Health Economics* 11 (5): 431–46.

Preker, A. S., G. Carrin, D. Dror, M. Jakab, W. Hsiao, and D. Arhin-Tenkorang. 2002. "Effectiveness of Community Health Financing in Meeting the Cost of Illness." *Bulletin of the World Health Organization* 80 (2): 143–50.

Preker, Alexander S., Cristian Baeza, Melita Jakab, and John C. Langenbrunner. 2000. "Arrangements that Benefit the Poor and Excluded Groups." Concept Note. World Bank/ILO/WHO Resource Allocation and Purchasing (RAP) Project, Washington, DC.

Preker, Alexander S., and Guy Carrin, eds. 2003. *Health Financing for Poor People: Resource Mobilization and Risk Sharing.* Washington, DC: World Bank.

Preker, Alexander S., and John C. Langenbrunner, eds. 2005. *Spending Wisely: Buying Health Services for the Poor.* Washington, DC: World Bank.

Rannan-Eliya, R. P. 2001. *Strategies for Improving the Health of the Poor—The Sri Lankan Experience.* Colombo: Institute of Policy Studies Health Policy Programme.

Ranson, M. 2002. "Reduction of Catastrophic Health Care Expenditures by a Community-Based Health Insurance Scheme in Gujarat, India: Current Experiences and Challenges." *Bulletin of the World Health Organization* 80: 613–21.

Ravallion, M. 1994. "Poverty Comparisons: A Guide to Concepts and Methods." Living Standards Measurement Study (LSMS) Working Paper LSM 88, World Bank, Washington, DC.

Ravallion, M., and B. Bidani. 1994. "How Robust Is a Poverty Profile? Vol. 1." *World Bank Economic Review* 8 (1): 75–102.

Rawlings, Laura B. 2004. "A New Approach to Social Assistance: Latin America's Experience with Conditional Cash Transfer Programs." Social Protection Discussion Paper 0416, World Bank, Washington, DC.

Rice, T. 2006. "The Physician as the Patient's Agent." In *The Elgar Companion to Health Economics,* ed. Andrew Jones, 261–68. Cheltenham, UK: Edward Elgar.

Rodwin, V. G., and C. Le Pen. 2004. "Health Care Reform in France—The Birth of State-Led Managed Care." *New England Journal of Medicine* 351 (22): 2259–62.

Rosa, R. M., and I. C. Alberto. 2004. "Universal Health Care for Colombians 10 Years after Law 100: Challenges and Opportunities." *Health Policy* 68 (2): 129–42.

Safaei, J. 2006. "Is Democracy Good for Health?" *International Journal of Health Services* 36 (4): 767–86.

Savedoff, W. D., and R. Levine. 2006. "Learning from Development: the Case for an International Council to Catalyze Independent Impact Evaluations of Social Sector Interventions." Center for Global Development, Washington, DC.

Schieber, G., C. Baeza, D. Kress, and M. Maier. 2006. "Financing Health Systems in the 21st Century." In *Disease Control Priorities in Developing Countries,* 2d ed., ed. Dean Jamison, George Alleyne, Joel Breman, Mariam Claeson, David Evans, Prabhat Jha, Anthony Measham, Anne Mills, and Philip Musgrove, pp 255–42. Oxford and New York, NY: Oxford University Press for World Bank.

Schieber, G., L. Fleisher, and P. Gottret. 2006. "Getting Real on Health Financing." *Finance and Development* 43 (4): 46–50.

Schieber, G., P. Gottret, L. Fleisher, and A. Leive. 2007. "Financing Global Health: Mission Unaccomplished." *Health Affairs* 26 (4): 921–34.

Schieber, George, ed. 1997. *Innovations in Health Care Financing.* Washington, DC: World Bank.

Schieber, George, and Nicole Klingen. 1999. "Islamic Republic of Iran—Health Financing Reform in Iran: Principles and Possible Next Steps." Prepared for Social Security Research Institute, Health Economic Congress, October 1999. World Bank, Washington, DC.

Schieber, George, and Akiko Maeda. 1999. "Health Care Financing and Delivery in Developing Countries." *Health Affairs* 18 (3): 193–205.

Soares, R. R. 2007. "On the Determinants of Mortality Reductions in the Developing World," NBER Working Paper 12837, National Bureau of Economic Research, Cambridge, MA.

Somanathan, Aparnaa. 2003. "Beneficiaries from Public Health Care in Five Asian Countries: Equity in Asia-Pacific Health Systems Network." Presentation at World Bank conference on Reaching the Poor, February 18–20, 2004, Washington, DC.

Sriratanaban, J. 2002. "Civil Servant Medical Benefit Scheme: Unregulated Fee-for-Service and Cost Escalation." In *Health Insurance Systems in Thailand,* ed. P. Pramualratana and S. Wibulpolprasert, 43–50. Nonthaburi, Thailand: Health Systems Research Institute.

Suraratdecha, Chutima. 2003. "Thailand's Universal Insurance Coverage Initiative." Presentation at World Bank conference on Reaching the Poor, February 18–20, 2004, Washington, DC.

Szende A., and Z. Mogyorosy. 2004. "Health Care Provider Payment Mechanisms in the New EU Members of Central Europe and the Baltic States: Current Reforms, Incentives, and Challenges." *European Journal of Health Economics* 5 (3): 259–62.

Tabor, Steven R. 2005. "Community-Based Health Insurance and Social Protection." Social Protection Discussion Paper 0503, World Bank, Washington, DC.

Tanahashi, T. 1978. "Health Service Coverage and Its Evaluation." *Bulletin of the World Health Organization* 56 (2): 295–303.

Tangcharoensathien, V., S. Srithamrongsawat, and S. Pitayarangsarit. 2002. "Overview of Health Insurance Systems." In *Health Insurance Systems in Thailand,* ed. P. Pramualratana and S. Wibulpolprasert, 28–38. Nonthaburi, Thailand: Health Systems Research Institute.

Tangcharoensathien, V., S. Wibulpholprasert, and S. Nitayaramphong. 2004. "Knowledge-Based Changes to Health Systems: The Thai Experience in Policy Development." *Bulletin of the World Health Organization* 82 (10): 750–56.

Taylor, Rob, and Simon Blair. 2003. "Financing Health Care—Singapore's Innovative Approach. Public Policy for the Private Sector." Note No. 261, World Bank, Washington, DC.

Thomas, S., and L. Gilson. 2004. "Actor Management in the Development of Health Financing Reform: Health Insurance in South Africa, 1994–1999." *Health Policy Plan* 19 (5): 279–91.

Towse, A., A. Mills, and V. Tangcharoensathien. 2004. "Learning from Thailand's Health Reforms." *British Medical Journal* 328 (7431): 103–5.

Trejos, Juan Diego. 2002. "La Equidad de la Inversión Social en el 2000." Octavo Informe sobre el Estado de la Nación en Desarrollo Humano Sostenible, United Nations Development Programme, San José, Costa Rica.

Trujillo, A. J., and D. C. McCalla. 2004. "Are Colombian Sickness Funds Cream Skimming Enrollees? An Analysis with Suggestions for Policy Improvement." *Journal of Policy Analysis and Management* 23 (4): 873–88.

UNDP (United Nations Development Programme). 2007. Human Development Database. http://www.undp.org.

van Doorslaer, E., O. O'Donnell, R. P. Rannan-Eliya, A. Somanathan, S. R., Adhikari, C. C. Garg, D. Harbianto, A. N. Herrin, M. N. Huq, S. Ibragimova, A. Karan, T. Lee, G. M. Leung, J. R. Lu, C. W. Ng, B. R. Pande, R. Racelis, S. Tao, K. Tin, K. Tisayaticom, L. Trisnantoro, C. Vasavid, and Y. Zhao. 2007. "Catastrophic Payments for Health Care in Asia." *Health Economics* 16 (11): 1159–84.

van Doorslaer, E., O. O'Donnell, R. P. Rannan-Eliya, A. Somanathan, S. R. Adhikari, C. C. Garg, D. Harbianto, A. N. Herrin, M. N. Huq, S. Ibragimova, A. Karan, B. R. Pande, C. W. Ng, R. Racelis, S. Tao, K. Tin, K. Tisayaticom, L. Trisnantoro, C. Visasvid, and Y. Zhao. 2006. "Effect of Payments for Health Care on Poverty Estimates in 11 Countries in Asia: Analysis of Household Survey Data." *Lancet* 368(9544): 1357–64.

van Doorslaer, E., O. O'Donnell, R. Rannan-Eliya, A. Somanathan S. R. Adhikari, B. Akkazieva, C, C. Garg, D. Harbianto, A. N. Herrin, M. N. Huq, S. Ibragimova, A. Karan, T. Lee, G. M. Leung, J. R. Lu, C. W. Ng, B. R. Pande, R. Racelis, S. Tao, K. Tin, K. Tisayaticom, L. Trisnantoro, C. Visasvid, and Y. Zhao. 2005. "Paying Out-of-Pocket for Health Care in Asia: Catastrophic and Poverty Impact." Equitap Project: Working Paper 2. Erasmus University, Rotterdam, and Institute of Policy Studies. Colombo.

Vasavid, C., K.Tisayaticom, W. Patcharanarumol, and V. Tangcharoensathien. 2004. "Impact of Universal Health Care Coverage on the Thai Households." In *From Policy to Implementation: Historical Events during 2001–2004 of Universal Coverage in Thailand*, ed. V. Tangcharoensathien and P. Jongudomsak, 129–149. Nonthaburi, Thailand: National Health Security Office.

Wagstaff, Adam. 2005. "The Economic Consequences of Health Shocks." Policy Research Working Paper 3644, Development Research Group, World Bank: Washington, DC.

Wagstaff, Adam, and Menno Pradhan. 2005. "Health Insurance Impacts on Health and Nonmedical Consumption in a Developing-Country." Development Research Group and East Asia Human Development Unit, World Bank, Washington, DC.

Wagstaff, Adam, and Eddy van Doorslaer. 2003. "Catastrophe and Impoverishment in Paying for Health Care: With Applications to Vietnam." *Health Economics* 12: 921–34.

Wagstaff, Adam, Abdo Yazbeck, and Mariam Claeson. "Poverty Reduction Strategy Framework." Adapted from Adam Wagstaff and Mariam Claeson. 2004. "The Millennium Development Goals for Health Rising to the Challenges." Washington, DC: International Bank for Reconstruction and Development/World Bank.

Waters, Hugh. 1999. "Measuring the Impact of Health Insurance with a Correction for Selection Bias—A Case Study of Ecuador." *Health Economics* 8 (5): 473–83.

Waters, Hugh, Gerard Anderson, and Jim Mays. 2004. "Measuring Financial Protection in Health in the United States." *Health Policy* 69 (3): 339–49.

Waters, Hugh, and Peter Hussey. 2004. "Pricing Health Services for Purchasers—A Review of Methods and Experiences." *Health Policy* 70 (2): 175–84.

Waters, Hugh, Laura Morlock, and Laurel Hatt. 2004. "How Healthcare Purchasers Can Influence Quality—A Conceptual Framework and Comparative Analysis of Contextual Factors." *International Journal of Health Planning and Management* 19 (4): 365–81.

Waters, Hugh, Axel Rahola, and Jennifer Hulme. 2005. "Health Insurance Expansion in Morocco." World Bank, Washington, DC.

Watson, N. 2004. "Poland's Broken Promises." *Lancet* 364 (9430): 235–38.

Webster, P. 2004. "Reforms Mean 25 Million Russians Lose Free Health Care." *Canadian Medical Association Journal* 171 (10): 1157.

Williamson, O. 1985. *The Economic Institutions of Capitalism.* New York, NY: Free Press.

WHO (World Health Organization). 2000. *World Health Report 2000—Health Systems: Improving Performance.* Geneva: WHO.

———. 2003a. *World Health Survey, Tunisia.* Geneva: WHO.

———. 2003b. "World Health Survey 2003 Results"; accessed at http://www.who.int/healthinfo/survey/whsresults/en/index.html.

———. 2007. WHO Statistical Information System (WHOSIS). Online database. http://www.who.int/whosis/database/core/core_select.cfm.

———. 2007. "WHO World Health Statistics." Geneva: WHO.

World Bank. 2002. "HNP Strategy Paper." World Bank, Washington, DC.

———. 2003. "Project Appraisal Document—Republic of Ghana Health Sector Program Support Project." Report No: 24842-GH. Human Development II. Africa Regional Office, Ghana. World Bank: Washington, DC.

———. 2004a. *World Development Report 2004: Making Services Work for Poor People.* Washington, DC: World Bank.

———. 2004b. "Croatia—Health Finance Study. Report No. 27151-HR." Human Development Sector Unit, Europe and Central Asia Region.

———. 2007a. *World Development Indicators 2007.* Washington, DC: World Bank.

———. 2007b. "Healthy Development: The World Bank Strategy for Health, Nutrition, and Population Results." Washington, DC: World Bank.

———. 2007c. *World Development Report 2007: Development and the Next Generation.* Washington, DC: World Bank.

Wouters, Annemarie. 1999. "Alternative Provider Payment Methods: Incentives for Improving Health Care Delivery." Partnerships for Health Reform, Primer for Policymakers 1. Bethesda, MD: Abt Associates Inc. http://www.phrproject.com.

Xu, Ke, D. Evans, K. Kawabatta, R. Zeramdini, J. Klavus, and C. Murray. 2003. "Household Catastrophic Health Expenditure: A Multicountry Analysis." *Lancet* 362 (9378): 111–17.

Yepes, F. 2001. "Health Reform in Colombia." In *Health Care Reform and Poverty in Latin America,* ed. P. Lloyd-Sherlock, 163–77. London: Institute of Latin American Studies, University of London.

Zurn, Pascal, and Orville Adams. 2004. "A Framework for Purchasing Health Care Labor." Health, Nutrition and Population (HNP) Discussion Paper 31597, World Bank, Washington, DC.

# Part II

# Nine Case Studies of Good Practice in Health Financing Reform

# 6

# Chile: Good Practice in Expanding Health Care Coverage—Lessons from Reforms

*Ricardo D. Bitrán and Gonzalo C. Urcullo*

*Chile, is a tricontinental country, with land in Latin America (756,950 sq. km), Antarctica, and Oceania. It is in the Latin America and Caribbean Region (LAC) of the World Bank. Chile has a population of 16.3 million, a total fertility rate of 1.98, and per capita income of $12,365 (PPP-adjusted). Total health expenditures equaled $282 per capita in 2005, 51.2 percent of this amount paid by private sources, including 23.7 percent paid directly by households as out-of-pocket expenditures. Health outcomes are among the best in the world: life expectancy is 78.2 years, and infant mortality is 7.6 per 1,000 live births.*

*In Chile, the expansion of a fiscally sound social security system, including health care coverage, has required considerable economic resources. An extended period of economic growth and an efficient tax collection system made this expansion possible. Chile also has a high degree of formality in employment. Chile's experience suggests that registration in social security systems and other formal labor market mechanisms is perhaps the single most important facilitator for extending health care coverage. The insurance system in place today in Chile, first implemented in 1981, covers more than 90 percent of the population. Although some questions remain regarding the equity and efficiency of the system, proposals for reform are aimed at improving the current system rather than replacing it.*

## Background

Sustained economic growth and a fiscally sound social security system provided the resources needed to extend health care coverage.

### Economic Context

Economic growth in Chile has, on the whole, been positive throughout its history (figure 6.1). Figure 6.2 provides a more detailed look at real GDP growth rates

**Figure 6.1  Chile: Economic Growth, 1810–2005**

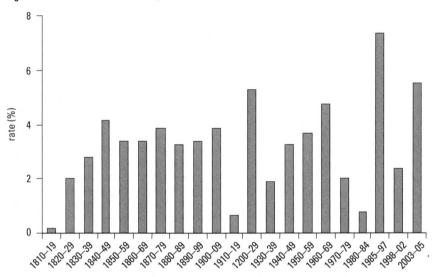

*Source:* Authors' elaborations based on data from the Central Bank of Chile.

from 1997 through 2005. As shown, only one year showed an economic downturn As a result of its sustained economic growth, Chile's GDP in international dollars has become one of the largest in Latin America (figure 6.3).

Chile has reported significant budget surpluses in recent years and continues to project surpluses for the future. These surpluses are due mainly to record prices for copper, Chile's main export product. As the global economy has grown, demand for minerals and metals has increased, especially in India and China. Chile's internal economy has also performed well. In 2005, for example, internal demand rose 10 percent and investments grew by 26 percent, representing a record 26 percent of the GDP.

In 2005, projected central government revenues were US$28.6 billion. The size of this figure is attributable in part to growing income from copper exports, but it is also due to increased tax revenues. Tax revenues, not including those related to copper exports, represent about 70 percent of the total central government revenues, while revenues related to copper exports represent about 10 percent of the total. The tax revenue structure is shown in table 6.1.

The fiscal surpluses noted above have gradually reduced the relative weight of the public debt and increased the resources available to the Collective Capitalization Fund of the social security system. Figure 6.4 shows the evolution of external debt in recent years. Debt has increased from year to year, although the rate of increase has decelerated. According to available reports, "the central government's debt has decreased from 11 percent of the GDP to around 8.4 percent, a record low."[1] Most of Chile's external debt is owed to private creditors (figure 6.5).

**Figure 6.2 Chile: Growth of Real GDP, 1997–2005**

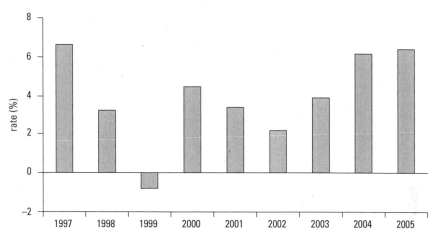

*Source:* Authors' elaboration based on data from the Central Bank of Chile.

**Figure 6.3 Chile: GDP per Capita, 2004**

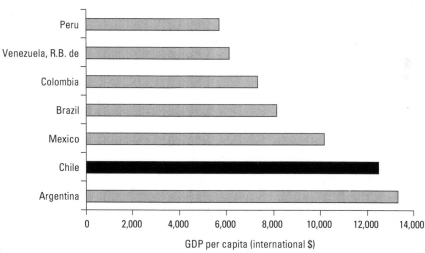

*Source:* World Health Organization 2006.

Chile enjoys striking macroeconomic stability, in terms of economic growth, external debt sustainability, internal capacity for savings, attractiveness to investors, and high import and export levels due to growing commercial and financial integration with the rest of the world. Table 6.2 shows the evolution of the major macroeconomic variables of the Chilean economy from 2000 to 2005. The years

Table 6.1   Chile: Net Tax Revenue Structure, 1996–2004 (percent)

| Type of tax | 1996 | 1997 | 1998 | 1999 | 2000 | 2001 | 2002 | 2003 | 2004 |
|---|---|---|---|---|---|---|---|---|---|
| Income tax | 23.59 | 22.95 | 24.05 | 22.60 | 24.97 | 26.70 | 27.74 | 27.07 | 25.72 |
| Value-added tax | 47.90 | 48.07 | 47.81 | 48.44 | 48.46 | 47.12 | 48.37 | 50.48 | 51.50 |
| Taxes on specific products | 11.03 | 11.79 | 12.43 | 14.09 | 13.72 | 13.74 | 13.67 | 13.41 | 12.17 |
| Taxes on legal documents | 3.81 | 4.12 | 3.85 | 4.22 | 3.64 | 4.10 | 4.39 | 4.46 | 4.36 |
| Import taxes | 11.86 | 10.86 | 10.30 | 9.22 | 8.28 | 7.02 | 5.67 | 3.91 | 2.85 |
| Other | 1.81 | 2.20 | 1.56 | 1.43 | 0.92 | 1.32 | 0.17 | 0.68 | 3.40 |

*Source:* Author's elaboration based on data form the Central Bank of Chile.

Figure 6.4   Chile: External Debt, 1996–2005

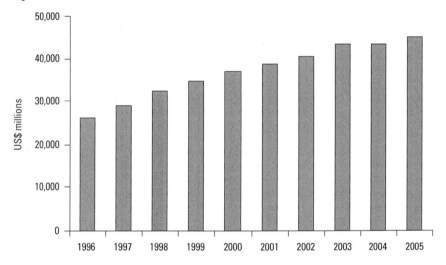

*Source:* Central Bank of Chile.

2004 and 2005 were especially outstanding, particularly in terms of gross capital as a percentage of GDP and import and export levels. The increased trade is due in part to increases in the price of copper. Furthermore, the budget moved from deficit to surplus.

## Demographic, Epidemiological, and Social Context

Until 1930, Chile's population lived mainly in rural areas. By 2002, the 2,026,322 people living in rural areas represented only 13.40 percent of the country's total population.

**Figure 6.5    Chile: Composition of External Debt, 2004**

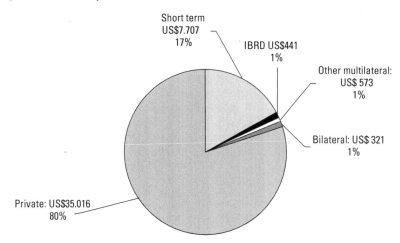

Short term
US$7.707
17%

IBRD US$441
1%

Other multilateral:
US$ 573
1%

Bilateral: US$ 321
1%

Private: US$35.016
80%

*Source:* World Bank 2004.

**Table 6.2    Chile: Macroeconomic Performance, 2000–05**

| Macroeconomic variable | 2000 | 2001 | 2002 | 2003 | 2004 | 2005 |
|---|---|---|---|---|---|---|
| GDP (% real annual variation) | 4.5 | 3.4 | 2.2 | 3.9 | 6.2 | 6.3 |
| Internal demand (% real annual variation) | 6.0 | 2.4 | 2.4 | 4.9 | 8.1 | 11.4 |
| National income (% real annual variation) | 4.4 | 2.4 | 2.8 | 3.9 | 8.6 | 9.1 |
| Investment (% GDP) | 21.9 | 22.1 | 21.7 | 22.0 | 21.4 | 23.0 |
| National savings rate (% GDP) | 20.6 | 20.6 | 20.7 | 20.7 | 23.0 | 23.6 |
| Inflation (December of each year) | 4.5 | 2.6 | 2.8 | 1.1 | 2.4 | 3.7 |
| Unemployment rate (%) | 9.2 | 9.1 | 8.9 | 8.5 | 8.8 | 8.0 |
| Real salaries (% annual variation) | 1.4 | 1.6 | 2.1 | 1.0 | 1.8 | 1.9 |
| Exports (US$ billions) | 19.2 | 18.3 | 18.2 | 21.7 | 32.2 | 40.6 |
| Imports (US$ billions) | 17.1 | 16.4 | 15.8 | 18.0 | 23.0 | 30.4 |
| Budget deficit or surplus (US$ millions) | −897 | −1,100 | −580 | −964 | 1,586 | 702 |
| Price of copper (US$ cents /pound) | 82.3 | 71.6 | 70.7 | 80.7 | 130.0 | 166.9 |

*Source:* Central Bank of Chile, INE Cochilco.

Two features define the Chilean demographic situation, categorized as in the advanced transition stage. First is the projected decrease in gross reproductive rate from 18.2 per 1,000 population in 2000–05 to 13.4 per 1,000 population in 2045–50. Second is the growth of the elderly population. In 2000, 36.9 percent of

Chileans were under the age of 19; by 2050, only 22.6 percent of the population will be under 19.

During the 20th century Chile experienced a 45-percent decrease in birth rate and an 85-percent decrease in the mortality rate. In the first half of the century, population growth increased at a moderate pace, accelerating in the 1950s. After 1960, the birth rate quickly began to decline, finally stabilizing in the 1980s. This shift was due to changing marriage trends, as well as increased individual control over family planning. This latter phenomenon occurred more rapidly than in developed countries. Between 1971 and 1992, the number of children per woman dropped from 3.80 to 2.39. The decrease was most pronounced in rural areas, even though historically this population has had higher fertility rates than urban areas.

Figure 6.6 illustrates the aging of the population structure.

In the middle of the twentieth century, Chile was a young country, with 40 percent of its population under the age of 15 and only 3 percent over the age of 65. By the end of the century, only 29 percent of the population was younger than 15, and 7 percent were 65 or older, marking it as an aging country. In a half century, the average age of the population increased by nearly five years, from 26 in 1952 to 31 in 2002.[2]

Other markers of the changing structure of the Chilean population are the indices of dependency and of aging.[3] In the last 50 years, the dependency index has decreased by nearly a fourth, reaching 50 percent. Meanwhile, the index of aging has increased by over half, reaching nearly 20 percent. Furthermore, the latest census data indicate that there are more women than men in Chile and that the gender ration (number of males per 100 females) is greater in rural than in urban areas.

*Epidemiological context.* The latest available study on Chile's disease burden was published in 1996 using 1993 data. At the risk of ignoring epidemiological changes that might have occurred after 1993, the authors selected this study as the most reliable reflection of Chile's epidemiological context (Chilean Ministry of Health 1996). The results of this study showed that Chile lost 1,769,557 years of healthy life (DALYs), 128.5 DALYs per 1,000 population. The disease burden varies by age and gender. The disease burden in Chile was 1.25 times higher for men than for women. In men, most of the disease burden was attributable to premature death, while for women most was attributable to disability. In both genders, the disease burden was highest for the very young and very old, and men lost more DALYs than women at all ages. Disease burden was mainly attributable to premature death among the very young and very old, and mainly to disability among those of intermediate ages. Table 6.3 lists the 15 diseases the produced the greatest death and disease burden in Chile in 1993, by DALYs lost, the percentage of lost DALYs attributable to that disease versus the total DALYs lost in Chile that year, and the DALYs lost attributable to that disease per 1,000 population.[4]

**Figure 6.6    Chile: Population, 1990, 2005, and 2020**

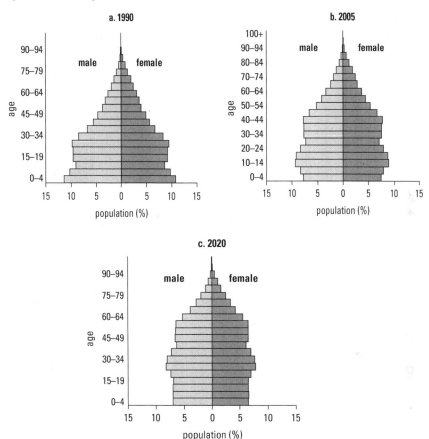

*Source:* National Statistical Institute of Chile (http://www.ine.cl).

These rankings vary by gender and age. In men, alcohol dependence places second, followed by traffic accidents and ischemic heart disease. In women, depression places second, followed by bile duct disorders and acute lower respiratory infections. Neoplasms do not make the top 15 due to low life expectancy. Cervical uterine cancer produces the most lost DALYs. However, among those over the age of 45, various cancers begin to rank higher on the list, including gallbladder, breast, and stomach cancer in women, and stomach, lung, and prostate cancer in men.

Among the very young and the old—those under the age of 5 or over the age of 60—the disease profile is similar among males and females. The largest gender differences in disease profile occur between the ages of 15 and 44, mainly due to the higher rates of injuries and alcohol dependence and abuse among men.

Table 6.3    Chile: Disease Burden, 1993 (DALYs lost)

| Illness | DALYs | % | Ratio/1,000 |
|---|---|---|---|
| Congenital anomalies | 103.654 | 5.86 | 7.53 |
| Acute lower respiratory infections | 73.234 | 4.14 | 5.32 |
| Ischemic heart disease | 67.534 | 3.82 | 4.90 |
| Hypertensive disease | 60.172 | 3.40 | 4.37 |
| Cerebrovascular disease | 57.700 | 3.26 | 4.19 |
| Asthma | 55.118 | 3.11 | 4.0 |
| Traffic accident | 53.692 | 3.03 | 3.90 |
| Alcohol dependence | 53.498 | 3.02 | 3.88 |
| Bile duct disorders | 53.361 | 3.02 | 3.87 |
| Major depressive disorder | 53.279 | 3.01 | 3.87 |
| Arthritis and similar diseases | 48.452 | 2.74 | 3.52 |
| Alzheimer's and other dementias | 42.889 | 2.42 | 3.11 |
| Perinatal infections | 41.710 | 2.36 | 3.03 |
| Psychosis | 32.474 | 1.84 | 2.36 |
| Cirrhosis | 32.172 | 1.82 | 2.34 |
| Total | 828.941 | 46.84 | 60.19 |

*Source:* MOH.

*Health indicators.* Infant mortality has gradually decreased. The most dramatic advances occurred between 1940 and 1950, when the infant mortality rate decreased by 58 percent. The rate continued to decrease from 1960 to 2002, although at a decelerated pace (figure 6.7). The Chilean infant mortality rate decreased from 234 to 8 per 1,000 live births from 1930 to 2003, a 96.6 percent reduction. The decreased infant mortality rate correlates with a number of other factors: improved living conditions, especially in terms of basic sanitation, availability of potable water, and sanitary waste disposal systems; better delivery of public services; better education; greater availability of food; and better access to medical care.

In 2000–05, life expectancy was 74.8 years for males and 80.8 years for females. This represents a 21.9-year increase in life expectancy for males and 24.03-year increase for females since the mid-20th century. The difference in life expectancy by gender held constant throughout all periods studied (figure 6.8).

Chile enjoys one of the lowest infant mortality rates and highest life expectancies in Latin America. Figure 6.9 shows 2004 data for infant mortality and life expectancy for several Latin American countries, listed in order of GDP per capita in international dollars. The two trend lines show that, as economic development increases, infant mortality decreases and life expectancy increases. Chile, the second-most-developed country, has the longest life expectancy and the second-lowest infant mortality rate of the Latin American countries shown here.

**Figure 6.7   Chile: Infant Mortality, 1960–2002**

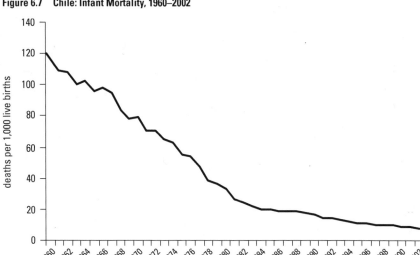

*Source:* National Statistical Institute of Chile.

**Figure 6.8   Chile: Life Expectancy, by Historical Period and Gender, 1950–2025**

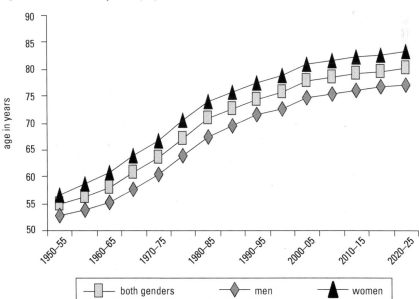

*Source:* National Statistical Institute of Chile.

**Figure 6.9  Poverty Compared with Other Latin America Countries, 1999**

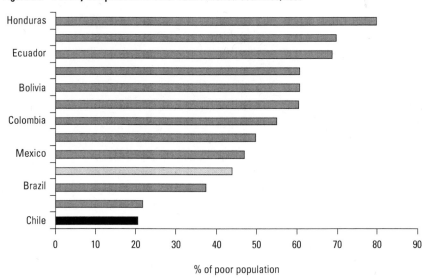

% of poor population

*Sources:* Universidad Emilio Máspero (http://www.utal.org/economia/hogaresypoblafcion.htm).

*Social context.* Chile's solid economic performance throughout its history, and especially in recent years, has allowed the country to make significant gains in alleviating poverty. According to data from the 2003 socioeconomic census (CASEN), 80 percent of the population is classified as "not poor." The number of people in Chile living on less than US$1 per day was 843,000, about 5.6 percent of the total population. Between 1987 and 2003, the population living below the poverty line in Chile decreased from 45.1 percent to 18.8 percent. Poverty in Chile is much less severe than in most other Latin American countries. Figure 6.10 shows that in 1999, only 20 percent of the Chilean population was poor, as compared with 40 percent in most other Latin American countries, and 43 percent for the region.

Although Chile has made important strides against poverty, the country's wealth remains inequitably distributed. Chile is considered one of the most inequitable countries in Latin America. According to 2003 CASEN census data, average income in the richest quintile was 16 times higher than that of the poorest quintile. The richest 10 percent of the population earned 41.2 percent of the country's total income, while the poorest 10 percent earned only 1.2 percent, 34.3 times less.

## Political Context

During the 19th and 20th centuries, Chile slowly consolidated a highly stable democratic political system (box 6.1).

Figure 6.10   Chile: Infant Mortality and Life Expectancy Compared with Other Latin American Countries, 2004

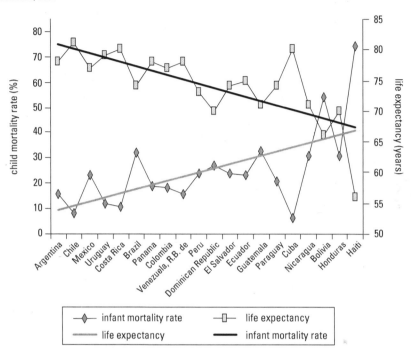

*Source:* National Statistical Institute (www.ine.cl).

---

**BOX 6.1** *Chile: Key Political Milestones*

| | |
|---|---|
| 1810 First elections held | 1925 Fourth Constitution drafted |
| 1822 First Constitution drafted | 1935 Women given right to vote in municipal |
| 1828 Second Constitution drafted | elections |
| 1833 Third Constitution drafted | 1949 Women given right to vote in |
| 1871 Presidents prohibited from running for | presidential and parliamentary elections |
| a second consecutive term | 1972 Illiterates given right to vote |
| 1874 Voting rights expanded | |
| 1890 Secret ballot established | *Source:* http://www.memoriachilena.cl. |

---

From 1835 to 1888, candidates put forth by the State Party regularly won presidential and parliamentary elections. After 1888, the electoral process became more transparent. However, while government intervention in elections decreased, irregularities in the electoral process remained common, and political power remained concentrated in one party. After 1920, social movements began to erupt; more of the population began to participate in elections; and leftist political parties developed, including a Communist Party (1922) and a Socialist Party (1933). The political mobilization of the population in the 1960s and early 1970s, in a highly polarized political climate, came to an abrupt end after the 1973 coup d'état. The autocratic government ended in 1990, followed by a series of democratically elected administrations. The latest election was in 2006.[5]

Chile's current system of government is tripartite. The executive branch is directed by the president of the republic, who is also the chief of state; the legislative branch consists of a two-chamber congress (representatives and senators); and the judicial branch is led by the Supreme Court. Functions of each branch are clearly delineated among the three branches, each of which operates independently.

Chile is divided into 13 regions, 51 provinces, and 342 communities. Each region is led by a superintendent, who represents the president of the republic in that region. The regional governments also include a regional council, which approves regional development plans and allocates regional investment resources, among other duties.

Within the regions, each province is led by a governor, who is subordinate to the superintendent, but functions in a decentralized manner. The governor presides over an economic and social provincial council.

Finally, at community level, a mayor presides over the economic and social municipal council, which allocates resources and makes community-level decisions. Local leaders are chosen by popular election to serve four-year terms.[6]

## Overview of Health Care Coverage and Financing in Chile

The defining feature of Chile's health care system is the mandatory social security system, which covers about 90 percent of the population. This section provides an overview of the Chilean social security system, as well as a discussion of health care financing, social security coverage, basic package coverage, and the equity and efficiency of the Chilean social security system.

### Chile's Mandatory Health Insurance System

Chile's mandatory health insurance (MHI) system consists of a single nonprofit public insurer (Fondo Nacional de Salud, FONASA) and multiple for-profit or nonprofit private insurers (Instituciones de Salud Previsional, ISAPREs), all operating in competition (figure 6.11). By law all formal sector workers who are not self-employed, retired workers with a pension or self-employed workers with a retirement fund must enroll with the MHI by making a monthly contribution equal to 7 percent of their income or pension, up to a monthly ceiling of US$2,000.[7] Other individuals may enroll as well. They include independent workers, who can voluntarily enroll with the FONASA or an ISAPRE conditional on their 7 percent contribution; and legally certified indigent citizens and legally unemployed workers, who are entitled to free coverage by the FONASA. ISAPRE beneficiaries may voluntarily make an extra contribution to their insurer to purchase additional coverage. Until

**Figure 6.11  Chile: The Mandatory Health Insurance System, 2006**

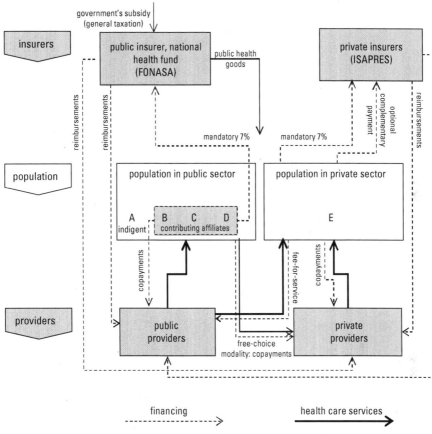

*Source:* Authors.

2005 no such thing as a basic benefits package was required of the FONASA or ISAPREs, although the latter could not provide less financial coverage than the former. Starting in 2005, a set of new laws collectively known as Explicit Health Guarantees (Garantías Explícitas de Salud, GES) mandated the public and private MHI insurers incrementally to provide coverage for 56 legally defined health problems, starting with 25 of them in July 2005 and encompassing all 56 problems in 2007. The FONASA must by law purchase most of its covered health services from public hospitals and health centers, although it also provides a modest subsidy to its beneficiaries willing to purchase private health care. Public health care providers must by law sell most of their services to the FONASA and are subject to tight limits on the kinds and volume of services they may sell to private patients and ISAPRE beneficiaries.

The National Health Superintendence is responsible for regulating the FONASA and the ISAPREs. Main regulatory functions include beneficiary protection, financial solvency of ISAPREs, and compliance by both the FONASA and ISAPREs with the provision of benefits stipulated in the GES law. Chile's MHI system is also characterized by a split between financing and delivery. In the public sector, the FONASA acts solely as a financing agent, and delivery is left in the hands of the Ministry of Health (MOH). In the private sector, by law ISAPREs are not allowed to provide health services directly (i.e., they cannot be vertically integrated). This split has widened beneficiaries' choice of provider alternatives. FONASA beneficiaries may choose to seek care from any provider, public or private, as long as they are registered with the FONASA. If the provider is public (called Modalidad de Atención Institucional, MAI) copayments are small or nil. If the provider is private (called Modalidad de Libre Elección, MLE) copayments are larger. ISAPRE beneficiaries have similar choices but almost always opt for private care.

## Key Indicators

Health care spending in Chile amounts to 6 percent of the GDP and is financed by both public and private sector entities.[8] As shown in table 6.4, public sector health spending has increased, but, until 2004, was lower than private spending. Spending decreased between 1999 and 2003 and then increased again in 2004 to over the 1998 amount. Spending as a percentage of GDP dropped about 1 percent from 1998 to 2004.

**Table 6.4  Chile: Key Health Spending Indicators, 1998–2004**

| Indicator | 1998 | 1999 | 2000 | 2001 | 2002 | 2003 | 2004 |
|---|---|---|---|---|---|---|---|
| Health spending (US$ billions) | 5.6 | 5.2 | 4.6 | 4.3 | 4.2 | 4.5 | 5.7 |
| Health spending as a percentage of GDP | 7.1 | 7.1 | 6.1 | 6.2 | 6.2 | 6.1 | 6.1 |
| Public health spending (US$ billions) | 2.1 | 2.2 | 2.1 | 2.0 | 2.0 | 2.2 | 2.7 |
| Private health spending (US$ billions) | 3.6 | 3.2 | 2.5 | 2.2 | 2.2 | 2.3 | 3.1 |
| Percentage of health spending by public sector | 36.7 | 39.0 | 46.4 | 48.1 | 48.0 | 48.8 | 46.4 |
| Percentage of health spending by private sector | 63.3 | 61.0 | 53.6 | 51.9 | 52.0 | 51.2 | 53.6 |
| Out-of-pocket spending (US$ billions) | 2.2 | 1.9 | 1.2 | 1.1 | 1.0 | 1.1 | 1.4 |
| Out-of-pocket spending as a percentage of total health spending | 38.9 | 37.0 | 25.2 | 24.9 | 24.6 | 23.7 | 24.6 |
| Spending on private health plans (US$ billions) | 1.4 | 1.2 | 1.3 | 1.1 | 1.1 | 1.2 | 1.7 |
| Spending on private health plans as a percentage of total health spending | 24.4 | 24.0 | 28.4 | 27.0 | 27.4 | 27.5 | 29.0 |
| Total per capita health spending (US$) | 375.0 | 342.0 | 299.0 | 272.0 | 265.0 | 282.0 | 355.0 |

*Source:* Authors' elaboration based on World Bank data (http://www.worldbank.org).

**Figure 6.12 Chile: Structure of Health Spending, by Source, 1998–2004**

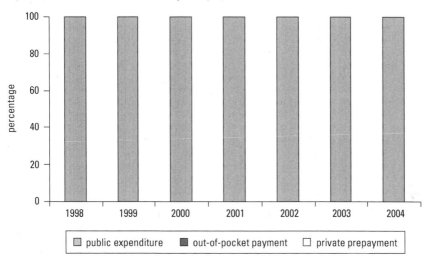

*Source:* Authors' elaboration based on World Bank data.

Private health spending consists of out-of-pocket payments on health care and payments for health insurance premiums. In 1998, out-of-pocket spending was 59 percent higher than spending on premiums, but this trend had reversed by 2000. The decrease in private health spending relative to public spending, therefore, can be explained as a decrease in out-of-pocket spending on health care.

Figure 6.12 shows how public spending and private spending on health insurance premiums have increased relative to out-of-pocket spending on care.

Private spending on health as a percentage of total health spending is greater in Chile than in most other similarly developed Latin American countries. Compared with Brazil, Costa Rica, and Mexico, Chile has the lowest level of public spending on health as a percentage of GDP and the highest level of private spending (table 6.5).

In 2002, public spending on health as a percentage of total public spending was 10.2 percent. From 2000 to 2005, public spending on health increased relative to total public spending on social welfare programs by about 2 percent, reaching almost 15 percent. This amounted to an average annual increase of US$100 million.

**Table 6.5 Chile: Health Spending as a Percentage of GDP, 2004 (percentage)**

| Source | Brazil | Costa Rica | Mexico | Chile |
|--------|--------|------------|--------|-------|
| Public | 3.6 | 4.9 | 2.8 | 2.6 |
| Private | 3.6 | 3.4 | 3.2 | 3.8 |
| Total | 7.2 | 8.3 | 6.0 | 6.4 |

*Source:* PAHO (http://www.paho.org).

**Table 6.6  Chile: Composition of Spending on Social Welfare Programs, 2000–05 (percentage)**

| Function | 2000 | 2001 | 2002 | 2003 | 2004 | 2005 |
|---|---|---|---|---|---|---|
| Health | 12.8 | 13.3 | 13.4 | 14.0 | 14.5 | 14.9 |
| Education | 16.7 | 17.4 | 17.8 | 17.8 | 18.5 | 18.8 |
| Social protection | 35.5 | 35.5 | 34.7 | 34.5 | 34.1 | 33.6 |
| Other social welfare programs[a] | 2.2 | 1.9 | 1.9 | 1.8 | 1.5 | 1.6 |
| Total spending on social welfare programs | 67.2 | 68.2 | 67.8 | 68.1 | 68.6 | 68.9 |
| Other | 32.8 | 31.8 | 32.2 | 31.9 | 31.4 | 31.1 |

*Source:* Ministry of the Interior, Budget Office (http://www.dipres.cl).

a. Includes environmental protection, housing and community services, recreational activities, culture, and religion.

Public spending on education also increased over this period, while spending on social protection and other social welfare programs decreased (table 6.6).

## The Basic Benefits Package

In 2005, Chile developed a benefits package with four basic guarantees: *guaranteed coverage* for eligible public and private sector beneficiaries; *guaranteed quality* of care, achieved through accreditation of participating health providers; *guaranteed access* to care, achieved by establishing maximum wait times and processes for enforcement; and *guaranteed financing* for care, achieved through a government fund to cover specified serious health conditions.[9] These promises, "the Explicit Health Guarantees" (GESs), contain the following specific provisions[10]:

- *Primary care.* The GESs follow the Integrated Family Care Model, continuing the coverage provided as part of the previous Family Health Plan. Coverage includes certain preventative and curative care provided by a family medicine team led by a physician. The GES covers acute illnesses, preventative health care, health screenings, and special programs for mental health, cardiovascular health, specialist referrals, and home visits.

- *Emergency care.* The GESs guarantee an emergency care network, covering the entire country, that provides prehospital care, transportation, diagnostic care, stabilization, and treatment for life-threatening or serious emergencies.

- *Targeted diseases.* The GESs guarantee effective treatment, according to current standards of practice, for certain targeted diseases in Chile. These diseases are selected according to the seriousness of the illness, the disease burden produced, the cost of care, considerations regarding equity, and other factors.

The GESs began by guaranteeing coverage for 25 health problems in 2005 (table 6.7, col. 1). Coverage was expanded to 40 health problems on July 1, 2006, and as of July 1, 2007, coverage was set to expand to 56 problems.

**Table 6.7  Chile: Health Problems Covered under the GES, 2005–07**

| No. | 2005 Health problem | No. | 2006 Health problem | No. | 2007 Health problem |
|---|---|---|---|---|---|
| 1 | End-stage renal disease | 26 | Preventative cholecystectomy for gallbladder cancer | 41 | Hearing loss in individuals over 65 years |
| 2 | Operable congenital cardiopathies in children under 15 years | | | 42 | Leukemia in adults |
| 3 | Cervical uterine cancer | 27 | Gastric cancer | 43 | Eye trauma |
| 4 | Pain relief and palliative care for advanced cancer | 28 | Prostate cancer | 44 | Cystic fibrosis |
| 5 | Acute myocardial infarction | 29 | Refractive disorders in individuals over 65 years | 45 | Severe burns |
| 6 | Type I diabetes mellitus | 30 | Strabismus in children under 9 years | 46 | Drug and alcohol dependence in adolescents from 10 to 19 years |
| 7 | Type II diabetes mellitus | 31 | Diabetic retinopathy | 47 | Complete prenatal and delivery care |
| 8 | Breast cancer in individuals over 15 years | 32 | Detached retina | | |
| 9 | Spinal defects | 33 | Hemophilia | 48 | Rheumatoid arthritis |
| 10 | Surgical treatment for scoliosis in individuals under 25 years | 34 | Depression in individuals over 15 years | 49 | Mild and moderate osteoarthritis of hip in individuals over 60 years; mild and moderate osteoarthritis of knee in individuals over 65 years |
| 11 | Surgical treatment for cataracts | 35 | Benign prostatic hyperplasia | | |
| 12 | Total hip replacement for advanced osteoarthritis in individuals over 65 years | 36 | Acute cerebrovascular accident | 50 | Ruptured aneurysms; ruptured ateriovenous malformations |
| 13 | Cleft palate | 37 | Chronic obstructive pulmonary disease | 51 | Central nervous system tumors and cysts |
| 14 | Cancer in children under 15 years | 38 | Bronchial asthma | 52 | Herniated disks |
| 15 | Schizophrenia | 39 | Infant respiratory distress syndrome | 53 | Dental emergencies |
| 16 | Testicular cancer in individuals over 15 years | 40 | Orthotics and technical support for individuals over 65 years | 54 | Dental care for adults over 65 years |
| 17 | Lymphoma in individuals over 15 years | | | 55 | Multitrauma |
| 18 | Acquired immunodeficiency Syndrome (AIDS) / HIV | | | 56 | Traumatic brain injury |
| 19 | Outpatient treatment for acute respiratory infection in children under 5 years | | | | |
| 20 | Walking pneumonia in individuals over 65 years | | | | |
| 21 | Primary (essential) arterial hypertension in individuals over 15 years | | | | |
| 22 | Nonrefractory epilepsy in children 1 to 15 years | | | | |
| 23 | Complete oral health care for children under 6 years: prevention and education | | | | |
| 24 | Prematurity – Retinopathy of Prematurity – Hypoacusia Prematurity | | | | |
| 25 | Major conduction disorders requiring a pacemaker in individuals over 15 years | | | | |

*Source:* Bitrán & Asociados 2005.

## Social Security Coverage

The social security system covers a large proportion of the population, 90 percent in recent years. Over two thirds of the population is covered by public health insurance (FONASA); a fifth to a sixth, by ISAPREs. A tiny percentage is covered by private insurance through the armed forces or universities. Table 6.8 shows the Chilean social security system's health coverage in 2005, by insurer.[11]

The public system is the main provider of health insurance in Chile. All the ISAPREs combined have never covered more than 26 percent of the total insured population. Average ISAPRE membership from 1984 to 2005 was 17.8 percent of the population. Figure 6.13 shows the evolution of coverage under the Chilean social security system. As seen, the public system has many more beneficiaries than the private. For a time, the number of ISAPRE beneficiaries was increasing and the number of FONASA beneficiaries was decreasing. This trend peaked in 1995–97 then reversed. The number of beneficiaries of other systems peaked in the late 1980s, then dropped by about half in succeeding years.

When the system was established in 1981, there were only five participating ISAPREs. Many more ISAPREs quickly entered the market, peaking at 35 in the 1990s. Later, the number of participating ISAPREs began to drop back down. In 2006, there were 15 ISAPREs, 7 of them closed and 8 open. Figure 6.14 shows the number of beneficiaries (subscribers plus dependents) in the ISAPRE system in April 2006. Over two-thirds of the total beneficiaries belong to three ISAPREs: Banmedica, Consalud, and ING Salud.

*Type care provided.* The most common type care provided to both FONASA and ISAPRE beneficiaries were diagnostic exams.

Table 6.9 shows the services provided to FONASA beneficiaries. As seen, although diagnostic exams and clinical support services are the most common types, physician visits and days hospitalized account for a larger proportion of the cost.

Table 6.8   Chile: Health Coverage Provided by Social Security System, 2005

| Insurer | Individuals covered | Population covered (%) |
|---|---|---|
| FONASA | 11,329,481 | 69.65 |
| Open ISAPREs | 2,521,444 | 15.50 |
| Closed ISAPREs | 138,894 | 0.85 |
| Uninsured | 1,701,648 | 10.46 |
| Others | 575,771 | 3.54 |
| Total population | 16,267,278 | 100.00 |

*Source:* Superintendence of Health (http://www.supersalud.cl).

**Figure 6.13    Chile: Coverage of Social Security System, 1984–2005**

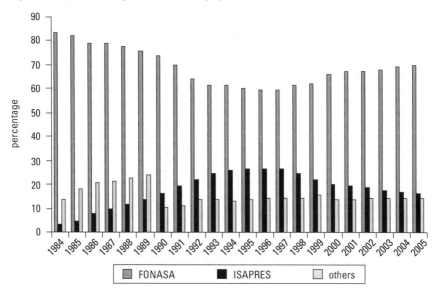

*Source:* Superintendence of Health (http://www.supersalud.cl).

**Figure 6.14    Chile: Coverage of Open ISAPREs, 2006 (number of beneficiaries and % of total beneficiaries)**

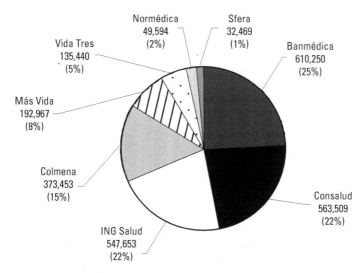

*Source:* Superintendence of Health.

**Table 6.9   Chile: Services Provided by the FONASA and Average Annual Spending per Beneficiary, 2004**

| Type of service provided | Number of services provided | (%) | Spending (US$ millions) | (%) |
|---|---|---|---|---|
| Physician visits | 5.14 | 33.7 | 20.15 | 24.0 |
| Diagnostic testing and clinical support services | 6.65 | 43.6 | 16.79 | 20.0 |
| Diagnostic and therapeutic procedures | 1.38 | 9.0 | 7.97 | 9.5 |
| Hemodialysis and peritoneal dialysis | 0.16 | 1.0 | 5.74 | 6.8 |
| Surgical interventions | 0.10 | 0.7 | 10.16 | 12.1 |
| Days hospitalized | 0.14 | 0.9 | 1.88 | 2.2 |
| Deliveries and obstetric surgeries | 0.65 | 4.3 | 19.21 | 22.9 |
| Other services | 1.04 | 6.8 | 1.97 | 2.3 |
| Total services | 15.26 | 100 | 83.87 | 100 |

*Source:* FONASA.

Table 6.10 shows the evolution of services provided by ISAPREs. Most striking is the nearly 50-percent increase in average annual services per beneficiary from 1996 to 2004, especially the number of laboratory tests.

Table 6.11 shows the number of hospital admissions by type of insurance. In 2003, FONASA patients accounted for 78 percent of hospital admissions. Given that in 2003 the FONASA covered 68 percent of the population, FONASA beneficiaries seem more likely to be hospitalized than the rest of the population. This may be because the FONASA has a greater proportion of elderly and poor beneficiaries than do the ISAPREs. For example, according to 2003 CASEN census data, 18.1 percent of ISAPRE beneficiaries were 20 to 39-year-old females and only 5.9 percent were females over the age of 65. Furthermore, ISAPREs cover only 3.2 percent of the poorest quintile of the population. Table 6.11 also shows that the num-

**Table 6.10   Chile: Average Number of Health Services Provided by ISAPRES per Beneficiary, 1996–2004**

| Type of service provided | 1996 | 1997 | 1998 | 1999 | 2000 | 2001 | 2002 | 2003 | 2004 | 2004 (%) |
|---|---|---|---|---|---|---|---|---|---|---|
| Physician visits | 3.34 | 3.42 | 3.62 | 3.96 | 4.13 | 3.82 | 3.97 | 4.00 | 4.53 | 26.8 |
| Diagnostic testing | 3.74 | 3.84 | 4.01 | 4.68 | 5.35 | 5.25 | 5.39 | 5.54 | 6.48 | 40.9 |
| Clinical support services | 1.87 | 1.86 | 1.97 | 2.44 | 2.80 | 2.98 | 2.70 | 2.72 | 3.22 | 20.3 |
| Surgical interventions | 0.09 | 0.09 | 0.09 | 0.10 | 0.11 | 0.11 | 0.11 | 0.11 | 0.12 | 0.8 |
| Other services | 1.26 | 1.36 | 1.47 | 1.41 | 1.17 | 0.91 | 0.88 | 0.85 | 0.85 | 5.4 |
| Not classified | n.a. | n.a. | n.a. | n.a. | n.a. | 0.96 | 0.69 | 0.57 | 0.66 | 4.2 |
| Total services | 10.30 | 10.56 | 11.16 | 12.58 | 13.56 | 14.03 | 13.74 | 13.78 | 15.86 | 100 |

*Source:* Superintendence of Health.
*Note:* n.a. = not applicable.

**Table 6.11   Chile: Number of Hospital Admissions, 2001–03**

| Insurer | 2001 | 2002 | 2003 |
|---|---|---|---|
| FONASA | 1,117,826 | 1,139,727 | 1,248,869 |
| ISAPRE | 245,553 | 261,579 | 252,879 |
| Private | 62,884 | 62,875 | 28,201 |
| Other | 121,343 | 128,926 | 68,599 |
| Unknown | 18,581 | 5,968 | 732 |
| Total | 1,566,187 | 1,599,075 | 1,599,280 |

*Source:* Authors, based on information from the MOH (http://www.misal.cl).

ber of hospital admissions for individuals with unknown insurance status dropped significantly from 2001 to 2003, likely due to improved registration systems. Finally, the table shows that the number of individuals belonging to other insurance companies dropped by nearly half between 2001 and 2003.

## Funding Sources

In Chile, the entire population is guaranteed access to the public health system, whether or not they have the resources to pay premiums. By law, dependent workers must enroll in the FONASA or an ISAPRE by contributing 7 percent of their income to the health system, up to a ceiling of 60 UF (an inflation-indexed unit) per month.[12] These monthly contributions account for about a third of FONASA funding. About half of FONASA funding comes from the state. The ISAPREs, in contrast, are funded mainly by their beneficiaries' monthly contributions. Funding for social security health benefits in Chile, not including copayments, comes from contributions to ISAPREs (35 percent), contributions to the FONASA (24 percent), and government subsidies (41 percent).

Funding for health care in public facilities comes from four main sources: government subsidies, monthly contributions, operational income, and copayments. The percentage of funding for health care in public facilities from government subsidies increased by 10 percent from 1990 to 1993. In the following years, this figure remained constant at about 55 percent, before dropping to about 50 percent by 2002 and 2003. Operating income and copayments represented a low proportion of funding throughout the period studied, and the proportion represented by copayment decreased slightly (figure 6.15). For example, in 2003, the public sector spent US$2.3 billion on health care, 51 percent of it from government subsidies, 35 percent from monthly contributions, 6.4 percent from operating income, and 7.3 percent from copayments.

## Equity

The following series of characteristics show the existing equity or inequity in the Chilean health system.

**Figure 6.15   Chile: Structure of Financing for Public Health Spending**

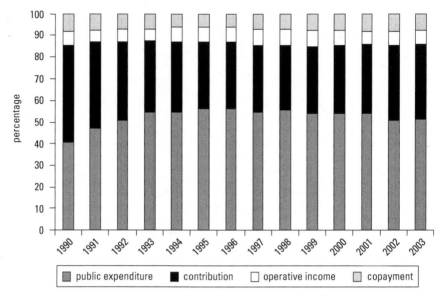

*Source:* Superintendence of Health.

*FONASA and ISAPRE membership vary by income.* Most lower-income individuals subscribe to the FONASA; those with higher incomes, an ISAPRE. Within the FONASA, beneficiary services also vary according income. FONASA Group A contains the poorest beneficiaries, while those with progressively higher incomes belong to FONASA Groups B, C, or D.

Figure 6.16 shows the different levels within the system. Some of the key attributes of this system include

- The social security system in Chile provides broad coverage (9 out of 10 Chileans are covered), which is uniform across levels of income. Only 2 percent of individuals in each decile of income are not covered.
- Likelihood of belonging to an ISAPRE increases with income. Only within the highest income decile do more individuals belong to an ISAPRE than to the FONASA.
- Low-income individuals are unlikely to subscribe to an ISAPRE, because FONASA A beneficiaries do not have to pay monthly contributions or copayments.
- Only 1 in 10 of individuals in the poorest decile is not covered by FONASA A or B (not including the uninsured).
- The percentage of high-income individuals covered by FONASA A is low.

**Figure 6.16** **Chile: Social Security System Beneficiaries, by Income Decile and Insurance Type, 2000**

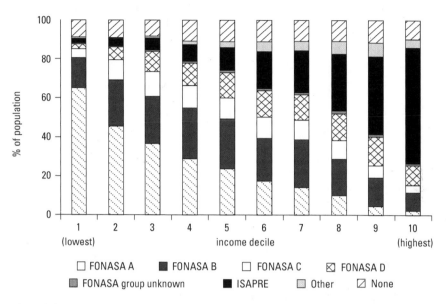

Source: CASEN Census 2000.

Across all income levels, the FONASA and the ISAPREs cover a large proportion of the population. The FONASA covers about two-thirds of the population. The FONASA and the open ISAPREs together cover 86 percent of the total population, or 96 percent of individuals with health insurance. Ninety-six percent of the poorest individuals are covered under FONASA A and B.

The FONASA is internally equitable. According to a study of equity within the FONASA in 1995 (Bitrán, R. 1997), nearly 41 percent of FONASA beneficiaries are indigent (Group A) and make no payments. Government subsidies for health are well targeted, with 90 percent of funds reaching the indigent and 7.5 percent reaching low-income individuals in Group B. Between 32 percent and 40 percent of the contributions of higher-income FONASA beneficiaries cross-subsidize care for the poorer beneficiaries, indicating that the FONASA's internal funding structure is progressive.

Indigents receive the most benefits per capita each year (US$116.63), followed by Group B beneficiaries (US$52.80). Public subsidies targeted to public health measures amounted to US$475.6 million, while government spending on public health measures was US$127.5 million, US$9.20 per capita. Groups C and D beneficiaries derive negative net benefits from the system, their contributions helping to subsidize those in Group B, and elderly beneficiaries receive a positive cross-subsidy from younger beneficiaries.

**Table 6.12 Chile: Contributions, Benefits, and Subsidies within the FONASA, 1995 (1995 Chilean pesos, millions)**

| Group | Contributions | (%) | Benefits | (%) | Net benefit |
|-------|--------------|------|----------|------|-------------|
| A | 27,344 | 10.26 | 202,594 | 44.35 | 175,250 |
| B | 111,664 | 41.88 | 172,408 | 37.74 | 60,744 |
| C | 60,915 | 22.85 | 41,661 | 9.12 | −19,254 |
| D | 66,707 | 25.02 | 40,139 | 8.79 | −26,568 |
| Total | 266,630 | 100.00 | 456,802 | 100.00 | 190,172 |

*Source:* Bitrán 1997.

Table 6.12 presents more data from this study, showing the contributions made and net benefits received by beneficiaries of each FONASA group. Benefits considered include primary, secondary, and tertiary levels of care, services provided under the free choice modality, the maternity subsidy, and health benefits provided through contracts with the private sector. The contributions considered include monthly premiums, copayments for publicly provided services, and copayments for services provided under the free choice modality. The lowest-income groups (A and B) received a positive net benefit; the higher-income groups derived negative net benefits. Group A received the greatest net benefit, followed by Group B, indicating that net benefits are distributed equitably within the FONASA. Group B contributed nearly double the amount contributed by Groups C and D, but received four to five times the amount in benefits. Forty-two percent of the benefits were subsidized by the government.

*ISAPREs discriminate among beneficiaries.* According to one study, most of the population above 50 years of age (even within the highest quintile of income) subscribes to the FONASA. This phenomenon is attributed to discrimination by the insurance companies against older beneficiaries, either by increasing prices or reducing coverage. Risk discrimination also affects the low-income individuals at high risk of illness (Titelman 2000). This type of discrimination can occur because the ISAPREs are able to decide whether to accept an individual as a beneficiary after gathering information about the person. The FONASA, in contrast, accepts anyone paying the monthly contribution or classified as poor. Figure 6.17 shows ISAPRE and FONASA membership by age group at two time points, illustrating how the ISAPREs discriminate against the elderly. As shown, the beneficiary population of the two types of insurers has changed little in 15 years, and the FONASA's beneficiary population is "older" than that of the ISAPREs.

*The benefits derived by ISAPRE members are proportional to their contributions.* The variety of plans offered by the ISAPREs allows them to assign beneficiaries to a plan that corresponds to their risk and income. The GES defines a basic benefits

**Figure 6.17   Chile: FONASA and ISAPRE Beneficiaries, by Age, 1990 and 2005**

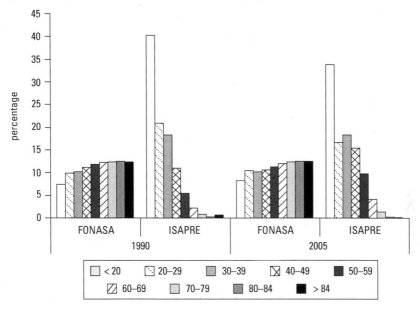

*Source:* Bitrán & Asociados 2006.

package that all plans must provide. Therefore ISAPRE beneficiaries receive all the benefits covered under the GES, as well as any provided by additional coverage that they may choose to purchase under their individual plan. The benefits provided by these individual plans are proportional to the cost of the plan. Premiums are equal to the amount specified by law plus the cost of any additional coverage.

## Efficiency

Some aspects that determine the degree of efficiency of the Chilean health system are described next.

*Moral hazard.* Having insurance coverage can influence an individual's behavior. First, knowing that their financial losses will be covered, insured individuals may be less careful to avoid injury or illness. Second, as the insured do not pay for the full cost of their treatment, they may visit the doctor more frequently and consume more medications than they would were they not insured. This phenomenon, called *moral hazard,* occurs with all types of insurance. To reduce the impact of moral risk, Chile has implemented copayments. Furthermore, the ISAPREs require a waiting period before insurance becomes active and before certain benefits are available. The waiting lists for certain services provided FONASA beneficiaries also reduce problems associated with moral hazard.

*Risk selection.* There is an asymmetry of information between the insured and the insurer. When the beneficiaries possess better information about their own risk than do the companies, given that the premiums charged do not necessarily reflect individual risk, the beneficiaries may choose not to subscribe (*adverse selection*). In other cases, companies may be better able to discriminate between high- and low-risk individuals than the individuals themselves and selectively enroll low-risk individuals to maximize profits (*cream skimming*).[13] In Chile, the mandatory system and set premiums protect against risk selection and allow greater diversification of risk. Similarly, the basic package is a tool to minimize cream skimming. The health authorities also work to reduce asymmetries of information.

*The system requires a minimum health expenditure, reducing the efficiency of society.* Chilean law requires all formal sector workers to contribute 7 percent of their income to enroll in an individual insurance plan. Since beneficiaries have different personal and family characteristics and preferences, some beneficiaries are compelled to purchase more insurance than they need. This diminishes the efficiency of the economy. A counterargument to this position is that, if free market forces are allowed to govern the social security system, a lower-than-optimal amount of insurance will be consumed. In general, individuals underestimate their future health risks and fail to take externalities into account. Fixed premiums based on income also pose a problem in that plans for high-income and low-risk beneficiaries include benefits that emphasize comfort and amenities in the settings in which the interventions are carried out.

*A wide variety of health plans are available, which minimizes some losses of efficiency but generates others.* The ISAPREs have created a wide variety of plans to fit individuals at various income and risk levels. This minimizes efficiency losses, because beneficiaries can choose the plan that best fits their needs and preferences. However, the inability of much of the population to determine which plan offers them the most advantages limits this potential advantage.

*High spending on sales and marketing.* Because the private insurance market is highly competitive, the ISAPREs spend a great deal of resources to attract members. For example, the companies mount intense marketing campaigns to position their products and deploy a large network of salespeople.

*The FONASA rations the services it provides.* The FONASA allocates health services using quantity rationing (lines and waiting lists) rather than price rationing. The entity has also tended to fund standard care without regard to health outcomes or member preferences.

*The salary scheme does not encourage efficiency.* Salaries for health professionals in public facilities are predetermined according to certain variables (professional degree, years of experience, location) rather than performance, effort, or results.

## Overview of the Health Care System

The supply capacity, regulatory features and the social security system of the Chilean health system are presented below.

### Public Hospitals, Physicians, and Health Programs

The supply capacity of the Chilean health system is described in terms of the available number of hospitals, beds, doctors, nurses, drugs and medical equipment, and the main health programs being implemented.

*Hospitals.* The public health sector provides outpatient facilities and various types of hospitals. In 2003, of the 191 public hospitals, 56 of them provided primary and secondary-level care, 31 tertiary-level care, and 104 quaternary level care. In addition, more than 500 outpatient facilities and nearly 2,000 rural health posts provided primary care.

*Beds.* According to the WHO, Chile had 25 hospital beds per 10,000 population in 2003, one bed for every 400 people. Eighty percent of these were public beds. Figure 6.18 shows the average number of beds available within the National Health Services System (SNSS, Sistema Nacional de Servicios de Salud). The department of social assistance and investment at the Chilean Ministry of Health estimates that about 80 percent of these beds are used for primary and secondary-level care. The MOH also estimates that existing hospital stock in 2003 represented an investment of US$1.8 billion, of which US$1.1 billion was attributable to infrastructure and

**Figure 6.18   Chile: Available Beds in the SNSS System, 1990–2002 (annual average)**

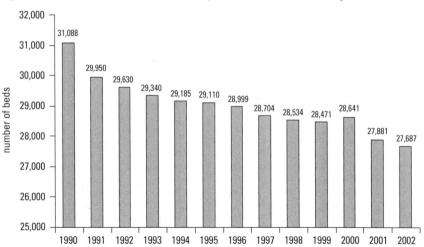

*Source:* Superintendence of Health.

US$700 million to equipment. The projected investment for 2004–08 was US$523 million (US$523 million for equipment and US$296 million for infrastructure).

*Physicians and nurses.* According to the 1992 Population and Housing Census, there were 13,897 physicians in Chile. Based on this statistic, as well as data on degrees earned, net income of foreign-born physicians in Chile, mortality rates, and retirement rates, one study estimated that there were 18,548 physicians in 2000 and a projected 25,704 physicians for 2007 (Bastías, Marshall, and Zúñiga 2000). MOH estimates put the number of physicians at 15,000 and medical support staff members at 60,000 in 2003. According to 2003 WHO data, there were 17,250 physicians, 10,000 nurses, and 6,750 dentists in Chile.

*Medications.* Data for 1999 indicated 16,000 registered pharmaceutical products. However, companies sometimes register a brand-name and generic version of the same product. Medications sold without a prescription represented 14 percent of total sales, while generic medications represented 38 percent of the pharmaceutical market. The total medications sold amounted to US$632 million, US$42 per capita each year.

*Medical equipment.* Investment in the public network has been heavy, especially during the 1990s. Thirteen hospitals were built or renovated during that time, at a cost of US$260 million. An additional 53 hospitals and 13 specialist facilities were modernized, at respective costs of US$180 million and US$105 million. Regional studies indicated that the care network acquired equipment valued at US$571 million in 1999. Thirty-two percent of the installed equipment is obsolete.

*Programs.* In July 2006, the MOH was executing various programs targeting specific segments of the population (programs for adolescents, older adults, women, and children), preventing illnesses (immunization campaigns, campaigns on preventing and managing acute respiratory infections in children), fighting diseases (programs for cancer, cardiovascular disease, schizophrenia, mental health, and tuberculosis), rehabilitation (integrated treatment for depression, integrated health and human rights services), and nutrition (free meal program).[14]

## Regulatory Issues

In a perfect market, no regulation is required. Market failures in the health insurance and health care markets in Chile, however, have led to a series of regulations. Health services are provided by the Regional Secretaries of the MOH (Secretarías Regionales Ministeriales de Salud, SEREMIS). When the ISAPRE system was launched in 1981, the insurance market was unregulated. Regulation of private insurers began in 1991, and in 2005 regulations were developed for public insurance providers. This has made the process more symmetrical, although different regulations apply to public providers and to private providers. For example, the

Superintendent of Health requires private insurers to provide extensive information regarding their financial stability, which is not required of the public insurer. However, many other requirements are symmetrical, such as compliance with the GES.

The earlier absence of insurance regulations for part of the market created two types of problems. First, beneficiaries had trouble understanding and comparing the products offered by the FONASA with the ISAPRE products. Second, the ISAPREs had complete freedom in screening their beneficiaries and dismissing them when they become too costly. Beneficiaries had no recourse.

The Superintendent of Health is responsible for: authorizing the creation of new ISAPREs, applying the laws and regulations on ISAPREs, specifying the guidelines and standards for the application of regulations and reporting procedures, arbitrating conflicts between ISAPREs and beneficiaries, and monitoring the financial solvency of ISAPREs.

The number of accountability mechanisms in the hands of the SIS (Superintendencia de Salud) has grown over time. At present, the SIS is responsible for carrying out the following supervisory procedures: inspecting all operations, goods, accounting books, files, and documents from ISAPREs and requesting any necessary clarifications; accessing ISAPRE financial balances at any time; and defining what information should be always available at the ISAPRE central office.

Health system regulations are intended mainly to protect consumers and create transparency of information. Asymmetries of information and adverse selection are the biggest and most complex problems within the health insurance market, and regulation is aimed at reducing the attendant risks.

## Systemic Strengths and Weaknesses

Below is an evaluation of the regulatory framework under which the health social security system operates and some observations about the main characteristics of the ISAPRE market.

*Market concentration.* About 15 ISAPREs, covering a quarter of the population, operate in Chile. The three ISAPREs with the largest memberships (Banmedica, Consalud, and ING) cover about 60 percent of this market, meaning that there are high levels of concentration within the ISAPRE market. However, concentration is not necessarily a negative characteristic as long as competition is sufficient to minimize service costs. Some authors argue that in risk administration markets (insurers) concentration is beneficial, because risk pooling reduces volatility and minimizes the size of the assets that the insurer must maintain. Other authors feel that high market concentrations lead to anticompetitive practices.

*Product homogeneity.* The health care sector offers diverse plans and products. Currently about 10,000 plans are available. The mandatory 7-percent-of-salary contribution means that a wide range of premiums are paid, so insurers offer a wide range of products. This feature of the system also creates an additional asymmetry of information that the insurer could exploit by appropriating excess contributions.

*Market transparency.* Market transparency has improved with increased regulation of ISAPREs. However, the heterogeneity of the insurance products offered makes it impossible to guarantee adequate market transparency.

> The way that prices and benefits are listed, along with the fee schedules and coverage limits, makes it difficult to compare health plans. These features vary not only from ISAPRE to ISAPRE but also within the same insurer. Furthermore, the fee schedules that the ISAPREs use as a reference in creating their health plans do not necessarily reflect real market prices for the services covered, making it difficult for consumers to evaluate health plans.
>
> —Superintendent of ISAPREs (1999)

*Barriers to entry.* There are no legal restrictions to make entry to the insurance market difficult. Legally, capital requirements are relatively low: companies must have at least US$160,000. The main barriers to entry are the accumulated power of established brands and the investment of physical capital. The first factor is important because of both product heterogeneity and asymmetries of information in the insurance market. Confidence in the ISAPRE is a major factor in choosing an insurer. Such confidence is created by establishing powerful brands, meaning expensive marketing and sales campaigns. The second barrier is the sheer amount of office space and the large sales, administrative, and specialized staff necessary for interacting with consumers and health providers. Finally, the economies of scale enjoyed by existing insurers could be considered a barrier to new entrants.

*Market behavior.* This market is characterized by clear segmentation or target marketing of high-income, low-risk members. Price is not the endogenous variable in the competition model for this market. In fact, the 7-percent-of-salary premium represents an exogenous variable determined by government regulations. Equilibrium should be achieved by offering the best plans in terms of coverage and quality in exchange for the above premium.

Yet selecting a health plan is problematic. The information regarding the content of the programs offered is difficult to process, and therefore some uncertainly is involved in selecting the best plan.

## Health Insurance Reforms

In the history of health care in Chile, there have been two pivotal moments:[15] the 1952 reform, which culminated in the creation of a National Health System, and the 1980s reform, which redefined the role of the state within the health care framework, created the ISAPREs, and transferred responsibility for primary care services to the municipal corporations.

**Figure 6.19  Chile: Chronology of Health Reforms, 1917–2006**

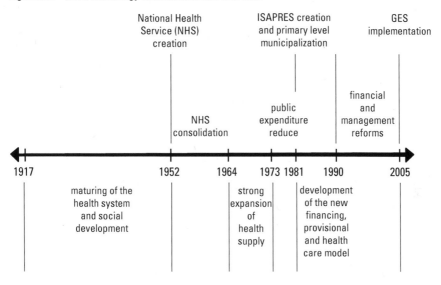

*Source:* Authors.

Figure 6.19 provides a timeline for the major developments in the history of the Chilean health system, including the two landmark moments described above followed by the establishment of the GES in 2005. Developments that did not occur on a specific date are depicted as occurring over a continuum. Six major periods of reform can be identified over the time frame examined here (1917–2006).

## The 1952 Reform

The health and social security system entered a period of maturation in 1917. That year, all the social welfare agencies and insurance providers participated in a national congress convened to improve organization within the health and health insurance system. In 1924, Chile established a Ministry of Hygiene, Social Assistance, and Social Protection; Mandatory Worker Insurance; and a Workers' Insurance Fund to cover risks of disability, aging, and death. In 1938, the pioneer Law of Preventive Medicine was drafted. SERMENA (Employees' National Medical Service) was created, covering public and private sector employees, and in 1948, the Medical Association of Chile was established.

*Creation of SNS.* The National Health Service (SNS) was created in 1952, uniting various public entities that provided health services. These included the General Health Office, hospital services provided by the Central Association of Beneficence and Social Assistance; the medical department of the Workers' Insurance Fund; the Office of Protection for Mothers, Children, and Adolescents; and certain municipal medical services. With the creation of SNS, nearly 90 percent of public resources for health were concentrated in one entity. Other coverage was provided by universities, public companies, the armed forces, and police departments.

SNS was led by a general director, with two suboffices (one technical, the other administrative) and emphasized centralized planning. SNS divided its efforts across three geographic territories, each covering one or more provinces (Palma, Friedmann, and Heyermann 1995).

*Evolution of the reform.*  In 1964, Chile initiated a variety of social reforms, including investment in health centers, training for medical personnel, and extension of geographic coverage. SNS eventually employed 120,000 functionaries, in a health network covering a large part of the geographic terrain and population. Centralized planning dominated political, economic, and organizational development in the health sector. From 1964 to 1973, health care was closely associated with social development by Chile's social and political leadership. From 1973 to 1980, social spending and funding for SNS declined significantly. The organizational framework of SNS was maintained but was controlled by the authoritarian regime. After 1979, the state health sector was restructured. The Ministry of Health and related institutions were reorganized, and the National Health Services System (SNSS) was established.

## The 1980s Reform

In 1981, the private sector entered the health insurance market.

*ISAPREs and decentralization.*  In 1985, the Health Law created a framework for health care provision, including the current model for financing, insurance, and health services. Between 1981 and 1986, various legal initiatives created the ISAPREs and transferred responsibility for most primary care facilities to the municipalities.

*Validation of the model with minor adjustments.*  Since 1990, the elected Coalition of Parties for Democracy administrations has assumed responsibility for the health system they inherited. The current health system maintains many of the same financing, organizational, and functional characteristics of the model established during the military period, especially in terms of health care provision (governed by the Health Law), the legal-normative configuration of the SNSS, and fiscal financing of the public system, the municipal administration of health facilities, the role of the ISAPREs in insurance provision, and the model for worker compensation claims.

However, recent administrations have implemented some reforms mainly to: increase investment in the health sector, with the support of international loans and researching proposals to improve and reform the sector; to improve public sector administration; and to accelerate the decentralization process. Some changes have been made in the primary care statute and the laws governing medicine, ISAPREs, and the FONASA. The major reform has been the introduction of the GES, as described above.

## Evaluation of the Insurance Reforms

Many of the changes in the health system were closely tied to the economic, social, and political context in which they occurred. Therefore, to evaluate the principal Chilean health system reforms, a chronological analysis covering three periods is provided: centralized planning under the SNS (1952–73); 1980s reform under the military government (1973–90); and adjustments during the current democratic period (1990–2006).

*Centralized planning under the SNS, 1952–73.* The SNS operated for 27 years and developed five important national programs: Program for Maternal Health, Program for Child and Adolescent Health, Program for Senescent Adults, Program for Social Health, and Program for Environmental Health. Most of the country and population groups were covered by these programs.[16]

In the mid-1960s and early 1970s, society became increasingly polarized, dividing the political-social arena into two diverging approaches. From 1964 to 1970, the state was involved in the market, but social policy was secondary to other concerns. Between 1970 and 1973, the market was closely regulated by the state, with the explicit goal of achieving certain social objectives. Public spending on social programs as a percentage of gross global product (GGP) increased during both periods, from 16.3 percent in 1963 to 25.8 percent in 1971. Public spending on health also increased as a percentage of GGP, from 3.1 percent to 4.0 percent over the same period.

From 1964 to 1970, the SNS attempted to cover as broad a segment of the population as possible, with the goal of having only one health provider. Health provision entities specific to certain sectors or unions were dissolved.

In the early 1970s, the government created the Single Health Care Service (Servicio Único de Salud, SUS), in an attempt to consolidate health care provision into one egalitarian, effective, coherent, and free service provider. However, these changes did not have the intended effect, and the SUS's functions were eventually absorbed by other public and private institutions.

To expand coverage, in 1968 the Curative Medicine for Employees law was drafted, bringing 2.5 million public and private employees into the socialized health system. By the mid-1970s, the health system had broadened its coverage, continuing the process initiated 20 years earlier. By 1920, the beneficiary population of the main health providers included the SNS—dependent workers and laborers (both active and retired), the indigent, the unemployed, and their families; SERMENA—employees (both active and retired) enrolled in various insurance funds (state and private) and their families; and Security Assistance Institutions (Mutuales de Seguridad)—active workers whose companies carry workers' compensation insurance.

The insured population consisted of workers covered by SNS (50 percent), employees covered by SERMENA (20 percent), and independent workers who paid for coverage through either SNS or SERMENA (7 percent). Between 18 and 20 percent were not covered by any of those institutions.

According to Palma, et al (1995), global health indictors continuously improved under the SNS, and faster than elsewhere in Latin America. The number of professional medical services provided also increased—as did health spending. However, the SNS had a number of flaws: excessive centralism and a swelling bureaucracy; inefficiency in the use and distribution of resources; administrative inefficiencies; inequitable payment and benefit schedules; and inadequate targeting of subsidies.

*1980s reform under the military government.* The military government's health policies were based on three principles: a limited role for the state; free market policies; and support for private business as the key to economic development.[17] The military regime developed new health policies in four stages:

- *Initial attempts to restructure the public health sector (1974–78).* This phase was characterized by strong inertia within the public health system, punctuated by the announcement in 1975 that services would no longer be provided free of charge, except in cases of extreme indigence.
- *Definitive restructuring of the system (1979–80).* SNS beneficiaries were allowed free choice among public and private providers. The Ministry of Health was reorganized into three branches with clearly defined responsibilities: the Ministry of Health (regulation of the health system); Health Services (execution of health services); and the FONASA (financing of health services).
- *Participation of the private sector and municipalization of primary-level care (1980–84).* In 1981 the private sector entered the health insurance market in the form of ISAPREs. These companies collected workers' mandatory health premiums and in exchange provided the services that would have fallen to the Health Services department and the FONASA. Service contracts covered inpatient care, intensive care, and emergency care. As part of the decentralization process initiated in 1981, responsibility for primary-level care (general urban and rural health posts and facilities) was transferred to the municipalities.
- *Conclusion of the health sector reform (1985–90).* The fourth stage ended with the Health Law, which had the following goals: equity in the health system, eliminating the disparities in quality of care; distributive justice, establishing a mechanism through which the consumer pays according to ability; and improved access, guaranteeing free or egalitarian opportunities for health care through a free choice system.

Health indicators measured during the military regime showed that the system was effective; however, there were gaps in efficiency and equity. In terms of efficiency, the main problems were ineffective management of resources by health facilities and providers and failure to fully implement certain reforms (especially the restructuring and decentralization of the system). In terms of equity, the reforms channeled Chileans by income into one of two health systems. Spending per capita and services provided per beneficiary were quite different under each system (Oyarzo, César 1993).

*Adjustments during the democratic period.* After the military government ended, the new administrations tried to accelerate decentralization of the Chilean health system. However, the SEREMIS were weak, had poorly defined responsibilities, and had many organizational flaws, including lack of collaboratively generated plans, objectives, and goals, lack of internal coordination, and poor flow of information.

Despite these weaknesses, the public sector sought to transform its health service providers and hospitals into autonomous entities through a series of actions intended to strengthen local administration. The government also sought to create technical, legal, and administrative conditions at other levels of the state to support this process. During this period, the state increased the MOH budget as a percentage of total fiscal budget. Along with the international loans, this increase represented a strong investment in health services.[18] It also established free health care for all FONASA beneficiaries (about 70 percent of the population at that time) and supported primary care facilities by establishing Regional Funds, creating a network of emergency primary-level services and increasing the real salaries of public health sector workers. At the same time, it explored new ways of financing the health system at the operational level.

Despite these measures, the CEP-Adimark survey carried out in the mid-1990s indicated that the public perceived a health sector in crisis. Some of the perceived flaws included insufficient decentralization of the system, inefficiency of the bureaucratic-administrative system, poor management of the public health system, and inadequate funding (Palma, Friedmann, and Heyermann 1995).

Aedo (2000) reported in the late 1990s:

> Chile has achieved better global health indicators than predicted for a country at this level of development. However, the public indicates low levels of satisfaction with their health system. The public sector suffers from funding and administrative limitations. The ISAPRE system is perceived as providing good health services, but under an inequitable funding model. There are few good alternatives, then, for the elderly or chronically ill.

Table 6.13 summarizes Chile's global health indicators.

Aedo (2000) also identified some factors that have limited the development of the post-reform Chilean health system. They include

- *Imperfections in the health insurance market.* The FONASA charges a monthly premium on a sliding scale according to beneficiaries' income and provides net

**Table 6.13  Chile: Global Health Indicators: 1960 and 1995**

| Indicator | 1960 | 1995 |
| --- | --- | --- |
| Infant mortality | 120/1,000 live births | 11.1/1,000 live births |
| Maternal mortality | 3/1,000 live births | 0.4/1,000 live births |
| General mortality | 12/1,000 population | 5.5/1,000 population |
| Mortality from tuberculosis | 53/1,000 cases | 5/1,000 cases |
| Mortality from infections | 193/1,000 cases | 5/1,000 cases |
| Life expectancy | 58 years | 74.8 years |

*Source:* MOH http://www.minsal.cl.

benefits inversely proportional to income. ISAPRE beneficiaries, in contrast, receive net benefits that are proportional to their contribution. Furthermore, price schedules, promptness of delivery of care, and level of income vary between the two systems. This disparity has created tension between the two systems.

• *Mandatory contributions for health care and the design of the mandatory insurance policy.* Making participation mandatory reduced opportunism (deriving unearned benefits from the system) and partially counterbalances the information asymmetries. However, the mandatory 7-percent-of-salary payment creates two problems. First, a number of people will be overinsured relative to their risk and income. Second, allowing individuals to design their own insurance plan can lead individuals to focus on outpatient rather than hospital care. This thwarts the function of insurance and of mandatory participation.

• *Spending on health care for older adults.* Chile is in a transitional phase in which the population is aging. Some studies have indicated that there should be adequate funds to finance care for the older adult, both because they have fewer dependents than younger people and because many will have a pension. However, social security coverage has decreased steadily since the 1980s, which may open funding gaps.

• *Increasing costs in the health sector.* The cost of medical services and products has increased for various reasons. Although the population is healthier than ever before, individuals are demanding better quality of care. New technologies and developments in health care mean more effective treatment for illnesses but require more highly trained personnel; and new medications are more sophisticated and effective, but also more expensive. Moreover, increased life expectancy increases not only the length of time for which a persona will require medical care, but also increases the likelihood of developing a chronic disease.

In the mid-1990s, the only changes were modifications in financial and administrative aspects of the FONASA. This was not because the government failed to recognize the profound epidemiological changes that had occurred over the past 20 years, but because a political decision had been made to postpone major changes until a minimum consensus could be reached. In any case, these changes represented important advances in the operational and conceptual framework of the system, for example, the separation of functions within the public sector, the purchase of services, and the establishment of new payment mechanisms to progressively replace the old procedures for allocating resources.

The administrations were also successful in increased public sector coverage of the population. These were the highlights (Acuña 1998):

- Increased coverage for low-income groups, accomplished by providing a full subsidy (no copayments) for specific health services.
- Establishment of a catastrophe insurance fund for public system beneficiaries, designed to cover all the costs of treating the most common catastrophic illnesses (including cervical uterine cancer, breast cancer, prostate cancer, coronary disease, renal insufficiency, bone marrow transplants for children under 16 with leukemia, and kidney, liver, and heart transplants).
- Establishment of a special program to provide 100 percent coverage for health problems common among adults over 65, including joint replacement surgeries.
- Drafting of a Beneficiaries' Bill of Rights defining the rights and responsibilities of public sector consumers. This Bill of Rights was well received by the population but created problems for public hospitals in that it imposed 25 demands in terms of access to information and standards of care, some of them beyond the facilities' capabilities.

The final important reform in the Chilean health sector has been the establishment of the Explicit Health Guarantees System Act by which the state guarantees the entire population coverage, access, financing, and quality of care for a variety of health problems, without discriminating by insurance plan, gender, or income. The GES Act represents an important change in the health system, making beneficiaries consumers with enforceable rights.

According to FONASA data, some public providers cannot satisfy all the GES requirements. In fact, the FONASA estimates that the first 25 health problems covered under the GES created a supply deficit among public providers that compelled the system to purchase services from public providers at a cost of about $35 billion in 2005 (about US$60 million). The FONASA estimates that services purchased from public providers in 2006 will cost about $50 billion; no estimates are yet available for 2007.

The cost of observing the GES is highly concentrated in specific health problems. Figure 6.20 displays the cumulative cost of the GES, starting with the most expensive health condition covered (arterial hypertension, type II diabetes mellitus, depression in individuals over the age of 15, and so forth) (Bitrán & Asociados 2005).

**Figure 6.20  Chile: Cumulative Cost of the 56 GES-Covered Health Conditions, estimates for 2007**

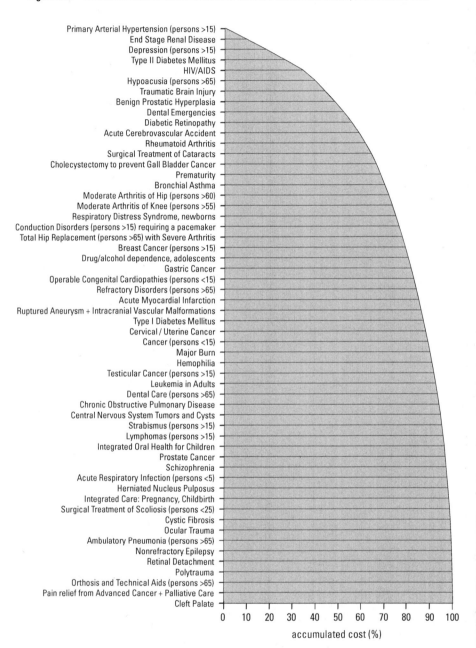

## Future Reforms: Characteristics and Conditions for Success

Chile has reached a socioeconomic level that allows it to provide a large segment of its population with care comparable to that available in developed nations, while also providing at least basic health coverage for practically its entire population. Within this framework, the major challenge is to keep the cost of health care from growing at a rate faster than the country's economic growth can sustain.

Below is a summary of priorities identified by health sector specialists and 10 proposals that a group of analysts have suggested as approaches to achieving these priority goals (Health Engineering Commission 2005). Priorities identified by health sector specialists include

- Increase funding for investment in hospital equipment for public facilities. Government studies indicate a US$600 million deficit in funds to cover investment needs over the next 10 years.
- Contain the growing cost of medical leave claims. Currently the system reimburses for 100 percent of lost salary, with no maximum length of leave.
- Spread the economic risk of health care among insurers and providers.
- Allow beneficiaries to allocate their own subsidies.
- Improve public services or lose beneficiaries, who, now free to choose providers, seek care in the private sector.
- Increase investment in research and development.
- Move from a supply-side subsidy to a demand-side subsidy.

The 10 proposals identified by analysts are

- Establish an explicit minimum level of coverage for the entire population, identifying the specific benefits an individual insurer may exclude. Priority should be given to preventive and coverage for catastrophic illness.
- Improve management of public hospitals, introducing competition and flexibility. Also, raise private funds for hospitals requiring major investments, contract services out to private facilities, including the Security Assistance Institutions, and change the Worker Compensation law so that employers rather than the public sector provide this coverage.
- Incorporate information technology tools to support health sector administration, for example, by incorporating the use of open communications standards between information systems and incorporating systems that allow for the development of networks.
- Shift from supply-side to demand-side subsidies; that is, give subsidies directly to the individuals that need them and allow the individuals to freely select the health provider that they prefer.
- Encourage the use of managed care, standardizing diagnostic and treatment procedures and establishing protocols for care "packages" at set prices and other mechanisms to transfer per capita risks.

- Open construction projects and administration of primary care facilities to private companies.
- Create special programs for the elderly and chronically ill. The health landscape is changing, and the system is experiencing more and more pressure from older adults. Priority should be given to primary care and chronic and degenerative diseases that affect older adults. To cover the increased costs that their care represents, insurers should be permitted to charge higher premiums than the 7-percent-of-salary contribution.
- Control the cost of paid medical leave. Suggested changes to this subsidy include: establish a maximum duration of paid leave; provide support to workers without replacing their entire salary (a form of copayment); establish sanctions for workers who abuse the system; allow for some flexibility in the levels of benefit paid and conditions for receiving the benefit.
- Update prevention programs to fight the spread of modern diseases such as obesity, diabetes, hypertension, tobacco addiction, high cholesterol, AIDS, drug addiction.
- Link premiums to coverage and cost of care. The mandatory contributions for health care were established in 1986 and have never been modified, even though health care has changed significantly in the intervening years.

## Potential Problems in the Short and Medium Term

Some potential short- and medium-term problems that the Chilean health system may present are described next.

*Public insurer, public providers.* The FONASA provides most of its beneficiaries' care in public facilities, which operate on fixed budgets. This situation has allowed the system to provide adequate coverage and quality of care, because operating and management costs are more moderate for public than private facilities (Bitrán & Asociados, 2005). If the FONASA had to buy all its services from private providers, its costs would increase.

*Asymmetrical regulation.* The Superintendent of Health regulates the ISAPREs and FONASA asymmetrically. For example, the information that the two types of providers must report is different. Moreover, the Superintendent of Health may be more lenient with the FONASA than with the ISAPREs in terms of enforcing the GES.

*Asymmetrical obligations.* The ISAPREs and FONASA are not required to follow the same rules in terms of enrollment. ISAPREs are permitted to practice risk selection, but the FONASA must accept any applicant fulfilling its requirements. The risk, due to adverse selection, is that the highest-risk beneficiaries may flock to the FONASA. Furthermore, moving to another ISAPRE is difficult for high-risk

ISAPRE beneficiaries. They remain captive members, facing ever-increasing premiums, which makes them more likely to leave the private system and enroll in the FONASA.

*Financing the GES.* The GES was drafted after reviewing studies estimating its implementation costs. However, the cost may be higher than anticipated, leaving the system inadequate resources to finance the guarantees. If funds do not cover the cost of the GES, what will happen is unclear.

*The GES and politics.* It is tempting for politicians to add illnesses to the list of covered conditions as a way of gaining popularity, but adding new guarantees without conducting cost studies could jeopardize the sustainability of the system. Another latent risk is that that so many conditions will be added to the GES that the cost of health spending will escalate, and the guarantees will be impossible to meet.

*The system and politics.* The ISAPREs are perceived as elite institutions by the common citizen. Therefore, there is a risk that, in the name of equity, the system will be dismantled in favor of channeling more resources to the public system.

*Changes in public hospital administration.* There have been trends toward reforming public hospital administration and governance, for example by introducing competition for contracts or providing facilities with greater autonomy to produce an atmosphere of greater accountability. However, these changes will probably occur slowly, if at all, because of resistance from various interest groups.

*Lack of coordination and moral hazard.* Primary care is managed at municipal level, while hospital care is administered centrally. At times, coordination among levels has been poor, reducing the effectiveness of care. In other cases, this disconnect has meant that a public hospital provides care that could have been provided at a primary facility. This is significant, because the municipalities receive capitated payments (according to the municipality's population).

*Focus of the GES.* The GES does not give preventive care a priority, nor does it necessarily encourage the most cost-effective public health measures. This decreases the efficiency of health spending in Chile.

*Price increases.* Traditionally, the ISAPREs have reimbursed providers per service provided. This system is inflationary. Now, the system is making a transition to a managed care scheme that will better contain costs.

## Health Coverage Reforms: Lessons for Other Countries

The Chilean health system is characterized by broad coverage under its social security system, with only 10 percent of the population not covered by any insurer. Some of the factors that have allowed this system to function adequately are described below.

## Conditional Factors

Implementing a social security system requires considerable economic resources, especially in the early years, because of moral hazard, or the likelihood that an insured population will use more health services than the uninsured population. Therefore, implementation is easier when public finances are adequate to bear these costs. Implementation of such systems typically occurs during periods of expansion, when economic growth is strong. Furthermore, because the state subsidizes the health social security system for about a quarter of its population, it must have adequate resources to do so. The greater the economic growth, the more taxes the state can collect to fund these costs.

The greater the concentration of the population in urban areas, the broader is the coverage of a social security system, due to reduced administrative costs. In Chile, the rural population amounts to just over 10 percent of the total population, a facilitating factor in coverage reforms.

The higher the income level within an economy, the greater is the probability of its being able to bear the high administrative and operational costs of a social security system with wide coverage. In Chile, the income level is considered medium-high. Income per capita was about US$7,700 in 2005, which partially explains the success of the social security system.

## Necessary Institutional Arrangements

"Institutional agreements are the overall rules that allow the actors, through political negotiation, to make economic and political deals," according to José Ayala Espino (2001).[19]

Chile has always had credible, independent, efficient institutions, and it has one of the lowest international risk ratings among Latin American countries. Its strong institutions have played a vital role in its health reforms.

*Existence of a competent, independent regulatory entity.* Because the private sector provides services within an imperfect market (e.g., with information asymmetries), a regulatory entity must ensure that the market behaves as if it were perfectly competitive. This entity must enforce general and sector-specific legal regulations and protect the rights of beneficiaries. Although the Superintendent of Health did not begin to regulate private insurers until 10 years after the system had been implemented, and did not begin to regulate the FONASA until 10 years after that, the creation of this entity at the start of the system provides a lesson learned for other countries.

*Clear rules of the game.* The three branches of government—executive, legislative, and judicial—must provide regulatory tools and mechanisms that allow insurers to understand their rights and obligations and protect their investments. At the same time, the state needs to provide the Superintendent of Health with a framework that will allow it to carry out its fiscal responsibilities. Chile's institutional solidity has fostered competition among private insurers and encouraged high standards to maintain their solvency and prestige.

*A predominantly formal labor market.* A health social security system is easier to implement where the institutional and legal framework fosters formality, particularly a formal labor market. Administrative processes are simplified in such a situation, as is the collection of contributions. The Chilean economy in general and the labor market in particular are fairly formal in comparison with those in other Latin American countries.

*Competition among insurers.* A pillar of the Chilean social security system's efficiency is competition among insurers, not least because markets in other sectors of the Chilean economy are competitive. In Chile, one public insurer and various private insurers, in theory, compete for beneficiaries. In practice, however, the only true competition within the health social security system takes place at the level of certain socioeconomic groups. The great majority of the poor are FONASA beneficiaries; most of the rich are ISAPRE subscribers.

*Existence of a public insurance system.* If the social security system were dissolved in favor of a completely free market system with only private insurers, it is likely that the adverse selection process would leave only the lowest-risk, highest-income individuals insured (with complete coverage). To forestall this problem, the public insurer in Chile is not permitted to employ discriminatory practices, making it possible to achieve broad coverage of the population.

## Key Factors in Financing a Social Security System for Health Care

Cost, equity, efficiency, and sustainability are the key factors in financing a social security system for health care.

*Escalating costs.* Providing such health care coverage usually triggers a burst of consumer spending, partly due to moral hazard. For example, the insured consult a physician more frequently, take more medicines, and generally use more health care the uninsured. To contain public health spending, the Chilean reform set budgetary ceilings, based on previous years' spending. This has provided a constant supply of health services, with demand controlled via rationing mechanisms.

*Adequate supply of health services.* The greater the supply of public and private health services, and the greater the efficiency of those provider facilities, the better an extensive social security system will be able to function. Chile had the advantage of adequate health services from the beginning, although there have been difficulties in supplying less-populated and less-accessible areas with services.

*Adequate funding sources.* A social security system should be financed through various sources. In Chile, these sources include monthly contributions from beneficiaries, public funds (used mainly to cover the medical costs of the indigent), copayments from beneficiaries, and other income from health services.

*Private funding support is essential for a sustainable system.* In Chile, private support comes from two main sources: copayments, which vary according to services consumed, and monthly contributions, which are set at 7 percent of the beneficiary's income. The average salary in Chile was US$490. Countries with lower income levels will likely need to charge the beneficiaries higher rates to beneficiaries to offer a comparable benefits package. The required contribution in Chile has risen over time, from 4 percent in 1981 to its current rate of 7 percent.

*Efficient tax collection agencies.* A third to a half of the health care provided in Chile is funded by public spending. Efficient tax collection and low evasion help ensure that the money will be there to pay for public spending.

*Mandatory membership.* Membership in the Chilean social security system is mandatory for formal workers and voluntary for independent and informal workers. The problem of adverse selection, present in any insurance system, is minimized when membership is mandatory. Risk diversification—spread across a broad and diverse membership—reduces the costs of providing insurance.

## Key Political and Economic Factors in Reform Success
Many political and economic factors influence the outcome of reform. They include a country's form of government, social solidarity, subsidy system, social and political accord, administrative system, and governmental credibility.

*Type of government system enacting the reform.* The 1980s health sector reform transferring many health functions from the public to the private sector in Chile was carried out under an autocratic government, reducing the potential for resistance from involved parties. Other countries enacting such a reform under a democratic government would likely have to contend with social conflicts. Such resistance might jeopardize the success of the reform or result in only partial implementation.

*Solidarity.* As a rule, the greater the tradition of solidarity within a country—that is, the more accustomed systems and institutions are to working together toward social consensus—the better are the chances of a successful social security system founded on risk pooling. In Chile, however, it may be argued, social security system relies less on solidarity than other systems, because the cross-subsidies provided are smaller than in other systems.

*Subsidy system.* A quarter of the Chilean population receives free social security benefits through subsidies provided mainly by the state, supplemented by small cross-subsidies contributed by other members. Therefore, although health care is ostensibly provided under the social security modality, the system functions by financing health care through tax revenues.

*Social and political accord.* The Chilean system includes two administrators, one public and one private. These administrators are linked to public and private providers. To work, this system depends on a certain level of social and political accord. Many other countries prefer an entirely public or an entirely private system.

*Capable administrators.* The more capable the system administrators and the better the public's confidence in them, the more efficient and reliable is the system.

*A capable and credible government.* As with the administrators, the more capably the government manages the system, the better is the system's chance of success.

## Replicability in Low-Income Countries

In light of the lessons noted above, replicating the Chilean model in low-income countries may be difficult. Many low-income countries also have additional challenges: a highly informal labor market, large rural population, too small a part of the population with sufficient income to cofinance the costs of a system offering an attractive benefits package, public lack of confidence in the reforming authorities and institutions, insufficient human resources and institutions capable of managing the changes, high resistance from interest groups, inability to limit fraud due to information gaps, shortages of health services to satisfy increased postreform demand, and insufficient budget to cover implementation costs.

## Replicability in Middle-Income Countries

Middle-income countries are better situated to implement a social security system similar to the Chilean system. Where lower-income countries have challenges, middle-income countries usually have advantages: a larger formal labor market, a smaller rural population, a broader population base of people with enough income to bear the costs of a system offering an attractive benefits package, better credibility on the part of the authorities and institutions that would execute the reforms, more human resources and institutions capable of managing the changes, experienced coalitions to negotiate with interest groups to achieve the required reforms, better ability to limit fraud within the system, a better supply of health services to meet increased postreform demand, and enough money to pay for it all.

## Endnotes

1. In 2005 the Collective Capitalization Fund amounted to US$1.1 billion.

2. The data used to describe Chilean demographics in the mid-20th century were taken from the 1952 census, and the data to describe the end of the 20th century were taken from the 1992 census.

3. The dependency index is expressed in terms of unproductive population (those under 15 and over 65 years of age) divided by the productive population (those between the ages of 15 and 65). The index of aging represents the number people over 65 divided by the number of children under 15.

4. A DALY, disability-adjusted life year, represents one lost year of healthy life, due to premature death or disability.

5. This historical timeline is based on http://www.memoriachilena.cl "Elecciones, sufragio y democracia en Chile (1810–2005)."

6. See http://www.gobiernodechile.cl.

7. The maximum legal monthly contribution to FONASA or an ISAPRE is therefore US$140.

8. Some experts feel that official data on health spending as a percentage of GDP underestimate out-of-pocket spending on medications and that the true figure is closer to 8 percent of GDP.

9. Before the GESs were established, there was no national benefits package. FONASA did not guarantee specific rights to its beneficiaries.

10. Before the GESs were established, a Family Health Plan covered certain preventative and curative care in municipal facilities. This plan became part of the GHS.

11. There are two types of ISAPREs, open and closed. Open ISAPREs are available to anyone working in a given sector, while closed ISAPREs are available only to workers in certain companies, both public and private.

12. UF [*unidades de fomento*] are units of account linked to the Chilean consumer price index. UF are used to set a price that will not devalue over time as a result of inflation. One UF is about US$35.

13. In Chile, the ISAPREs allow members to self-select by offering a variety of health plans. The ISAPREs also screen members for preexisting conditions, whereas by law FONASA may not reject applicants.

14. For more information, visit the Chilean Ministry of Health's Web page: http://www.minsal.cl.

15. Source: http://www.colegiomedico.cl.

16. This section is based on findings reported by Palma, Friedmann, and Heyermann (1995).

17. A limited role for the state means here that the state should assume direct control only of functions serving the common good and not addressed by the private sector. This principle leaves the free market to allocate economic resources through supply and demand, assigning the state the role of regulating the markets as needed.

18. Investment in health services increased from US$10 million in 1986–90 to US$540 million in 1990–97.

## References

Acuña, Cecilia. 1998. "Evolución y reforma de los sistemas de protección de la salud, en los países del MERCOSUR y en Chile." http://www.fes.org.ar/.

Aedo, Cristian. 2000. "Las reformas en la salud en Chile." In *La transformación económica de Chile*. Felipe Larraín and Rodrigo Vergara, ed. Santiago: Centro de Estudios Públicos. http://www.cepchile.cl/dms/archivo_3267_1620/ 14_aedo.pdf

Ayala Espino, José. 2001. "Políticas de estado y arreglos institucionales para el desarrollo de México." *Revista Planeación y Desarrollo* 8/9 http://dialnet.unirioja.es/servlet/articulo?codigo= 298394.

Bastías, G., G. Marshall, and D. Zúñiga. 2000. "Número de médicos en Chile: estimaciones, proyecciones y comparación internacional." *Revista médica de Chile* 128(10). http://www.scielo.cl/scielo.php?pid=S0034-98872002000500015&script=sci_arttext.

Bitrán & Asociados. 2006. "Coyuntura del sistema de salud en Chile: oportunidades y desafíos para clínica Las Condes." Documento elaborado para la Clínica Las Condes.

———. 2005. "Verificación del costo esperado por beneficiario del conjunto priorizado de problemas de salud con garantías explícitas 2005–2007." Documento elaborado para el Ministerio de salud de Chile. http://www.minsal.cl/ici/destacados/estudio_verificacion/Resumen_Ejecutivo_GES_30_Noviembre_2005_Corregido.pdf.

Bitrán, Ricardo (1997). "Equity in the Financing of Social Security for Health in Chile." Partnerships for Public Health, Abt Associates, Inc., Bethesda, MD. http://ideas.repec.org/a/eee/hepoli/v50y2000i3p171-196.html.

Health Engineering Commission. 2005. "El sistema de salud de Chile: Análisis, 10 propuestas de cambios." Instituto de ingenieros de Chile, Santiago, Chile. Documento elaborado para el Ministerio de Planificación de Chile.

Melis Jacob, Fernanda. 2000. "La situación de la mujer en Chile." *Revista Occidente 56* http://www.revistaoccidente.cl/374/reportajes/SituacionMujer/lasituacion374.act.

Concha, Marisol. 1996. "La carga de la enfermedad." Documento elaborado para el MOH. http://epi.minsal.cl/epi/html/sdesalud/carga/Inffin-carga-enf. pdf.

Oyarzo, Cesar. 1993. "La mezcla pública privada: una reforma pendiente." Estudios Públicos 55, Santiago. http://www.cepchile.cl/dms/archivo_1635_169/rev55_oyarzo.pdf.

Palma, E., R. Friedmann, and B. Heyermann. 1995. "El sistema de salud en Chile ante la descentralización política." Latin American and Caribbean Institute for Economic and Social Planning, World Health Organization, and Ministry of Health, Santiago.

Superintendent of ISAPREs. 1999. "Sistema de salud privado en Chile." In L. Figueroa, and V. Lazén. "Propuestas de políticas de salud privada en Chile, 2001." http://www.perseo.cl/Politicas_de_salud.pdf.

Titelman, Daniel. 2000. "Reformas al sistema de salud en Chile: desafíos pendientes." En Reformas, crecimiento y políticas sociales en Chile desde 1973. Ricardo French-Davis, ed. Santiago: Comisión Económica para América Latina.

# 7

# Colombia: Good Practices in Expanding Health Care Coverage

*Diana Masis Pinto*

## Background

*Colombia is a 1,038,700-km², lower-middle income country in the Latin America and Caribbean Region of the World Bank. Its population numbers 41.2 million, with a per capita income (PPP-adjusted) of US$7,769. The country is divided into four capital districts corresponding to major cities and into 32 administrative departments, subdivided into 1,098 municipalities. The concentration of more than 60 percent of the population in the six largest urban municipalities facilitates health insurance coverage in those areas. Seventy percent of the other municipalities are rural and have fewer than 20,000 inhabitants, posing challenges for insurance expansion and implementation of the managed competition model.*

*In 1993, Colombia introduced one of the most ambitious health care reforms in Latin America, creating a National Social Health Insurance (NSHI), organized as a model of "managed competition." Two insurance schemes were implemented, the contributory regime (CR), for people who could pay, and the subsidized regime (SR), for those who could not. To expand health insurance coverage to all Colombians, the reforms mobilized a substantial amount of resources and undertook simultaneous changes in the organization of the health care delivery system and the administrative structure.*

*Total health expenditures were $136 per capita in 2003—7.8 percent of GDP. The health system is largely publicly financed—with 15.9 percent of this amount paid by private sources, including just 7.5 percent paid directly by households as out-of-pocket expenditures. Life expectancy is 72.5 years, and infant mortality is 17.5 per 1,000 live births.*

# Introduction

## Economic Environment

Until the mid-1990s Colombia had one of the most stable economies in Latin America. Economic growth was good until 1996, when a period of economic recession began. In 1999, unemployment hit 20.1 percent, and poverty reached a peak of 58.2 percent of the population. Social public expenditure as percentage of GDP decreased from 15.3 percent in 1997 to 13.6 percent in 2000 (Lasso 2004), which had a negative impact on enrollment in the National Social Health Insurance (NSHI). Since 2000, the economy has been on a path to recovery, which, if continued, will be likely to favor current health insurance expansion policies. Table 7.1 presents current selected macroeconomic indicators.

## Demographic and epidemiologic profile

The key demographic indicators for Colombia are shown in table 7.2. Total life expectancy at birth in Colombia was 72.5 years in 2004. Life expectancy for males was six years less than for females, a likely result of male mortality due to violence. Colombia has moderate birth, mortality, and fertility rates. Large disparities in child mortality persist between urban and rural areas.

According to the 2005 census, the population is 49 percent male and 51 percent female. Age-specific fertility rates have been decreasing for all age groups since 1985 (figure 7.1). The population pyramid (figure 7.2) shows fewer people in the younger age categories as the population has shifted to more conservative birth rates.

**Table 7.1    Colombia: Selected Economic Indicators**

| Indicator | Value |
|---|---|
| GDP per capita, Colombia, 2004 (constant 2004 US$)[a] | 2,099 |
| GDP per capita, Latin America, 2004 (constant 2004 US$) | 2,835 |
| GDP growth, annual, 2004 (%)[a] | 7,256 |
| Annual GDP growth rate (2004)[b] | 4.3 |
| Population under living under poverty line, 2005 (%)[b] | 49.2 |
| Population living under US$1 per day, 2004 (%)[b] | 2.4 |
| Population living under US$2 per day, 2004 (%)[b] | 7.6 |
| National unemployment rate, 2006 (%)[c] | 11.3 |
| Revenue, excluding grants (% of GDP)[a] | 17.1 |
| Tax revenue (% of GDP)[a] | 13.8 |
| External debt (% of GDP)[a] | 37.1 |
| Aid (% of GNI)[d] | 0.5 |

*Sources:* a. World Bank 2006; b. MERPD 2006; DNP 2006; c. DANE 2006; d. IMF 2006.

Table 7.2   Colombia: Demographic Profile

| Indicator | Value |
|---|---|
| Total population (2005)[a] | 41,200,000 |
| Percentage urban population (%)[a] | 75 |
| Life expectancy at birth, total, 2004 (years)[b] | 72.5 |
| Life expectancy at birth, females, 2004 (years)[b] | 75.7 |
| Life expectancy at birth, males, 2004 (years)[b] | 69.6 |
| Mortality rate for children under five years per 1,000 live births, 2005[c] | |
| Urban | 19 |
| Rural | 30 |
| Infant mortality rate per 1,000 live births, 2005[c] | |
| Urban | 17 |
| Rural | 24 |
| Total mortality rate per 100,000, 2002[d] | 438.6 |
| Male total mortality rate per 100,000, 2002[d] | 535.5 |
| Female total mortality rate per 100,000, 2002[d] | 343.7 |
| Maternal mortality rate per 100,000 newborns, 2002[d] | 99.8 |
| Total fertility rate per woman, 2005[c] | |
| Urban | 2.1 |
| Rural | 3.4 |
| Total dependency rate dependents to working-age population[a] | 57.6 |
| Age dependency ratio (dependents to working-age population), 2004[b] | 0.57 |

*Sources:* a. DANE 2005; b. World Bank 2006; c. Profamilia 2005; d. DANE 2002.

Colombia has a double burden of disease: an increasing incidence of chronic and degenerative diseases typical of developed countries and persistence or resurgence of infectious and parasitic diseases such as malaria and tuberculosis. Main causes of mortality for 2002 are summarized in table 7.3. Tables 7.4 and 7.5 show the top five conditions by contribution to the total burden of disease (DALYs).

This profile poses several challenges for the National Social Health Insurance System (NSHIS). For example, the contents of the benefits packages need to be revised and updated to include the key interventions for the prevention and control of these diseases. The system also needs to anticipate measures to deal with a trend toward rising costs for treatment of diseases of aging. Provision of incentives for preventing these diseases by health insurance plans and articulation of private and public programs is another key implication.

## Government and Political Environment

Colombia has been a republic since 1810, when it declared its independence from Spain. The government structure is divided in three branches: the executive, the legislative, and the judicial. The executive branch is represented at the national level by a president elected by popular vote for four-year terms with the possibility of reelection and at the departmental and municipal levels by governors and

**Figure 7.1   Colombia: Age-Specific Fertility Rates**

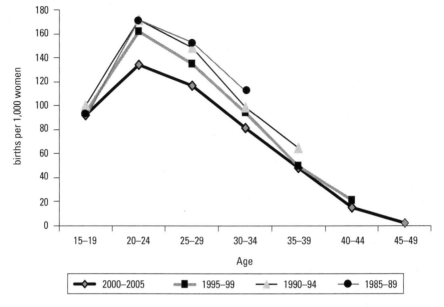

*Source:* ORC Macro, 2006. MEASURE DHS STATcompiler (http://www.measuredhs.com).

**Figure 7.2   Colombia: Population Pyramid, 2005**

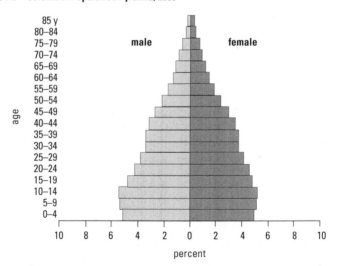

*Source:* DANE 2005.

Table 7.3 Colombia: Main Causes of Mortality, by Age Group and Gender, 2002

| Age (years) | Top three causes of mortality | |
| --- | --- | --- |
| | Males | Females |
| < 1 | Specific perinatal respiratory diseases<br>Genetic and congenital malformations<br>Other perinatal conditions | Same as males |
| 1–4 | Acute respiratory infections<br>Nutritional deficiencies and anemia<br>Accidental drowning | Nutritional deficiencies and anemia<br>Acute respiratory infections<br>Intestinal infections |
| 5–14 | Motor vehicle accidents<br>Homicides<br>Accidental drowning | Motor vehicle accidents<br>Homicides<br>Lymphoma and leukemia |
| 15–44 | Homicides<br>Motor vehicle accidents<br>Accidental drowning | Homicides<br>Motor vehicle accidents<br>Pregnancy, childbirth, and puerperium |
| 45–64 | Homicides<br>Ischemic heart disease<br>Cerebrovascular disease | Ischemic heart disease<br>Cerebrovascular disease<br>Diabetes |
| > 65 | Ischemic heart disease<br>Cerebrovascular disease<br>Chronic respiratory disease | Same as males |

*Source:* DANE 2002.

Table 7.4 Colombia: Top Five Health Conditions, by Burden of Disease and Cause, 2002 (DALYs)

| Rank | Health condition | Total estimated DALYs (thousands) |
| --- | --- | --- |
| 1 | Intentional injuries | 1,882 |
| 2 | Neuropsychiatric conditions | 1,825 |
| 3 | Infectious and parasitic diseases | 800 |
| 4 | Unintentional injuries | 651 |
| 5 | Cardiovascular diseases | 575 |

*Source:* WHO 2002.

Table 7.5 Colombia: Burden of Disease, by Disease Category and Cause, 2002 (DALYs)

| Rank | Disease category | Total estimated DALYs (thousands) | % total |
| --- | --- | --- | --- |
| 1 | Communicable, maternal, perinatal, and nutritional conditions | 1,499 | 17.8 |
| 2 | Noncommunicable diseases | 4,380 | 52.1 |
| 3 | Injuries | 2,533 | 30.1 |
| | Total | 8,412 | 100.0 |

*Source:* WHO 2002.

majors, respectively, both elected for three-year terms. The legislative branch is a bicameral congress, composed of the Senate and the House of Representatives.

Colombia's 1991 Constitution assigned the state the responsibility for directing, coordinating, and regulating a universal social security service, thus establishing a legal framework for National Social Health Insurance. In 2006, a center-right president was reelected, whose agenda for the next four years regarding health policy is centered on achieving universal health insurance coverage (Departamento Nacional de Planeación 2006). The head of the health sector is the Ministry of Social Protection (MPS), created in 2003 by merging the former Ministries of Health and Labor.

Colombia has had a long history of armed conflict between guerrilla groups and military forces, initially motivated by leftist ideology. In the past decade, conflict has been increasingly led by economic interests in control of drug traffic zones, with increased participation of paramilitary groups. Armed conflict has implied large losses for the Colombian economy—estimated at between one and two percentage points a year through losses in human and physical capital and productivity (Cárdenas 2006). Additionally, the opportunity costs of expenditures on public and private defense, repair of losses in infrastructure, and compensation of victims could amount to 2 percent of GDP per year, the approximate current total cost of NSHI for the poor.

The health toll of armed conflict is also high (Pinto, Vergara, Lahuerta 2005). Armed conflict is likely to have: reduced life expectancy (by an estimated 1.7 years in life expectancy at birth for all Colombian citizens); increased mortality (10 times greater probability of dying for populations displaced by conflict than for the general population and a 6 times higher probability of dying for men than for women); reduced fertility (due to premature female deaths and widowhood); and increased disease (reemergence of vector-transmitted diseases such as malaria, dengue, and yellow fever in conflict zones due to security obstacles for reaching this population by government programs). Besides the expenditures on medical care necessitated by violence-related events, additional resources have had to be allocated to attend to the special needs of the growing numbers of displaced people.

To end this problem, Colombia has implemented a combination of strategies and policies. They include cease-fires and negotiations with armed groups, investments in national security and drug traffic control, and implementation of pro-poor economic policies such as provision of the NSHI as a strategy to protect vulnerable groups.

## Overview of Health Financing and Coverage

The NSHI was introduced by the 1993 health care reforms as the key instrument for financing health care. It was designed as two separate insurance schemes according to ability to pay. This section describes each scheme in terms of its target population and coverage, sources of financing, and payment mechanisms for insurers and providers, and compares the benefits packages. It also explains how services not covered by the benefits package and services for the uninsured are financed. Finally, key health expenditure indicators and indicators of access and financial protection are presented.

## National Social Health Insurance Schemes

The *contributory regime* (CR) is the mandatory health insurance scheme for the formally employed (formal sector workers) and the self-employed[1] (informal sector workers) who can pay, and pensioners. The *subsidized regime* (SR) allocates public monies to pay individual insurance premiums for the poor.

*The contributory regime.* CR health insurance covers all first-degree family members as beneficiaries of contributing individuals. In the case of working couples, both must contribute to a premium, called the *Unidad de pago por capitación* (UPC, per capita *payment* unit). By mid-2006, 15.9 million people were enrolled in the CR (34 percent of total population); 46 percent were individuals contributing to the premium and 53 percent were their beneficiaries (MPS 2006).

Individuals contribute 12 percent of their total salary to the UPC. In the case of formal workers, 4 percent is contributed by the employee and 8 percent by the employer. Independent workers contribute the full 12 percent of their salary, starting from a floor of two minimum wages (around US$355 in 2006). Individuals choose to enroll in health plans[2] that serve the CR, called Empresas Promotoras de Salud (EPS, Health Promoting Companies), which collect the wage contributions and transfer them to a central fund that pools and distributes revenues among subfunds. This administrative fund is called the Fondo de Seguridad Social y Garantía (FOSYGA, Social Security and Guarantees Fund). The flow of funds of the CR takes place in the following way (figure 7.3):

- FOSYGA receives total wage contributions collected by health plans from employers and from individuals.
- To finance the SR, 1 percent of total revenues is transferred to a solidarity subfund.
- To finance health promotion and prevention activities, 0.41 percent of total revenues is transferred to a promotion and prevention subfund.
- For sickness leave payments, 0.25 percent of total revenues is set aside.
- For maternity leave payments, 0.25 percent of total revenues is set aside.

The remaining revenues are used for payment of UPCs to the EPS and for payment of claims filed by these health plans to the FOSYGA for medications and procedures not included in the benefits package. Surpluses are invested in government bonds and reserved for future contingencies.

The yearly final balance of the SSGF is determined mainly by the number and size of the wage contributions by enrollees (revenues), family density, and the level of the UPC (expenditures). The financial balance of the CR is closely related to macroeconomic and labor market conditions, as will be illustrated.

**Figure 7.3  Colombia: Flow of Funds in the Solidarity and Guarantees Fund**

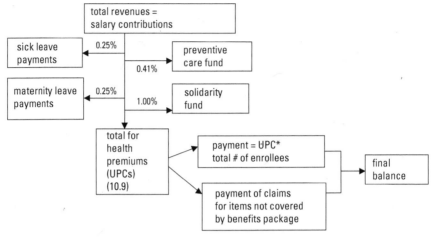

*Source:* Author.

***The subsidized regime.*** Colombia allocated 1.1 percent of GDP to the SR in 2005, nearly US$1.39 billion. The SR subsidizes individual insurance premiums for the poor according to a proxy-means testing index known as Sistema de Identificación de Beneficiarios (SISBEN, the Beneficiaries Identification System). SISBEN scores are calculated on a number of dimensions of poverty, including labor market participation, income, educational attainment, family structure, assets, housing material and crowding, and access to water and sanitation. Data for calculating scores are obtained through a household survey designed for this purpose and administered at the municipal level. The total SISBEN score takes values between 0 and 100 and is divided into six categories. The people with the lowest scores, 1 and 2, are eligible for the SR, as long as they are not enrolled in the CR. According to household survey data from 2003, about 28 percent of Colombia's population falls into SISBEN categories 1 and 2 (table 7.6).

Because of resource constraints, not all persons eligible for the SR can be given health insurance. Priority enrollment is given to the people with the lowest scores and within vulnerable groups such as pregnant and lactating women, children under five (U5), the handicapped, and displaced populations, according to rules set at the national level (Acuerdo 244). By mid-2006, 18.3 million persons (39 percent of total population) were enrolled in the SR.

The SR is financed from national government transfers (56.3 percent of total resources),[3] a 1 percent solidarity contribution from the CR (34.4 percent of total resources), local tax revenues from "sin taxes" (8.8 percent of total resources), and contributions from family benefits funds[4] (0.5 percent of total resources). Figure 7.4 depicts these sources of finance.

**Table 7.6 Colombia: Total Population, by SISBEN category, 2003**

| SISBEN category | % of total population |
| --- | --- |
| 1 | 7.2 |
| 2 | 21.1 |
| 3 | 32.1 |
| 4 | 22.5 |
| 5 | 15.9 |
| 6 | 1.3 |
| Total | 100.0 |

*Source:* Calculations by Panagiota Panopolou with data from DANE 2003.

**Figure 7.4 Colombia: Funding for the Subsidized Regime, by Source, 2005**

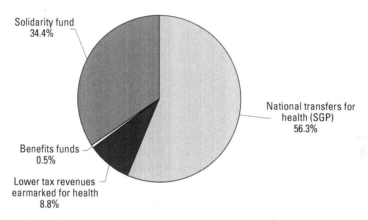

Solidarity fund
34.4%

National transfers for
health (SGP)
56.3%

Benefits funds
0.5%

Lower tax revenues
earmarked for health
8.8%

*Source:* Data from Grupo de Economia de la Salud 2006.

*Note:* Total resources in 2005 = Col$3.2 billion (US$1,390,000,000); 1 billion = 1x1012.

The allocation formula for the national government transfers includes population size, risk of malaria and dengue, immunization rates, and geographic dispersion of the population and local administrative capacity. The breakdown of total national government health transfers earmarked for health in 2005 was: 55.2 percent for health insurance coverage by the SR; 45.0 percent for the provision of health care services by public hospitals, or supply subsidies; and 11.9 percent for provision of collective public health activities (CONPES 2006).

Funds flow in the following way. National transfers for the SR are allocated yearly to municipalities for payment of their current SR enrollees' premium and for programmed gradual expansion of insurance coverage to the eligible population.[5] The allocation formula for the latter is defined by the National Department

Table 7.7 Colombia: UPC Premium Value, 2006

| Regime/age group | Value per year | |
| --- | --- | --- |
| | Col$ | US$ |
| CR | | |
| < 1 year | 955,597 | 415 |
| 1–4 years | 495,208 | 215 |
| 5–14 years | 263,079 | 114 |
| 15–44 years, males | 232,129 | 101 |
| 15–44 year, females | 479,733 | 209 |
| 45–59 years | 313,374 | 136 |
| > 60 years | 882,089 | 384 |
| SR | 215,712 | 94 |

*Source:* Acuerdo 322 de 2005, Consejo Nacional de Seguridad Social en Salud.

of Planning, as a function of a municipality's total uninsured population weighted by the municipality's share of uninsured with respect to total uninsured population in the country. Total funds for health insurance subsidies are channeled to each municipality, where the local health authority directly contracts health plans[6] serving the SR.

*Payment to insurer.* The EPSs and the ARS receive a UPC with a fixed value for each enrollee. The value of the UPC is adjusted by age group only in the case of the CR; higher premiums are paid for young children, women of childbearing ages, and the elderly. Values of the UPC for 2006 are shown in table 7.7. The value of the premium is around 20 percent higher for dispersed geographical areas for both the CR and SR (not shown).

As additional sources of revenue, health insurers can charge copayments for ambulatory and hospital services, set at the national level on a sliding, income-based scale. SR copayments apply only for hospital services. Ceilings are set for all copayments, and some services, such as preventive care, are excluded from cost-sharing.

Colombia's health system has not developed mechanisms for monitoring and adjusting the premium value. Decisions on the premium have been guided by the annual increments in the minimum wage summed to considerations regarding the FOSYGA balance at the end of the fiscal year. After 13 years of the reform, no actuarial studies have been done of the real cost of providing the benefits packages, mainly due to a lack of reliable information for these calculations. Acosta (2005) estimates that the UPC has lost its real value over time, about 20 percent for the SR and 10 percent for the CR. Poor information on the cost of the benefits package has serious implications: if the premiums are set above true costs, the system is wasting resources. If premiums are set below true costs, consumers will suffer, because health plans will have incentives to cut quality and access.

*Payment to providers.* Health plans are free to establish payment mechanisms and payment levels for services they purchase from providers. As benchmarks for its fees, the NSHI has used the fee schedules developed by prereform public health plans, adjusted for inflation. In actuality, few adjustments have been made for the real cost of services. These schedules are used as ceilings for price negotiations between health plans and providers. Provider associations are aggressively seeking price regulation by the MPS (setting floors), and several proposals for fee schedules have been issued.

Two patterns of payment are common to all health plans: preventive and primary care services are contracted mainly by capitation, and most specialist care and hospital care is paid on a fee-for-service basis or by service packages. The effects of these payment mechanisms on access and quality have not been evaluated.

*Other insurance schemes.* Although there were efforts to unify the insurance schemes existing in 1993, exceptions were made for the military and police forces, the education sector, and employees of the Colombian oil company (Empresa Colombiana de Petróleos, ECOPETROL), which remain autonomous in the organization and provision of health benefits. About 5 percent of Colombia's population is covered by these independent schemes.

In 2004 a subscheme known as Subsidios Parciales (Partial Subsidies, PS) was introduced in the SR. This subscheme provides temporary health insurance coverage to the urban SISBEN 2 and 3 populations not covered by the SR because of lack of funds to provide full subsidies. Financing for the program comes from local resources of departments and municipalities that opt to implement the program. The national government supplements those funds. Wealthier municipalities can receive up to 40 percent of the total value of the local program and the less wealthy up to 50 percent. The insurance premium for this subscheme is about half the "full" SR premium, because it provides a small subset of services covered by the SR benefits package. By December 2005, 2.8 million people were covered by PS.

*Supply-side subsidies.* To provide health care services for the uninsured or services not covered by the SR benefits package, there is a network of public providers. These services are financed mainly by supply subsidies from national tax revenue transfers to municipalities earmarked for health and local tax revenues from "sin taxes." Supply-subsidy expenditures represented about 0.5 percent of GDP in 2005. To receive these funds, public providers establish service provision contracts with the local health authority. Public providers are allowed to charge user fees, priced nationally on a sliding scale according to income. The uninsured population needing such services can also pay private providers out of pocket.

Table 7.8    Colombia: Summary of NSHI Schemes, December 2005

| Scheme | Target population | People covered (millions) | Percent of total population | Financing source |
|---|---|---|---|---|
| Contributory | Formal sector workers and people with ability to pay | 15.5 | 37 | Employee and employer contributions |
| Subsidized | Poor population (SISBEN 1 and 2) | 16.5 | 40 | National and local tax revenues earmarked for health, solidarity contribution from CR, contribution from benefits funds |
| Partial subsidies | Urban SISBEN 2 and 3 populations | 2.1 | 5 | Local tax revenues with matching funds from government |
| Supply subsidies | Uninsured and insured requiring services not included in benefits packages | 5.1 | 13 | National and local tax revenues earmarked for health |
| Special regimes | Military and police forces, education sector, oil company workers | 2.1 | 5 | Combinations of employer / employee contributions |

*Source:* MPS 2006.

The target population, coverage, and financing sources of the different schemes in Colombian Social Health Insurance are summarized in table 7.8.

## The Benefits Packages

The benefits packages—the "compulsory health plans" under the CR and the SR (*Planes Obligatorios de Salud,* POS and POS-S, respectively) are detailed lists of the covered interventions, issued in 1994. Interventions are grouped into three levels of ascending complexity of specialization, technology, and financial resources required for their provision. Table 7.9 summarizes these interventions by categories of medical care and levels of complexity. The first level of complexity includes preventive and emergency care, basic medical, dental, and diagnostic services. The second and third levels include specialized and rehabilitation care, hospitalizations and their corresponding diagnostic tests. For example, in the case of a person with diabetes, a general consultation would be provided at the first level, hospitalization for an infected diabetic foot at level 2, and diabetic coma at level 3. Catastrophe care is a subcategory for which interventions at all levels are included. Partial subsidies provide coverage only for prenatal and maternal services, services for children aged less than one, medications, and orthopedic and catastrophe care.

Table 7.10 shows a comparison of coverage breadth, by population group, of the benefits package under each regime. The CRS benefits package, POS, is the

**Table 7.9   Colombia: Classification of Medical Care Types, by Complexity**

| Type of care | Coverage description and examples | | |
| --- | --- | --- | --- |
| | Level 1. Low complexity | Level 2. Intermediate complexity | Level 3. High complexity and specialized centers |
| **Preventive care** | Age and risk groups specific screening, visual and ear screening, immunizations | Not eligible | Not eligible |
| **Ambulatory care (consultations)** | | | |
| General practitioner | Includes family planning, nurse practitioner | Not eligible | Not eligible |
| Basic medical specialties | Prenatal care by ObGyn | Pediatrician, ObGyn, Internal medicine, Orthopedics | |
| Visual care | Ophtalmology and optometry | Not eligible | Not eligible |
| Other medical specialties and subspecialties | Not eligible | Neurologist, ORL, Cardiologist, Infectious disease | |
| Dental | Fluoridation, prophylaxis, cavity occlusion | Not eligible | Not eligible |
| **Emergency care** | Provided at all levels | | |
| **Hospital care** | | | |
| Medical conditions | Conditions managed by general practitioner | Conditions requiring specialist or subspecialist care | |
| Obstetric | Uncomplicated birth attendance | Cesarean section | High risk obstetric care |
| Surgical conditions | Skin sutures, abscess drainage | General surgery (herniorrhaphy, appendectomy, cholecystectomy, histerectomy) | Neurosurgical, cardiovascular surgery |
| **Rehabilitation** | Not eligible | Physical, respiratory, occupational and language therapy, cardiovascular rehab, neurologic procedures | |
| **Lab tests** | Basic tests (hemoglobin, urine analysis, renal and liver function tests, glycemia, lipid profile, STDs), pap smear, biopsies | Bacterial cultures, pathology | Spirometry, immune function, hormones, toxicology, medication levels |
| **Radiology** | Bone and chest x-rays, obstetric echography | Mammography, special x-ray projections, endoscopies, ecographies | Arteriography, hemodynamic tests, MRI |
| **Catastrophic care** | | Treatment with radiotherapy and chemotherapy for cancer, dialysis and organ transplant for renal failure; surgical treatment of heart, cerebrovascular, neurological and congenital conditions; treatment of major trauma, intensive care unit, hip and knee replacement, major burns, treatment for AIDS | |

*Sources:* Elaborated by author based on Acuerdos CNSSS 72, 74, and 83; Resolución 5261 of 1994.

**Table 7.10  Colombia: Comparison of Breadth of CR, SR, and PS Benefits Packages**

| Age/Population Group | Preventive care | TYPE OF BENEFIT | | | | | | Excluded interventions |
|---|---|---|---|---|---|---|---|---|
| | | Level 1 care | Level 2 care | Level 3 care | Catastrophic care | Medications in National formulary | Transportation for referrals, catastrophic care cases | |
| < 1 year | Neonatal care and screening (Vit K, anemia, TSH), immunizations, well child care | All | All | All | All | All | All | Aesthetic surgery Infertility treatment Treatment for sleep disorders |
| 1–4 | Well child care, immunizations, anemia screening | All | Cataract and strabismus | Not eligible | All | All | All | |
| 5–19 years | Well child care, immunizations, anemia screening | All | surgery, herniorraphy, appendectomy, cholecystectomy, | Not eligible | All | All | All | Organ transplants (except renal, heart, chornea and bone marrow) |
| 20–60 years | Cardiovascular and renal disease risk screening, cervical and breast cancer screening | All | orthopedics, rehabilitation services and procedures | Not eligible | All | All | All | Psychotherapy and psychoanalysis |
| > 60 years | Cardiovascular and renal disease risk screening, cervical and breast cancer screening | All | | Not eligible | All | All | All | Treatments for end stage disease |
| Pregnant women | High risk screening, STD, prenatal care | All | Same as above plus obstetric care | Obstetric care | All | All | All | |

*Sources:* Elaborated by author based on Acuerdos CNSSS 72, 74, and 83; Resolución 5261 of 1994.

**Table 7.11   Colombia: CR and SR Enrollment Rules, Copayments, and Choice, 2006**

| Contents | Contributory regime, POS | Subsidized regime, POS-S | Subsidized regime, partial subsidy |
|---|---|---|---|
| Enrollment rules | Minimum weeks of enrollment required before full coverage of higher complexity care takes place; minimum period of 2 years' enrollment before switching plans | Minimum period of 2 years enrollment before switching plans | None |
| | No denial of coverage or preexclusions of conditions | No denial of coverage if eligibility criteria are met or preexclusions of conditions | No denial of coverage if eligibility criteria are met or preexclusions of conditions |
| | Risk adjustment of premium by age and gender | No | No |
| Cost sharing | No cost sharing for emergency care, preventive services, and services for conditions of public health interest (e.g., hypertension, diabetes). Sliding-scale copayments for ambulatory care and hospitalization up to yearly ceiling | | |
| Choice of insurer | Free choice within set of plans available in city where job is located | Free choice within set of SR plans operating in municipality | Free choice within set of SR plans operating in municipality and offering partial subsidy product |
| Choice of provider | Free choice within plan network, use of gatekeepers | Choice restricted to public network for low-complexity care, free choice within plan network; other care managed by gatekeepers | Same as POS-S |

*Sources:* Elaborated by author, based on Acuerdos CNSSS 72, 74, and 83; Resolucion 5261 of 1994.

most comprehensive, covering interventions at every level and complexity, a wide national listing of medications, and medical transportation expenses. It has few explicit exclusions. The SR benefits plan, POS-S, is equal to the POS in terms of coverage of first-level interventions, catastrophe care, medications, and transportation but less comprehensive in terms of preventive, ambulatory care, and levels 2 and 3 interventions. The PS covers orthopedic and catastrophe care and the necessary medications to render these services. Coverage for children aged less than one year and for pregnant women is equivalent in all plans.

*Other services.* Coverage of interventions that complement individual-level medical services included in the POS and POS-S is provided through different mechanisms (table 7.12).

- A set of community-level public health interventions, such as health educational and risk-prevention campaigns and control of vector-transmitted diseases are provided by local governments as part of a program known as the *Plan de Atención Básica* (PAB, Basic Care Plan). The Ministry of Social Protection issues national priorities and guidelines for interventions to be included in PAB which are adopted and adapted locally. PAB is financed from transfers earmarked for health from the national level to departments and municipalities.

- Medical interventions for motor vehicle–related accidents are financed through compulsory insurance policies for all vehicles, known as Seguro Obligatorio de Accidentes de Transito (SOAT, Mandatory Insurance for Motor Vehicle Accidents).

- Contributions by employers to insurance policies for work-related injuries, medical conditions, and disabilities are mandatory. Services are provided by specialized insurance carriers known as Administradoras de Riesgos Profesionales (ARP). As of March 2006. 5.2 million employees were enrolled in ARPs (MPS 2006).

- Private supplemental insurance policies can be purchased by individuals who want medical services not covered by the POS or more amenities (table 7.12). About 5 percent of the population purchases these policies.

*Appropriateness of coverage.* With the exception of psychiatric disorders for which coverage is very limited, the benefits packages of both regimes (except PS) include minimum preventive and curative interventions for uncomplicated cases. This coverage should address the most common conditions in Colombia (table 7.13). Neurological conditions such as epilepsy are covered by POS and POS-S.

However, as mentioned, there are no systematic mechanisms for revising the contents of the benefits packages. Few modifications have been made, and decisions to add medical interventions have frequently been a response to pressure by interest groups. Epidemiological information has not been updated systematically. Thus, further action is needed to evaluate the appropriateness of the benefits package to address Colombia's changing health priorities.

**Table 7.12   Colombia: Coverage of Services to Supplement the Benefits Packages**

| Type of health services | Provision |
| --- | --- |
| Individual | POS, POS-S |
| Public health, educational outreach | PAB |
| Motor vehicle accidents | SOAT |
| Work-related injuries and conditions | ARP |
| Additional medical services and amenities | Private supplemental health insurance |

*Source:* Author.

**Table 7.13    Colombia: Coverage of Minimum Interventions to Address 2002 Burden of Disease**

| Health condition by rank order (total DALYs) | Coverage of minimum interventions to control condition in uncomplicated cases | | | | |
|---|---|---|---|---|---|
| | POS | POS-S | PS | PAB | SOAT |
| Intentional injuries | √ | √ | √ | √ | |
| Neuropsychiatric conditions | | | | | |
| Infectious and parasitic diseases | √ | √ | √[a] | √ | |
| Unintentional injuries | √ | √ | √ | √ | √ |
| Cardiovascular disease | √ | √ | √[a] | √ | |

*Source:* Author.

a. Includes medications.

## Key Health Expenditure Indicators

Selected health expenditure indicators for 2003 are shown in table 7.14.

## Financial Protection and Access Indicators

There is evidence that NSHI has decreased financial barriers to access to health care (figure 7.5). According to a national household survey in 1992, the main reason for nonuse of health care in the lowest quintiles of the population was the cost of services. Responses to the same question in a subsequent household survey in 1997 showed a reduction in the percentage of people reporting nonuse of health care services for this reason, regardless of income level.

There are large differences by insurance status in the percentage of the population that reports out-of-pocket payment as the source of payment for consultations and hospitalizations (figure 7.6).

**Table 7.14    Colombia: Selected Health Expenditure Indicators, 2003**

| Indicator | Value |
|---|---|
| Absolute health expenditure (current US$) | 6,250,797,175 |
| Health expenditure, total (% of GDP) | 7.8 |
| Health expenditure per capita (current US$) | 136 |
| Health expenditure per capita (current international $) | 514 |
| Public health expenditure as % total health expenditure | 39.6 |
| Private health expenditure as % total health expenditure | 15.9 |
| Out of pocket health expenditure as % total health expenditure | 7.5 |
| CR expenditures as % of total expenditures in National Health Insurance | 58.5 |
| SR expenditures as % of total expenditures in National Health Insurance | 14.5 |
| Supply subsidy expenditures as % of total expenditures in National Health Insurance | 26.9 |

*Source:* Baron 2006.

**Figure 7.5    Colombia: Main Reasons for Not Using Health Care Services, by Income Quintile, 1992 and 1997**

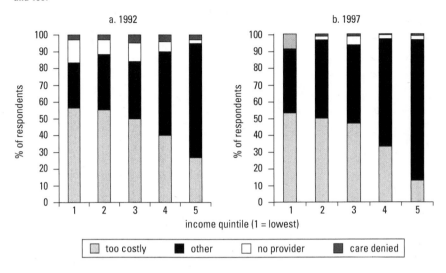

Source: Escobar 2005.
Note: "Other" includes perception.

**Figure 7.6    Colombia: Reported Sources of Payment for Consultations and Hospitalizations, by Insurance Status, 2000**

a. Consultations

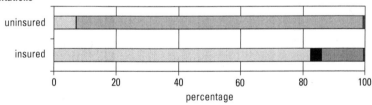

b. Hospitalizations

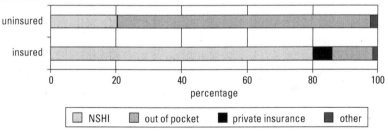

Source: calculations by Panagiota Panopolou, with data from DANE 2000.

**Table 7.15   Colombia: Households Experiencing Catastrophic Payments or Impoverishment Due to Ambulatory or Hospital Health Shock, by Insurance Status, 2003**

| Type of health shock and catastrophic health expenditure | | Percent of households | | | |
|---|---|---|---|---|---|
| | | Insurance status | | | |
| | | Contributory | Subsidized | Uninsured | Total |
| Ambulatory shock | Impoverishment | 0.4 | 0.9 | 0.7 | 0.6 |
| | Catastrophe (5%) | 4.6 | 7.5 | 8.8 | 6.4 |
| | Catastrophe (10%) | 2.1 | 3.9 | 4.6 | 3.3 |
| | Catastrophe (20%) | 0.9 | 1.6 | 1.7 | 1.3 |
| | Catastrophe (30%) | 0.3 | 0.8 | 0.9 | 0.7 |
| Hospital shock | Impoverishment | 1.5 | 1.2 | 2.0 | 1.6 |
| | Catastrophe (5%) | 8.2 | 11.6 | 12.1 | 10.0 |
| | Catastrophe (10%) | 5.5 | 9.1 | 9.3 | 7.5 |
| | Catastrophe (20%) | 3.5 | 5.8 | 6.1 | 4.9 |
| | Catastrophe (30%) | 2.4 | 4.5 | 4.8 | 3.7 |

*Source:* Calculations by Rodrigo Muñoz, based on DANE 2003.

*Note:* Poverty line based on definition by CEPAL 2002, adjusted for inflation.

Overall, 0.6 percent and 1.6 percent of households were impoverished[7] by a catastrophic ambulatory or a hospital health shock, respectively (table 7.15). Health expenditures greater than 30 percent of total consumption occurred in 0.7 percent of households experiencing an ambulatory shock and 3.7 percent of households experiencing a hospital shock. Overall, differences in rates of catastrophic expenditures and impoverishment by insurance status are observed for both types of shocks, and in every case the insured fare better than the uninsured.

Insurance coverage has made a difference in access to care for the Colombian population, according to data from household surveys. Figure 7.7 presents a comparison of treatment rates (the percentage of the population that had a health problem and were seen by a doctor) between 2000 and 2003. Being insured seems to be positively related to being seen by a doctor. In that period in both urban and rural areas, not only are treatment rates higher for the insured than for the uninsured, but they also increased more. The rural-urban gap in the percentage of the insured population with a problem and seen by a doctor also seems to have decreased.

Reports of use of preventive services are more frequent among the insured than the uninsured, although among the insured (figure 7.8), use of preventive services is less frequent among SR enrollees. The percentage of the insured population reporting use of preventive services also seems to have increased between 1997 and 2003, a trend not seen among the uninsured. These use patterns could be explained by the emphasis placed by the benefits packages on preventive services and also by differences in the breadth of coverage between the CR and SR.

**Figure 7.7 Colombia: Respondents with a Health Problem and Seen by a Doctor, by Insurance Status and Location, 2000 and 2003**

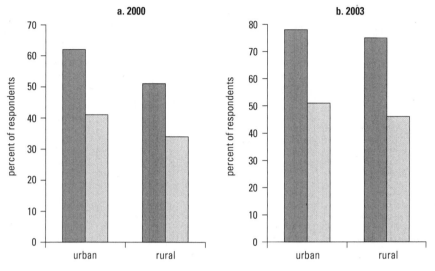

*Source:* Author's calculations with data from DANE 1992 and 2003.

**Figure 7.8 Colombia: Population Reporting Use of Preventive Services, by Insurance Status, 1997 and 2003**

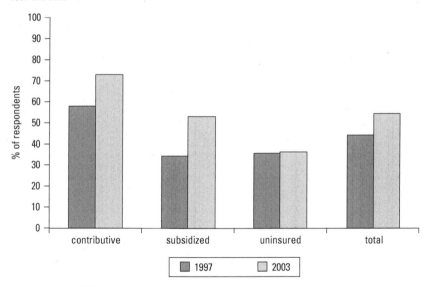

*Source:* Ramírez et al. 2005.

Figure 7.9   Colombia: Population Reporting Hospitalization in Last Year, by Insurance Status, 1997 and 2003

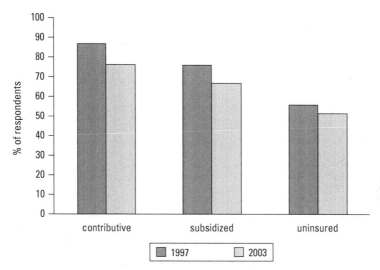

*Source:* Ramírez et al. 2005.

Hospitalization rates decreased for the entire insured population between 1997 and 2003 (figure 7.9). The decreases were highest for the CR insured and lowest for the uninsured. Although these differences could be due to increased access to hospital services through insurance, they might also be due to differences in population health status.

## Overview of the Health Delivery System

The 1993 reforms organized the CR and the SR health delivery systems following a two-market, managed-competition model that operates on two levels. On the first level, the insurance market, consumers have freedom to choose from among a set of public or private health insurance plans offering services covered by the POS/POS-S in exchange for a fixed premium, the UPC described above. Because the premium is fixed, theoretically health plans should compete for enrollees not through price, but through their distinctive service and quality features. Health plans act as group purchasers for their enrollees by arranging a network of providers they select based on the best price and quality. On the second level, the provider market, health care providers compete for inclusion in health plan provider networks and selection by enrollees on the basis of price and quality.

### The Health Insurance Market

Colombia's NSHI market is segmented into health plans serving the CR (EPS) and the SR (ARS). As of December 2005, 21 EPS plans operated in the CR, which are

**Figure 7.10   Colombia: Total Enrollees, by Type of Health Plan and Regime, 2005**

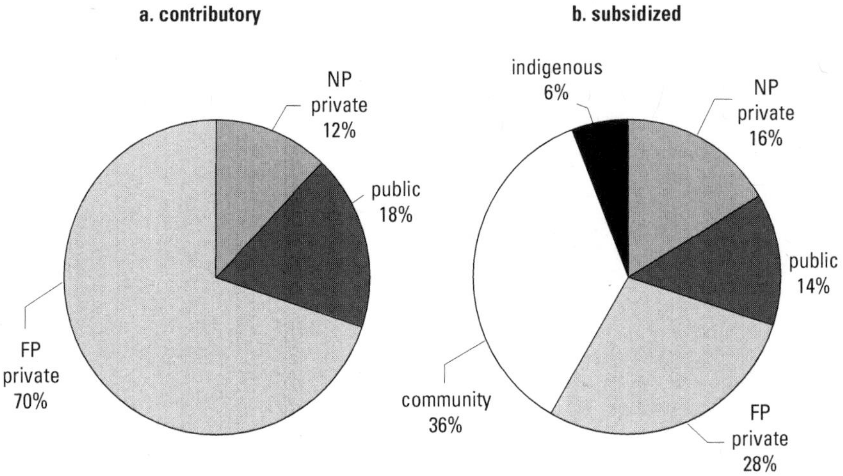

a. contributory                                      b. subsidized

*Source:* Enrollment data obtained from MPS 2005.

private for-profit and nonprofit, and public. Of the total enrollees, 82 percent belonged to private plans (for-profit, 70 percent, nonprofit 12 percent); the rest (18 percent) belonged to public plans.

The ARS insurance market has two other types of plans: community-based health plans (Empresas Solidarias de Salud, ESS) and health plans serving indigenous populations. In December 2005, ARSs totaled 43—44 percent of them private (28 percent for-profit and 16 percent nonprofit), 14 percent public, 36 percent community-based, and the remainder (6 percent) for indigenous populations. Figure 7.10 shows the distribution of health plans by percentage of total of enrollees in both regimes.

Private health plans can choose their own provider network structure. Most use private providers for first- and second-level care and a mix of public and private for tertiary care. In the last five years, there has been a trend toward vertical integration (ownership of first-level providers by insurance plans). The main administrative strategies used by health plans to control demand are the use of gatekeepers and utilization management for specialist, hospital, and diagnostic care (Restrepo, Arango, and Casas 2001). The characteristics of public health plans differ from those of private plans. Under their original organizational structure, financing and service provision were integrated, setting limitations on how much choice of provider they could offer and on their capacity to provide efficiency and quality incentives. Measures were taken to separate financing from provision in these organizations.

Health plans in the SR are required by law to contract at least 40 percent of their network with public providers, but they are free to structure the rest of their network. This has led the ARSs to contract with public institutions for most primary care and, for more complex levels of care, with public and private institutions They use payment methods and administrative strategies similar to those used by the EPS.

Although there are several health plans in most municipalities, most municipal markets have a dominant health plan, with more than 73 percent of enrollees. Only in major cities does the market appear to be competitive (Restrepo, Arango, and Casas 2001).

The Superintendencia Nacional de Salud (National Health Superintendency) is the government body in charge of health plan monitoring and oversight. Minimum quality, financial, and administrative standards for health plan operations have been defined by the Ministry of Social Protection, and health plans are required to demonstrate fulfilment of these requirements through a certification process begun by the superintendencia in 2005.

## The Health Care Provider Market

At the time of the reform, Colombia had developed an extensive public network as a result of policies to improve access to health services implemented in the late 1980s. A supply of private providers had grown to meet demand for services not satisfied by the public sector. The 1993 reform integrated the supply of public and private providers into the national health insurance regimes, allowing health plans to include both public and private institutions in their provider networks.

The supply of hospital services is organized by levels of care. First-level care comprises health posts, centers, and hospitals that offer general medicine. This level is expected to provide the most services needed. Second-level care includes providers of basic specialized medical and surgical services, both ambulatory and hospitalizations, and third-level care includes institutions that provide specialty and subspecialty care and high-complexity hospitalization.

In 2000, about 43,200 physicians were practicing in Colombia, a ratio of 10.4 physicians per 10,000. The average ratio for the Latin America and Caribbean Region that year was 13 (Ascofame 2000). Of these physicians, 57 percent were general practitioners (5.9 general practitioners per 10,000); the rest were specialists (4.4 per 10,000). General practitioners were concentrated in municipalities with more than 500,000 people, 23 times the number of physicians in municipalities with populations smaller than 20,000. With respect to other health care professionals, in 2003 there were about 24,800 nurses and 32,600 dentists, ratios of 0.56 and 0.80 per 10,000 residents, respectively (Cendex-Minsalud 2001).

In 2004, the MPS provider registry reported a total of 13,804 health care facilities of different levels of complexity, 68 percent of them private (MPS 2005). There are 1,039 public institutions.[8] More than half of all facilities, most of them private, are located in the Colombia's five major cities. Rural areas are served chiefly by public providers. Among public providers, 85 percent deliver primary care services, 13 percent deliver secondary care, and 2 percent deliver third-level

Table 7.16    Colombia: Services Offered by Health Care Facilities, by Type, 2004

| Type of service | % of total |
|---|---|
| Dental care | 18.9 |
| General medicine | 17.4 |
| Surgery | 15.0 |
| Physical therapy | 11.2 |
| Nursing | 10.7 |
| Internal medicine and subspecialties | 7.8 |
| Mental health | 5.7 |
| Emergency care | 5.1 |
| Other (pediatrics, immunization, anesthesia, intensive care unit) | 8.2 |

*Source:* MPS 2005.

care. Forty-three percent of hospital beds are devoted to primary care, 36 percent to secondary care, and 21 percent to tertiary care.

With respect to the type of services offered by both private and public providers, half are dental care, general medicine, and surgery. Types of services as percent of total services are shown in table 7.16.

To guarantee that providers meet minimum quality, financial, and administrative standards, the MPS issued a set of certification requirements in 2002. To operate, providers must register at the local health authority (Secretaría de Salud), which verifies that the requisites are met through an inspection visit and issues a three-year certification. In 2004, a hospital accreditation system was established. Accreditation is carried out by an independent organization, on a voluntary basis. So far five private and three public facilities have qualified.

## The 1993 Health Care Reforms

Law 100, the legal foundation of the Colombian health care reform, was approved in 1993. The main goals of this reform were to improve access, efficiency, and service quality, and equity. The key strategy of the reform—improving access to health care—is NSHI, together with changes in the financing, organization, and administration of health service delivery. Beginning with a description of the Colombian health sector before reform and its problems, this section explains how the reform strategies to increase health insurance coverage were designed and implemented and assesses their achievements. The milestones in the reforms between 1993 and 2006 are presented in table 7.17.

### *The Prereform Health System*

Prior to 1993, Colombia had a three-tiered health care system[9]. One tier consisted of the National Health System, designed after the primary care models in vogue in

**Table 7.17 Colombia: Milestones toward Achievement of Universal Health Insurance Coverage**

| Pre-reform period | 1993 | 1994 | 1995–1997 | 1998–2001 | 2002 | 2003 | 2004 | 2005 | 2006 |
|---|---|---|---|---|---|---|---|---|---|
| Decentralization legislation (Laws 10 and 60); New Constitution 1991; SISBEN targeting instrument; ESS development program | Law 100 enacted | Operation of CR begins; operation of National Health Superintendency and National Social Security Council | Application of SISBEN survey; operation of SR begins | Further development of rules and regulations; hospital restructuring program launched | Quality assurance legislation issued; subnational government resource allocation rules and responsibilities reform (Law 715) | New SISBEN targetting instrument issued; certification of providers begins; Ministries of Health and Labor merged to become Ministry of Social Protection | Partial subsidies program initiated; health plan certification begins | National-subnational government SR cofinancing strategies launched; regional operation of SR legislation passed | Universal health insurance plan announced in government agenda |

*Source:* Author.

the late 1960s and early 1970s. A network of public facilities for health care delivery financed from national revenues offered services to about half of the population. A private health care provider market grew in parallel to the public network, targeting the population that could pay and meeting the demand for services and quality not provided by the public sector. Analyses of the 1992 Household Survey showed that public hospitals dominated the provision of inpatient services in rural areas; in urban areas private hospitals were used for about a third of admissions, regardless of insurance status. In both urban and rural areas, private providers supplied a large proportion of ambulatory care use (42 percent and 36 percent of all contacts, respectively), regardless of income group (Harvard School of Public Health 1996).

A second tier was a mandated social insurance plan for workers in the public and formal sectors.[10] Financed by employee and employer contributions, this plan covered about 50 percent of salaried workers and about 18 percent of their families, for a total of 20 percent of the population. A few public agencies[11] held a monopoly for the provision of health insurance for this population group.

The third tier consisted of private insurance or health care services paid out of pocket for the upper-income group, about 11 percent of the population. This market was covered by private commercial health insurers, prepaid group health organizations, or worker cooperative organizations.

In the early 1980s, Colombia began to implement a nationwide fiscal, political, and institutional decentralization that sought to reassign functions and responsibilities between the national, departmental, and municipal governments. Although decentralization was not an explicit component of the 1993 health care reform, legislative mandates between 1990 and 1993 had introduced additional territorial functions and responsibilities and defined new sources of financing for health service provision and their respective allocation formula.[12] Administrative procedures to certify local governments as "decentralized" were established, which if met, shifted authority, responsibility, and budgetary control over these resources to departmental and municipal governments.[13] Within these laws, the legal basis for institutional decentralization of public hospital facilities was laid through provisions mandating separation of hospitals from administrative dependency on departments and conversion of these facilities to semipublic entities. Thus, they received the financial and managerial autonomy necessary to prepare for competition with the private sector under the new health insurance scheme.

## Motivation for the Reforms

In the pre-1993 Colombian health system, access to even basic health services was limited for a large part of the population, health spending was inequitable and inefficient, and quality was uneven. About 75 percent of the population had no health insurance, and one out of every six individuals in the first income quintile who fell ill in 1992 did not seek medical care because they could not afford to pay for it (Escobar 2005). About 19 percent of the population had no access to health services. According to national household surveys in 1992 health care expenditures were 2.4 percent of total household expenditures. The lowest income decile spent about 10 percent of their income on health, while the upper-income decile spent less than 0.5 percent. Cost was cited by more than 55 percent of the poorest people as a major access barrier to health care services.

Public resources were poorly targeted, as evidenced by the fact that 40 percent of the subsidies to public hospitals benefited the wealthiest 50 percent of the population, and allocation of health care resources was biased toward more expensive, curative care, despite evidence of low productivity. Allocation of resources followed historical hospital spending rather than people's needs. Large investments in hospital infrastructure with small correspondence to health service demand resulted in low occupancy rates and underutilization of services in secondary and tertiary hospitals. Finally, poor service quality was reflected in low use and acceptance of the public provider network.

## Key Strategies for Broadening Health Insurance Coverage

Law 100 established universal health insurance coverage for all Colombian citizens, to be provided by the CR for people who could pay and by the SR for the poor. Overall, the system sought solidarity between different population groups, from the rich to the poor, from the healthy to the sickly.

*The NSHI and coverage expansions, 1993–2005.* Social health insurance was initially designed as two separate schemes with target populations, financing sources, and benefits. This was to allow time for funds to become available to gradually expand insurance coverage and benefits for the population eligible for subsidies. Universal insurance and convergence of the two regimes in terms of benefits coverage was planned for 2001.

First, universal coverage for the CR-eligible population (about 70 percent of total population) was to be reached by 2001 through an increased number of mandatory affiliations of individuals who could contribute. This would be possible by an annual increase in formal and informal sector workers (3.5 and 2.1 percent, respectively), favored by projected annual economic growth of 5 percent and a 1.8 percent increase in average income. CR enrollment would also increase by extending coverage of health insurance to family members of contributing individuals.

Second, achievement of universal coverage for the poor (30 percent of total population) was sought by adding new sources of financing and directing existing public resources toward demand subsidies for the SR. The eligible population would be identified using SISBEN, an instrument designed to target social programs designed earlier. Application of SISBEN was initiated in 1994 in larger and more developed municipalities, under the responsibility of local majors and was extended to the rest of the country in 1997.[14] SISBEN was increasingly criticized as a targeting instrument because of its potential for classification error and because of many operational problems, including evidence of corruption in the calculation

**Figure 7.11    Colombia: Expansion of CR and SR Insurance Coverage, 1992–2006**

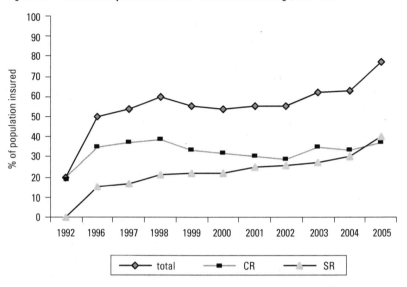

*Sources:* 1992–2004 (calculations with enrollment data provided by the MPS, percentage based on 1993 census projections); 2005 (MPS 2006, percentage based on 2005 census data).

of scores to favor enrollment of ineligible individuals for political purposes (BDO and CCRP 2000; DNP and MS 2003; Fresneda 2003). This motivated changes in the design of the original instrument in 2002 and of the processes and rules to identify, select, and prioritize health subsidy beneficiaries. Implementation of these changes began in 2003.[15]

In the last 13 years Colombia's health care reform has expanded insurance coverage from 20 percent to 74 percent of the total population.[16] Total growth of enrollment in each regime in 1992–2006 is shown in figure 7.11.

Growth of enrollees of the CR has been largely a result of affiliation of contributing individuals' family members (figure 7.12). Between 1993 and 1997, about 5 million beneficiaries entered this regime, for a total of about 7.3 million. Since then, the total number of beneficiaries has remained about the same. The number of contributors increased from 5 million in 1993 to 7.5 million in 1997, fell in 2000, and slowly recovered to 7.2 million in 2005. The percentage of contributors belonging to the informal sector increased little, from 2.5 percent in 1993 to 4 percent in 2005 (figure 7.13).

The growth of enrollment in the SR was amazing, from 0 percent to almost 40 percent of the total population in 13 years, 1993 to 2006. SR insurance coverage has reached the people most vulnerable to economic shocks. For example, a comparison of the proportion of insured individuals by income quintile in 1992 and 2003 shows an increase of 37 percentage points or a variation of 444 percent for the first quintile (9 percent in 1992 to 48 percent in 2003), whereas in the fifth

**Figure 7.12   Colombia: Total CR enrollment, Contributors, and Beneficiaries, 1993–2005**

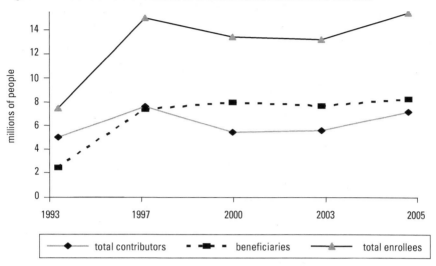

*Sources:* For 1993, Ministerio de Salud 1994; for 1997–2005, author's calculations with data provided from FOSYGA.

**Figure 7.13   Colombia: Employment of SR Contributors, 1993–2006**

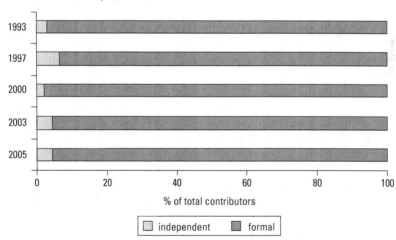

*Sources:* For 1993, Ministerio de Salud 1994; for 1997–2005, author's calculations with data provided from FOSYGA.

quintile the increase was 21 percentage points (60 percent in 1992 to 81 percent in 2003), as seen in figure 7.14.

Figure 7.15 illustrates how rural and urban disparities in insurance coverage have been progressively bridged. The top panel shows a rural-urban insurance coverage gap of 26 percent in 1993 that was narrowed to 13 points in 2003. The

**Figure 7.14 Colombia: Insurance Coverage, by Income Quintile, 1992–2003**

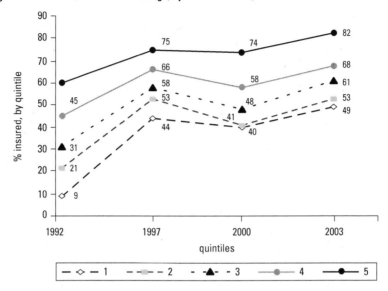

*Sources:* Based on MPS calculations DANE 1992 and 2003.

bottom panel, covering the same period, shows that health insurance coverage in rural areas is now mainly at the expense of the SR.

*Changes in financing.* These SR coverage trends were a response to the availability of resources as new sources were found and existing resources reallocated. The 1993 legislation opened new funding sources for each regime. Funds for the CR were obtained by mandating wage contributions for everyone who could pay and by increasing the of the contribution rate from 11 to 12 percent of salary. With the initially favorable macroeconomic and labor market assumptions, these resources would provide for CR expenditures and for SR solidarity funds.

To finance the SR, national and local resources allocated to health were to be increased and directed toward demand subsidies. For example, between 1994 and 2000, the share of total national revenues for health transferred to local governments would be raised from 8.7 to 10.5 percent, and supply subsidies to public providers would be gradually transformed into demand subsidies. New sources of funding for the SR were bundled into FOSYGA's solidarity subfund, which included: the solidarity point from the CR and contribution from Cajas, to be matched one to one by resources from the national budget; financial returns on FOSYGA surpluses; and expected revenues from taxes on oil exploitation. Together, national and local resources represented 40 percent of funding for the SR and solidarity resources 60 percent.

**Figure 7.15  Colombia: Growth of Insurance Coverage, by Regime and by Residence, 1993–2003**

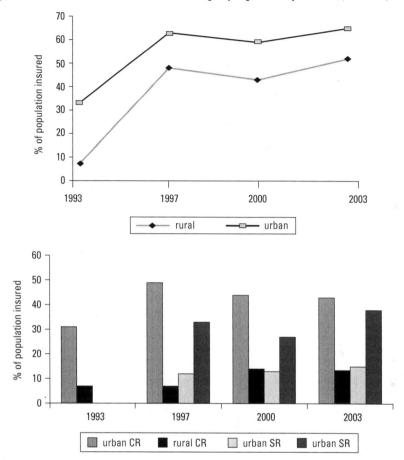

*Sources:* 1993: Ministerio de Salud (1994); 1997–2003 based on calculations by Panagiota Panopolou with DANE 1997, 2000, and 2003.

These changes had an impact on health spending and the CR financial balance. Total health expenditures as a share of GDP grew from 6.2 percent in 1993 to 7.8 percent in 2003, mainly as a result in increases in public expenditures (1.4 percent in 1993 to 3.1 percent in 2003). Social security expenditures grew from 1.6 percent in 1993 to 3.7 percent until 1999, when they began to decrease, to 3.0 percent in 2001. Total private expenditures remained around 3 percent from 1993 to 1997 and then decreased, to 1.2 percent in 2003. Direct out-of-pocket expenditures also decreased, from 2.7 percent to 0.6 percent over the period, most likely as a result of health insurance. Figure 7.16 summarizes these health spending distribution and trends.

**Figure 7.16    Colombia: National Health Spending Distribution and Trends, 1993–2003**

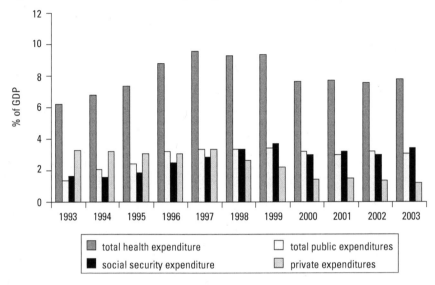

*Source:* Barón 2007.

*Note:* According to NHA methodology, total expenditure includes direct public expenditures and public expenditures on insurance (subsidized regime), social insurance expenditures, which are essentially contributory regime expenditures, and private expenditures (including both voluntary private insurance and families' out of pocket expenditures).

The financial equilibrium of the CR is reflected in the balance of the FOSYGA account, obtained by subtracting all yearly payments to EPS[17] from wage contribution revenues. Figure 7.17 shows the positive balance between 1996 and 1998, the deficits between 2000 and 2001, and the subsequent recovery (Restrepo 2006).

In 1996 to 2005, macroeconomic conditions had a direct impact on FOSYGA revenues and expenditures. Figure 7.18 shows unemployment rates, GDP real growth, and population in poverty between 1991 and 2005. The period began with favorable real GDP growth rates around 5 percent and unemployment rates below 10 percent, which explain health reformers' optimistic projections. However, between 1996 and 2001 average real GDP growth was only 1.1 percent, hitting negative values in 1999, and unemployment soared to 20 percent. By 2002, the economy began to recover and, although unemployment rates have decreased, employment has not returned to prerecession levels. The percentage of the population in poverty rose from values below 50 percent to a peak of 57 percent between recession years and has also been recovering.

Table 7.18 presents the values of key determinants of the FOSYGA balance for 1998 to 2002. Enrollment in the CR decreased, together with the ratio of contributors to beneficiaries. Family density increased, and average salaries decreased. The behavior of these variables are related not only to low employment during

**Figure 7.17  Colombia: Balance of FOSYGA Compensation Fund, 1996–2005**

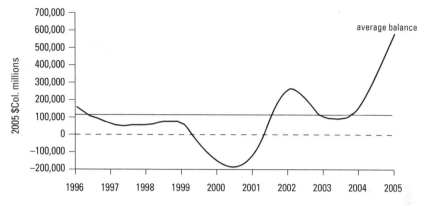

*Source:* GES 2006.

this period, but also to increased informality. All this resulted in an increase in payments to health plans that surpassed revenues from wage contributions, and in negative balances of the FOSYGA account, requiring use of the accumulated surplus. In subsequent years, the balance recovered, but its dependency on the behavior of factors not under control of the health sector shows the fragility of the balance.

Evasion of premium contributions, particularly by independent workers has also had a negative impact on FOSYGA revenues. Health plans collect premium contributions directly from this population and have no incentives to promote accurate income reporting or income-verification mechanisms. Bitrán (2002) estimates that, in 2002, only 65 percent of potential contributors actually paid their obligations, and that the contributors who did pay contributed much less than they owed. Evasion and elusion together decreased CR revenues, possibly by as much as 35 percent.

Without this problem in 2000, resources would have been available to enroll an additional 1.5 million people in the SR. As it was, the available funding amounted to only a third of the projected total needed to insure all eligible people in 2000 (figure 7.19).

The budget constraints to reach universal health insurance have several explanations. First, unfavorable macroeconomic conditions after the reform reduced the availability of SR funding from other sources, such as solidarity contributions and national tax revenues (figure 7.20). The solidarity point reached only 70 percent of its expected level in 2000, not only because contributions to the CR fell short of projections, but also because, for political reasons and fiscal pressures, other projected sources of funding such as matching government funds and oil revenues were not allocated to the SR.

**Figure 7.18   Colombia: Unemployment, GDP Real Growth, and Percentage of Population in Poverty, 1991–2005**

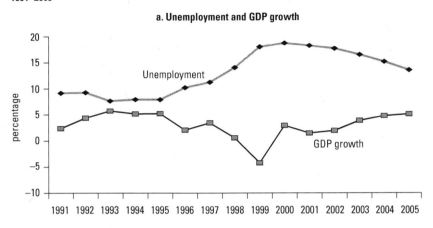

**a. Unemployment and GDP growth**

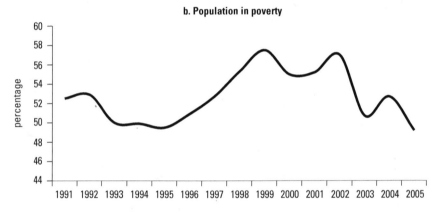

**b. Population in poverty**

*Sources:* Unemployment and growth, Lasso 2004 (data for years 1991–2000) and DANE (2000); population in poverty, calculations by DNP-SISD.

In addition, the transformation of supply subsidies into demand subsidies has taken place more slowly than expected. Political opposition has come from public hospitals, and the persistence of uninsured groups and the design of the POS-S thrust the public network into the role of satisfying demand for a large part of second- and third-tier care, which has been used justify payment of supply subsidies to public hospitals (Sáenz 2001; Giedion, Lopez, and Marulanda 2000; Giedion, Morales, and Acosta 2000).

Despite these constraints, the growth of resources for the SR has been substantial. Resources to finance SR premiums increased from 0.75 percent of GDP in 1995 to 1.1 percent in 2005. Growth of resources for the SR, halted during the eco-

**Table 7.18    Colombia: Selected Determinants of FOSYGA Balance, 1998–2002**

| Key determinant | 1998 | 1999 | 2000 | 2001 | 2002 |
|---|---|---|---|---|---|
| % total population enrolled in CR | 39 | 33 | 32 | 30 | 29 |
| Ratio of beneficiaries / contributors | 1.27 | 1.46 | 1.47 | 1.49 | 1.51 |
| Family density | 2.27 | 2.46 | 2.47 | 2.49 | 2.51 |
| Average salary (number or minimum wages) | 2.18 | 2.09 | 2.07 | 2.10 | 2.00 |
| Total revenues ($Col. millions) | 3,314,565 | 3,841,614 | 4,096,909 | 4,539,282 | 4,741,443 |
| Total expenditures ($Col. millions) | 2,980,795 | 3,845,181 | 4,159,935 | 4,497,739 | 4,594,324 |
| FOSYGA balance | 333,770 | –3,567 | –63,026 | 41,543 | 147,119 |

*Source:* Acosta, Ramírez, and Cañon 2004.

*Notes:* total revenues = contributions + financial returns, millions of pesos; total expenditures = premiums, maternity and sickness leaves, 1% solidarity, and prevention fund.

**Figure 7.19    Colombia: SR Projected Resources versus Actual Expenditures, 1994–2000**

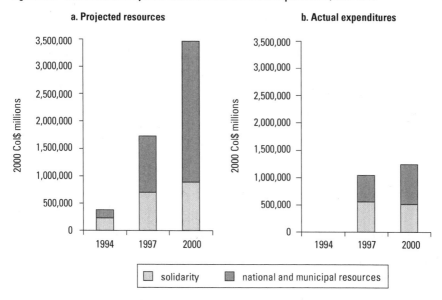

*Source:* Based on data in Martinez, Robayo, and Valencia 2002.

*Note:* No data are available for actual expenditures in 1994.

nomic crisis, have resumed growth. Sources of financing for the SR have also been changing, largely in response to the behavior of the solidarity account of the FOS-YGA. Also, in 2001, Law 715 was enacted, which sought to correct problems of previous decentralization policies and stabilize national resources available to local

**Figure 7.20    Colombia: SR Projected Resources versus Actual Expenditures of Solidarity Funding Sources, 2000**

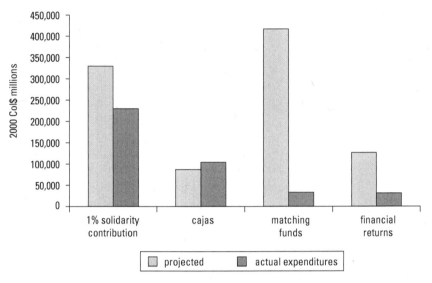

*Source:* Based on data in Martinez, Robayo, and Valencia 2002.

governments. This law reset the amount of national fiscal resources for health and replaced the parameters used for their distribution with territorial indicators of equity and efficiency. It also redefined and aligned responsibilities with territorial capacity, although it allows decentralized municipalities to maintain competences and authority over resources and service provision as long as they meet prescribed performance indicators. Table 7.19 shows how the solidarity contribution, originally the main source of financing, was gradually replaced with resources from the

**Table 7.19    Colombia: SR Funding Sources, 1995–2005 (percent of total resources)**

| Source | 1995 | 1996 | 1997 | 1998 | 1999 | 2000 | 2001 | 2002 | 2003 | 2005 |
|---|---|---|---|---|---|---|---|---|---|---|
| FOSYGA | 85.7 | 63.1 | 46.7 | 51.3 | 38.0 | 34.6 | 36.0 | 29.4 | 31.70 | 34.40 |
| National transfers | 14.3 | 36.9 | 44.0 | 37.2 | 50.0 | 51.9 | 51.0 | 67.9 | 62.0 | 56.3 |
| Local resources | — | — | 3.8 | 4.5 | 3.9 | 5.1 | 3.0 | 2.0 | 4.2 | 8.8 |
| Sin taxes | — | — | 1.8 | 2.2 | 3.4 | 2.1 | 9.0 | — | — | — |
| Cajas | — | — | 3.7 | 4.8 | 4.8 | 6.2 | 2.0 | 0.6 | 1.8 | 0.5 |

*Source:* GES 2006.

*Note:* — = not available.

national budget, amounting to 56 percent of total funding sources in 2005, about US$783 million.

In 2005, the MPS began to explore providing central government matching funds as an incentive for departmental and municipal governments to finance insurance premiums for the poor from their own resources. That year, 6 of the 32 departments, which include 250 municipalities and a total SISBEN 1 and 2 population of about 2 million, signed three-year commitments to provide resources to attain universal health insurance for SR-eligible people. Most of the participating local governments are the wealthiest ones or have just acquired new sources of revenues from exploitation of natural resources such as oil and coal.

Due to the complexity of the system, the administrative costs of health plans can be large and variable, ranging from 4 percent to 60 percent of the value of the premium (Cendex 2000). More than 50 percent of the administrative costs are spent on support activities for daily operations (financial, personnel, and information management) and enrollment processes; little is spent on risk management and quality assurance (Cendex 2000).

*Changes in the organization and administration of health care delivery.* The development of insurance markets, the integration of public and private providers, and the preparation of public providers to compete are the main changes in the organization and administration of public health care delivery.

Before 1993, public insurers, almost exclusively, provided employees with health insurance, mainly through the ISS, the largest insurer. Private insurance offered supplemental coverage or coverage for employees' family members. The reform ended the public health insurance monopoly by promoting the creation and entry of health plans (EPS and ARS) as organizations that would articulate the financing and delivery of services for CR and SR enrollees.

The CR health insurance market developed rapidly, because there was already a supply of commercial health insurers, prepaid group health organizations, and benefits funds, with infrastructure, established provider networks, and experience managing health care services that were ready to enter the CR as EPS. Between 1995 and 1998, the market share of private health plans increased from 11 percent to 30 percent of the population in the CR, a net increase of 261.1 percent (Céspedes, Ramírez, and Reyes 1998). Competition by private health plans dramatically reduced the public sector's CR market shares in terms of CR population covered, from 100 percent in 1993 to 18 percent in 2005.

Development of the ARS health insurance market was assisted by the implementation of a government program to support the creation of community-based insurance organizations, ESSs, which began before the passage of Law 100. Nongovernmental organizations (NGOs) were contracted to provide technical assistance to help local governments establish ESSs, and central government and local municipal funds were dedicated for this purpose. Between 1993 and 1994, 172 ESS contracts were established, covering 1.48 million people (Harvard School of Public

Health 1996). ARSs were authorized to operate in 1995, and by December 1999, 239 ARSs had entered the market, with a total of 9 million enrollees, 22 percent of the total population (Cardona 1999). Participation was not restricted to ESSs, and other types of health plans also entered the market. In 1999, SR enrollment was distributed among public (10 percent), private for-profit (30 percent), ESS (40 percent), and private not-for-profit (20 percent) firms. ARS size ranged between a couple hundred to a million enrollees.

However, there were too many ARSs to permit adequate risk pooling, their large transaction costs generated large inefficiencies, and oversight was difficult. Furthermore, some ARSs did not operate in some parts of the country. This situation motivated the government to start implementing measures to consolidate the ARS market in 2001, first by requiring a minimum membership size and then by requiring regional operation of ARS by November 2005 (MPS 2005b; 2005c). Through a public competitive process, ARSs were assigned to five different regions of the country to operate during a four-year period. Regions were defined to permit a maximum of 15 ARS, each serving a population of 200,000, depending on the potential number of enrollees. At the end of the four years, the results will be evaluated in terms of efficiency, financial stability, and improved access.

At the time of the reform, Colombia had a well-developed private supply of health services and a wide network of public providers set up during the 1970s as part of a national strategy to increase health service coverage. The NSHI model required the participation of both public and private providers.

As part of the reforms, public institutions were to transform their management and budgeting structure to improve efficiency and service quality. For this purpose since 1999 the MPS has been implementing a program to guide and support public institutions' efforts to improve productivity and sustainability.[18] So far 172 public institutions of all levels of complexity have voluntarily participated in the restructuring program. Among the observed program results, total expenditures and personnel expenditures have been reduced, and the number of services provided and bed-occupancy rates have increased. Some institutions had been on the verge of closure, but they managed to recover and maintain their operations. However, many of these providers are still struggling with liquidity due to cash-flow problems and have not been able to pay off previously acquired pension debts to their employees (MPS 2005).

In the managed competition model, the role of the government and its affiliated regulatory bodies is to provide information, to formulate, monitor, and enforce regulations to minimize market failures, and to devise mechanisms to guarantee equitable access to health care services. Thus, the 1993 reforms defined and assigned functions to the following governing institutions of the health sector:

- *Ministry of Health:* formulation and monitoring of national policies, regulations
- *Consejo Nacional de Seguridad Social en Salud (CNSSS, National Health and Social Security Council):* inspection and oversight of health plans and providers

- *FOSYGA:* pooling and management of the system's revenues
- *Consejo Nacional de Seguridad Social en Salud:* created and given regulatory and policy-making authority over benefits packages, premium payments, copayments and measures to avoid adverse selection, tariffs, SR operation rules, and management of the FOSYGA

These institutions have had to face the typical problems of public, bureaucratic institutions, including lack of qualified personnel and frequent rotation of upper-level management. These inconveniences affected the speed with which they were able to focus on priority tasks and develop the skills to carry out their assigned functions. For instance, many of the foundations of a quality assurance system were outlined in the reform, and the regulatory basis was formulated in 2002, but only in 2004 did the provider certification process begin. Thus, evaluation of results is in the early stages.

Lack of information systems has been a major handicap for all these institutions attempting to carry out their responsibilities. For example, it took FOSYGA almost 10 years and countless pesos to refine the procedures for detecting duplicate enrollees and multiple affiliations in its databases. There is still no reliable information for calculating the costs of providing the benefits packages to enable the CNSSS to make sound decisions about the affordability of premium adjustments and updates to the benefits packages.

Though not a formal part of the 1993 reform, since the transformation of the former Ministry of Health into the Ministry of Social Protection in 2003, NSHI has acquired new significance as a policy for achieving goals beyond the scope of the health sector, such as poverty alleviation.

## Challenges and Lessons for Other Countries

As a result of the 1993 health care reform, Colombia has achieved one of the most extensive health insurance systems in Latin America. This case study concludes by discussing major future challenges for the NSHI in Colombia, deriving lessons for other countries from the circumstances that contributed to the reform achievements, and discussing replicability in other low- and middle-income countries.

### Future Challenges

Multiple challenges still face Colombia in closing the remaining health insurance gap and achieving NSHI financial sustainability. First, with respect to the CR a major task is finding mechanisms to enroll the informal sector (58 percent of the working population in 2005) (DNP 2006). About a third of this population is known as the "sandwich population," which can be sorted into two groups: one includes people who earn less than two minimum wages, who are ineligible for subsidies, but for whom payment of the full contribution to the CR premium could be difficult; the other is people able to contribute to the premium but who lack incentives to become affiliated. According to a household survey in 2003, the total

**Figure 7.21 Colombia: Projections for Universal Health Insurance, 2005–2010**

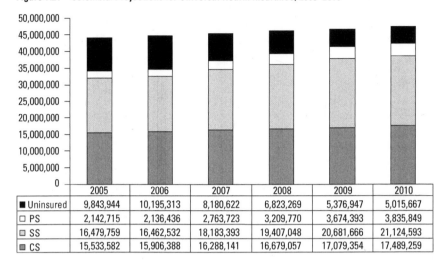

| | 2005 | 2006 | 2007 | 2008 | 2009 | 2010 |
|---|---|---|---|---|---|---|
| ■ Uninsured | 9,843,944 | 10,195,313 | 8,180,622 | 6,823,269 | 5,376,947 | 5,015,667 |
| □ PS | 2,142,715 | 2,136,436 | 2,763,723 | 3,209,770 | 3,674,393 | 3,835,849 |
| □ SS | 16,479,759 | 16,462,532 | 18,183,393 | 19,407,048 | 20,681,666 | 21,124,593 |
| ▣ CS | 15,533,582 | 15,906,388 | 16,288,141 | 16,679,057 | 17,079,354 | 17,489,259 |

*Source:* MPS calculations, 2005.

sandwich population numbered about 7.3 million (workers and their families), 17 percent of the population (calculations by Panopolou 2004). Of these, 2.5 million had some capacity to pay (Bitrán, Giedion, and Muñoz 2004). The administrative costs of enrolling, monitoring, and collecting contributions from this population can be substantial, and the potential for adverse selection is large. Among the alternatives being explored by the MPS are providing partial subsidies to individual contributions to the premium. A pilot program will be launched in 2007 to evaluate the feasibility of this strategy. Another alternative is to devise temporary income protection mechanisms, within the framework of an integrated social protection system that the MPS seeks to develop.

A second challenge for the CR is reduction of tax evasion. One of the antievasion strategies Colombia has started to implement is investment in improvements in the information system by establishing cross-links between pension system data and health insurance contribution data. Increased enrollment of informal workers could complement these measures.

Third, in the case of the SR, not only will it be necessary to finalize the transformation of supply subsidies, but it is also likely that alternative sources of financing will have to be found. For example, under current growth, employment, and poverty conditions and with the available resources, universal health insurance would not be reached by 2010 (figure 7.21).

As mentioned, reaching universal health insurance by 2010 is in the government's agenda, but at the time of writing, stable sources of funding for this purpose have not been lined up. For example, although there has been some success in engaging local governments to use their own resources to cofinance demand subsidies, issues have been raised regarding the risk of local government defaults and the subsequent need for central government bailouts.

Fourth, much still has to be done to design and activate of mechanisms for obtaining accurate information on enrollment, population eligibility, and cost and effectiveness of covered services. Evaluation of service quality is another priority. The affordability and sustainability of the NSHI could be improved by reducing the inefficiencies generated by these information gaps.

Finally, the equity and efficiency implications of maintaining two separate insurance schemes have to be evaluated and consideration given to feasible alternatives toward convergence. For example, due to the gaps in SR service coverage, the poor are likely to experience discontinuities in care that may reduce the effectiveness of treatment.[19] Also, since this population has access to health services both from health plans (covered services) and from local governments and public hospitals, the monitoring of access, quality, and efficiency has become especially cumbersome.

## Lessons from the Colombian Reform: Enabling Factors

Prescience, in the form of legal and institutional groundwork, good economic conditions, and political support combined with a generous measure of luck to make a success of the 1993 reform in Colombia.

*Prior legal framework.* The prereform decentralization laws, plus the formulation of the 1991 Constitution provided a legal framework for many of the strategies of the 1993 reform. Decentralization laws did the job of mobilizing national resources for health, which were then to be reallocated by Law 100 for the purposes of the reform. Decentralization increased local government autonomy to manage resources and set the stage for public hospitals to respond to market mechanisms, conditions that were necessary for insurance contracts. The 1991 Constitution gave political legitimacy for the provision of health services under a National Social Health Insurance (NSHI) scheme with the participation of the private sector.

*Institutional arrangements.* The NSHI was able to quickly sign up a large number of enrollees throughout the country because a reasonable number of private and public institutions already could meet the organizational requirements for delivering services under the managed competition model or could adapt to the fulfill these conditions. In addition, a program for the development of community-based health insurers in the rural areas had been implemented. Many of these networks already had a public-private mix of providers, which facilitated the NSHI response to demand for health care services. The availability of the SISBEN provided the reform with an instrument for identifying its target population and providing subsidies for the neediest.

*Financial aspects.* Positive economic growth conditions prior to and during the first four years of the reform smoothed acceptance of increases in contributions to the NSHI and mobilization of large sums of general revenues to finance the insurance expansions. The enrollment of a large part of the population through coverage of families of contributing individuals allowed the public sector to free additional resources to provide the poor with health care.

*Political support.* Anecdotal evidence suggests the potential to use the SR to gain electoral support played a role in local governments' uptake of the SR. Expansion of the NSHI has been a hot topic on the presidential agenda in the last two elections. There is also evidence from household surveys that people see the value of being enrolled in the SR, very likely a result of the expected learning curve about eligibility and benefits after 13 years of experience with it (Fresneda 2002).

## Replicability in Other Countries

The probability is low that Colombia's coverage expansion experience can be replicated in *poor countries*. The main obstacle would be that a large portion of the population would have to be subsidized and large sums of national resources would have to be mobilized, but these countries have small tax bases. This group of countries may have supply constraints that would have to be addressed, and the breadth of the SR benefits package would have to be reduced. The administrative costs of running the system might be better invested in improving the quality of public services.

*Middle-income countries* considering national social health insurance should evaluate whether they meet key conditions to replicate the Colombian experience successfully and avoid some of its problems. The key conditions that assisted Colombia include

- Favorable economic growth and a reasonable volume of general revenues and potential enrollee contributions to finance the desired benefits
- Existence of quality assurance regulations guaranteeing minimum safety and quality standards
- The existence of, or the possibility of setting up in a parallel with the reform, accurate and reliable information systems with population, financial, accounting, clinical, and service-use data
- Well-developed insurance and provider markets
- Institutional capacity for oversight and enforcement

## Endnotes

1. Among informal sector workers are salespeople, small business owners, taxi drivers, and agricultural and construction workers.

2. Health plans are health insurance companies that articulate financing and delivery of services, modeled after health maintenance organizations in the United States.

3. These resources are part of the social investment budget known as the Sistema General de Participaciones (SGP).

4. Cajas de Compensacion Familiar [family benefits funds] are companies that manage employer-provided benefits in addition to health care, such as recreational services.

5. Allocation rules for resources of the SR are established in Law 715, 2001; Law 812, 2003; Decree 159, 2002; and Decree 177, 2004.

6. These plans are called Administradoras del Régimen Subsidiado (ARSs, Subsidized Regime Administrating Companies).

7. *Impoverishment* is defined as falling below Colombia's poverty line.

8. The provider registry counts the number of services reported, so single facilities may appear more than once, inflating the number of facilities.

9. Most of the information in this subsection is derived from Ministerio de Salud (1994), unless specified otherwise.

10. At the time of the reform 46 percent of the working population belonged to the formal sector and the rest to the informal sector.

11. The largest was the Instituto de Seguros Sociales (Social Security Institute).

12. Ley 10 of 1990; Constitución Política de 1991; Ley 60 of 1993 (Competencias y recursos) y decreto reglamentario 1757; Ley 100 of 1993.

13. Ley 10 of 1990, Art. 37; Ley 60 of 1993 Arts. 14 and 16; Decreto 1770 of 1994.

14. For targeting purposes, municipalities where SISBEN was not available were allowed to use census listings of households with unsatisfied basic needs (another index of poverty used in Colombia) or socioeconomic categories used for definition of public service tariffs.

15. Acuerdo 244 of 2003.

16. This total percentage does not take into account that 5 percent of the population receives partial subsidies, which are a temporary measure, and another 5 percent is enrolled in exception regimes. This implies that 87 percent of the total population is covered by some type of insurance. A change in the denominator is important to mention between 2004 and 2005: the total population in 2004 was based on the 1993 census projection of 45 million; in 2005, on the 2005 census of 41.2 million.

17. Premium payments, maternity and sickness leave and payments to cover expenses of medications and procedures not covered by the POS.

18. This is known as "Programa de modernización de hospitales."

19. For example, a woman with a positive PAP smear for cervical cancer—covered by the POS-S—has to pay out of pocket to have the diagnosis confirmed by a colposcopy, which is not covered.

## References

Acosta, O. L., M. Ramírez, and C. I. Cañon. 2004. "Principales estudios sobre sostenibilidad financiera del SGSSS." Working paper, Corona Foundation [Fundación Corona], Bogotá.

Ascofame (Asociación Colombiana de Facultades de Medicina). 2000. *Recurso Humano en Medicina: formación, distribución y bases para una propuesta política*. Bogotá: Ascofame.

Barón, G. 2007. "Cuentas de salud de Colombia 1993–2003. El gasto nacional en salud y su financiamiento." Programa de Apoyo a la Reforma de Salud del Ministerio de la Protección Social, Bogotá.

Bitrán and Associates, Econometría and Superior School of Public Administration [Bitrán & Asociados-Econometría and Escuela Superior de Administración Pública]. 2002. *Propuestas de reestructuración de los procesos, estrategias y organismos públicos y privados encargados de la afiliación, pago y recaudo de aportes al SGSSS.* Health System Reform Support Program of the Ministry of Social Protection [Programa de Apoyo a la Reforma de Salud del Ministerio de la Protección Social.] Project 03–99, Bogotá.

Bitrán, R., U. Giedion, and R. Muñoz. 2004. *Risk pooling, ahorro y prevención: Estudio regional de Políticas para la protección de los más pobres de los efectos de los shocks de salud.* Washington, DC: World Bank.

BDO and CCRP (Corporación Centro Regional de Población). 2000. "Evaluación del Sisben. Eficiencia, Eficacia Institucional de los proceso de clasificación y selección de beneficiarios." Informe final, Ministerio de Salud, Bogotá.

Cárdenas, M. S. 2006. *Introducción a la Economía Colombiana.* Bogotá: Alfaomega-Fedesarrollo.

Cardona, A. 1999. "Participación de las entidades promotoras de salud (EPS) en el mercado de aseguramiento de salud." *Revista Facultad Nacional de Salud Pública* 17 (1): 52–62.

Cendex-Ministerio de Salud. 2001. *Los Recursos Humanos de Salud en Colombia: balance, competencias y prospectiva.* Bogotá: Editorial Javegraf.

Céspedes, J. E., M. Ramírez, and A. Reyes. 1998. "Análisis de la encuesta de calidad de vida del DANE." Santafé de Bogotá: Econometría S.A.

CONPES (Consejo Nacional de Política Económica y Social). 2006. "Distribución del Sistema Nacional de Participaciones Vigencia 2006." Documento 97, Departamento Nacional de Planeación. Bogotá.

DANE (Departamento Nacional de Estadística). 1992. *Encuesta de Hogares, 1992.*

———. 1997. *Encuesta Nacional de Calidad de Vida, 1997.* Bogotá: DANE.

———. 2000. *Encuesta de Hogares 2000, modulo de salud.* Bogotá: DANE.

———. 2003. *Encuesta Nacional de Calidad de Vida, 2003.* Bogotá: DANE.

———. 2002. *Vital Statistics Registry for 2002.* Bogotá: DANE. http://www.dane.gov.co.

———. 2005. *Census Results 2005.* Bogotá: DANE. http://www.dane.gov.co.

———. *Labor Statistics 1990–2005.* Bogotá: DANE. http://www.dane.gov.co.

DNP (Departamento Nacional de Planeación). 2006. *Bases del Plan Nacional de Desarrollo 2006–2010.* Bogotá: DNP. http://www.dnp.gov.co/paginas_detalle.aspx?idp=890.

DNP and MS (Ministerio de Salud). 2003. "Quien se beneficia del SISBEN. Evaluacion Integral." Government document. Bogotá.

Escobar, M.L. 2005. "Health Sector Reform in Colombia." *Development Outreach*, May 2005. World Bank, Washington, DC. http://www.worldbank.org/devoutreach/may05/article.asp?id= 295 - 28k

Fresneda, Óscar. 2003. "Focusing on the Subsidized Health Regime in Colombia." *Rev. salud pública* 5(3):209–45.

———. 2002. "La visión de la población sobre el sistema de salud. Ha mejorado el acceso en salud?" In *Evaluacion de los procesos del regimen subsidiado*, ed. D. Arevalo and F. Martinez. Bogotá: Universidad Nacional de Colombia.

González-Rossetti, A., and T. J. Bossert. 2000. "Enhancing the Political Feasibility of Health Reform: A Comparative Analysis of Chile, Colombia, and Mexico." Contract No. HRN-5974-C-00-5024-00. Harvard School of Public Health, Latin America and Caribbean Regional Health Sector Reform Initiative. http://www.hsph.harvard.edu/ihsg/publications/pdf/lac/PolicyProcessSynEng2.PDF.

GES (Grupo de Economia de la Salud). 2006. "Resultados financieros del seguro público de salud en Colombia 1996–2005." *Observatorio de la seguridad social* 13. Medellín, Colombia: Universidad de Antioquia, Facultad de Ciencias Económicas.

Giedion, U., H. R. Lopez, and J. A. Marulanda. 2000. "Desarrollo institucional del sector salud en Bogotá." *Coyuntura Social* 23: 57–81.

Giedion, U., L. Morales, and O. L. Acosta. 2000. "Efectos de la reforma en salud sobre las conductas irregulares en los hospitales públicos." *Coyuntura Social* 23: 98–126.

Harvard School of Public Health. 1996. "Colombia Health Sector Reform Project." Final Report, Boston, MA.

Lasso, F. 2004. "Incidencia del gasto público social sobre la distribución del ingreso y la reducción de la pobreza." Working paper, Mission for the Design of a Strategy for Poverty and Inequality Reduction, National Department of Plannning [Misión para el diseño de una estrategia para la reducción de la pobreza y la desigualdad, Departamento Nacional de Planeación], Bogotá.

IMF (International Monetary Fund). 2006. "Article IV Consultation, Poverty Reduction and Growth Facility Reports." IMF, Washington DC.

Martínez, F., G. Robayo, and O. Valencia. 2002. "Porqué no se logra la cobertura universal de la seguridad social en salud?" Bogotá, Fundación para la Investigación y Desarrollo de la Salud y la Seguridad Social (FEDESALUD).

MPS (Ministerio de la Protección Social). 2006. *Informe de Actividades al CNSSS 2005–2006.* MPS, Bogotá, Colombia.

———. 2005. *Politica Nacional de Prestacion de Servicios de Salud.* MPS, Bogotá.

MERPD (Misión para el Diseño de una Estrategia para la Reducción de la Pobreza y la Desigualdad). 2006. "Metodología de Medición y Magnitud de la Pobreza en Colombia." Departamento Nacional de Planeación, Bogotá.

ORC Macro. 2006. MEASURE DHS STATcompiler. http://www.measuredhs.com.

Pinto, M. E., A. Vergara, and Y. Lahuerta. 2005. "Cuanto ha perdido Colombia por el Conflicto?" Estudios Económicos, Documento 277, Departamento Nacional de Planeación, Bogotá.

Profamilia. 2005. "Salud Sexual y Reproductiva en Colombia. Informe de resultados de la Encuesta Nacional de Demografía y Salud." Profamilia, Bogotá.

Ramírez, M., A. Zambrano, F. J. Yepes, J. Guerra, and D. Rivera D. 2005. "Una Aproximación a la Salud en Colombia a Partir de las Encuestas de Calidad de Vid." Borradores de Investigación No. 72. Bogotá: Universidad del Rosario.

Restrepo, J. H. 2002. "El seguro de salud en Colombia. Cobertura Universal?" *Revista Gerencia y Políticas de Salud* 2: 25–40.

Restrepo, J. H., M. Arango, and L. Casas. 2001. "Estructura y conducta de la oferta del seguro de salud en Colombia." *Observatorio de la Seguridad Social* 1: 1–10.

Sáenz, L. 2001. *Modernización de la Gestión Hospitalaria Colombiana: Lecciones aprendidas de la transformación de los hospitales en Empresas Sociales del Estado.* Regional Initiative of Health Sector Reform in Latin America and the Caribbean, Document No. 46. http://www.lachsr.org/documents/187-modernizaciondelagestionhospitalaria colombianaleccionesaprendidasdelatransformac-ES.pdf.

WHO (World Health Organization). 2002. "Global Burden of Disease (GBD) Estimates, 2002." WHO, Geneva. http://www.who.int/healthinfo/bodestimates/en/index.html.

World Bank. 2006. *World Development Indicators.* Washington, DC: World Bank.

# 8

# Costa Rica: "Good Practice" in Expanding Health Care Coverage—Lessons from Reforms in Low- and Middle-Income Countries

*James Cercone and José Pacheco Jiménez*

## Background

*Costa Rica is a small (51,100 sq. km) republic in Central America in the Latin America and Caribbean Region (LAC) of the World Bank with a population of 4.3 million and per capita income of US$9,985. Total health expenditures equaled $305 per capita in 2005. In 2004, life expectancy was 78.7 years, and infant mortality was 11.3 per 1,000 live births. Costa Rica is an outstanding example of a middle-income country that provides its people, including the poor, with broad and deep health care coverage, considerable financial protection, and an extensive package of services. These good outcomes are the result of a century of efforts to improve living conditions.*

*In 1941, with the creation of the Caja Costarricense del Seguro Social (CCSS), a health insurance system began operations, one of the first such systems in Latin America. By 2006, 88 percent of the population was affiliated with the health insurance scheme, and around 93 percent of the people had adequate access to primary care services. Before the 1994 health care reform, access to primary care services was restricted to 25 percent of the population. To surmount obstacles to achieving its coverage objectives, Costa Rica revamped its organizational structure by redefining the network and bringing private and nongovernmental partners into the delivery system. These reforms were aimed at correcting the structural problems and further separating financing, purchasing, and provision within the vertically integrated CCSS model.*

## Introduction

This section provides a brief overview of Costa Rica in three main areas: economics, demographics and epidemiology, and the political environment. The main trends of the last 15 years are described as background information for issues addressed later in the chapter.

### Economic Profile

Between 1990 and 2005, the Costa Rican economy was characterized by a stable macroeconomic context with persistent problems that weakened over time, a stagnant poverty rate after the mid-1990s with increasing inequality after 1998, and decreasing dependence on external funds and declining external debt. Costa Rica has been classified as an upper-middle-income economy, with a GDP per capita of US$4,327 in 2004 (US$9,481 in PPP terms). Between 1990 and 2004, the GDP per capita grew at a 4.7 percent rate a year, but growth between 2000 and 2004 decelerated to an average rate of 3.3 percent. Between 1991 and 2005, real disposable income per capita grew 2 percent a year, but between 2000 and 2005, the annual rate fell to just 1 percent. Although the unemployment rate has risen during the last decade, it is still low, compared with regionally common rates close to 10 percent.

The part of the population that is poor declined from 32 percent in 1990 to 21.7 percent in 2004. Despite substantial progress on this issue, in the last 10 years poverty has been stuck at around 20 percent of the population.

Fiscal problems are constant in the Costa Rican economy. The gap between revenues and expenditures has been constant, with the fiscal deficit averaging 3 percent of GDP (table 8.1). The ratio of tax revenues to GDP has remained at between 12 percent and 13.5 percent. The ratio of expenditures to GDP has stayed in a 14 percent to16 percent range. Recurrent deficits are often blamed for causing higher inflation rates than international averages. For almost two decades, infla-

**Table 8.1   Costa Rica: Economic Indicators, 1990–2004**

| Indicator | 1990 | 1995 | 2000 | 2004 |
|---|---|---|---|---|
| GDP per capita PPP (current international US$) | 5,219.6 | 6,630.2 | 8,621.3 | 9,481.4 |
| GPD growth rate (%) | 3.6 | 3.9 | 1.8 | 4.2 |
| Headcount ratio | 31.9 | 20.4 | 20.6 | 21.7 |
| Revenue to GDP ratio (excluding grants) | 23.1 | 20.3 | 20.9 | 22.4 |
| Tax revenue to GDP ratio | 13.1 | 12.1 | 12.1 | 13.4 |
| Expenditures to GDP ratio | 14.2 | 16.1 | 15 | 15.9 |
| External debt to GDP ratio | n.a. | 36.6 | 19.9 | 21.1 |
| ODA as % of GDP | 4.2 | 0.3 | 0.08 | 0.07 |
| Unemployment (% of total labor force) | 4.5 | 5.1 | 5.2 | 6.5 |
| Inflation, consumer prices (annual %) | 19 | 23.2 | 11 | 12.3 |

*Source:* World Development Indicators 2006. Revenue-to-GDP ratio comes from MIDEPLAN.

tion in Costa Rica has been higher than 10 percent; in 2005 it was the second highest rate in Latin America.

External debt has shown steady signs of decline. By 2005, the ratio of external debt to GDP was less than half the ratio in 1990, not a significant threat to macroeconomic stability. Similarly, official development assistance (ODA) decreased in the overall context, to just 0.07 percent of GDP in 2004.

## Demographic and Health Profiles

The Costa Rican population is aging, a trend expected to continue for the next 15 years (figure 8.1). The number of children between 0 to 4 years old is expected to decrease from 13.4 percent of the population in 1990 to 7.2 percent in 2020. Similarly, the 0 to 14-year-old group is expected to shrink from 36 percent to

**Figure 8.1  Costa Rica: Population Pyramids, 1990, 2005, and 2020**

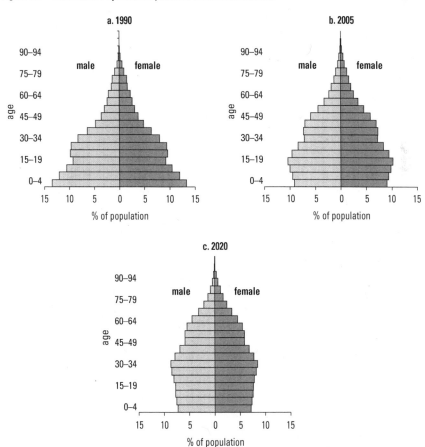

*Source:* United Nations Population Division 2004.

**Table 8.2   Costa Rica: Population Growth Rates and Projections, 1990–2020**

| Period | Annual average ( %) |
|--------|---------------------|
| 1990–95 | 2.4 |
| 1995–2000 | 2.4 |
| 2000–05 | 2.0 |
| 2005–10 | 1.5 |
| 2010–15 | 1.3 |
| 2015–20 | 1.1 |
| 2020–25 | 1.01 |

*Source:* United Nations Population Division 2004.

22 percent of the total population. Thus, older groups will make up an ever-increasing share of the population. For instance, while in 1990, women 60 years of age and older made up 7.2 percent of the female population, in 2020, women of this age will make up 14.2 percent of the female population. In other words, the number of older people will practically double between 1990 and 2020. By residence, the urban population accounts for 61 percent of the total population.

Accelerating the demographic transition, which will double the old age population by 2020, is the decline in fertility: total fertility rates declined from 3.5 in 1980-85 to 2.5 during the second half of the present decade. These two trends will decrease the population growth rate and produce dramatic changes in the child and old-age dependency ratios.

As shown in table 8.2, the population growth rate in the early 1990s was 2.4 percent but then began declining at the turn of the century. By 2020, the growth rate is expected to slow to 1 percent per year. The child dependency ratio will decline from 61 percent in 1990 to 31 in 2025 (figure 8.2). At the same time, the old-age dependency ratio will increase from 8 to 16 percent.

Overall, life expectancy and infant mortality rates have improved since 1990 (table 8.3). Although infant mortality has decreased, the maternal mortality rate has nearly doubled, partially explained by improvements in maternal death recording and registration. Almost 98 percent of all births were attended by skilled staff. Immunization rates showed a U-shaped pattern, falling from 95 percent coverage of children aged 12 to 23 months to 85 percent in 1995, and then rising to 90 percent in 2004.

The mortality and morbidity profile of Costa Rica shows the characteristic pattern of a developed economy (table 8.4). Half of the deaths in 2002 were due to circulatory diseases and cancers; noncommunicable diseases represented 76 percent of all deaths. In terms of disability-adjusted life years (DALYs), the top five causes accounted for 60 percent of all DALYs, led by neuropsychiatric conditions and unintentional injuries (38 percent of total DALYs). By disease category, around 70

**Figure 8.2    Costa Rica: Basic Demographic Indicators**

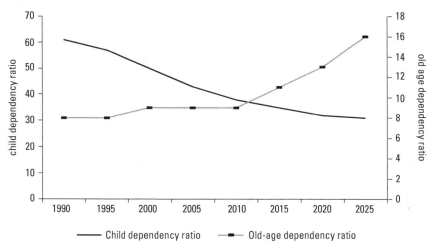

Source: United Nations Population Division 2004.

**Table 8.3    Costa Rica: Basic Health Information**

| Year | Life expectancy at birth | Infant mortality (per 1,000 live births) | Maternal mortality (per 10,000 live births) | Immunization, (% of children ages 12–23 months) |
|------|--------------------------|------------------------------------------|---------------------------------------------|--------------------------------------------------|
| 1990 | 76.8 | 16.0 | 1.5 | 95.0 |
| 1995 | 76.7 | 14.3 | 2.0 | 85.0 |
| 2000 | 77.7 | 12.5 | 3.6 | 88.0 |
| 2004 | 78.7 | 11.3 | 3.0 | 90.0 |

Sources: World Development Indicators 2006; for maternal mortality, MIDEPLAN (http://www.mideplan.go.cr/sides/social/index.html).

**Table 8.4    Costa Rica: Leading Causes of Morbidity and Mortality, 2002 (percent of total)**

| Top five burden of disease causes (DALYs) | | Top five causes of mortality | |
|-------------------------------------------|---------|------------------------------|---------|
| Cause | Percent | Cause | Percent |
| Neuropsychiatric conditions | 28 | Cardiovascular diseases | 31 |
| Unintentional injuries | 10 | Malignant neoplasms | 21 |
| Infectious and parasitic diseases | 9 | Unintentional injuries | 8 |
| Cardiovascular diseases | 7 | Infectious and parasitic diseases | 7 |
| Malignant neoplasms | 7 | Digestive diseases | 7 |

Source: World Health Organization 2004.

percent of the burden of disease was caused by noncommunicable diseases. Communicable and materno-infant diseases represented 14.5 percent of total episodes; injuries, one in seven cases of illness.

## Political and Administrative Profile

Costa Rica is administratively organized into seven provinces, 81 cantons, and 459 districts. The government is democratic and structured in three branches: executive, legislative, and judicial. The presidential term lasts four years, and reelection has been permitted since 2003. Costa Rica has a long tradition of political stability, and since 1889, elections have taken place normally except for two instances: the 1917 to 1919 tyranny and the 1948 to 1949 transitional period when a new Constitution emerged and the army was abolished. The last two elections (2002 and 2006) broke the hegemony of the two main political forces, and new actors emerged with solid voter support.

The political, administrative, and fiscal systems are centralized, and resources are allocated centrally, usually following historical patterns. The excessive number of regulations makes for a rigid budget and leaves the Ministry of Finance (MOF) little freedom to reallocate resources according to needs or to control the fiscal deficit. High centralization is evident from the low participation of the 81 municipalities in the total budget: just 2 percent of the funds are municipally managed.

The National Development Plan (NDP) elaborated by each new government is the main political, programmatic, and budgetary tool. The Ministry of Planning is in charge of monitoring plan implementation through the National Evaluation System. Social policies are also part of the NDP. Besides the three branches, the institutional framework is complemented by three key entities: the Controller General Agency, the Constitutional Court (Sala IV), and the Ombudsman's Office. The main function of the Controller General, the public auditing institution, is to evaluate administrative contracting processes (like purchasing). The Constitutional Court is empowered to revoke any unconstitutional decision by the Congress. The Ombudsman supervises the quality of public services and protects citizens against any abuse of power.

## Health Financing and Coverage

This section analyzes the main financing and coverage characteristics of the Costa Rican health system—health expenditure trends and distribution in the last decade. A brief analysis of the benefits package and payment mechanisms is also included, as well as an evaluation of the equity issues.

## Health Expenditures

Total health spending in Costa Rica amounted to US$1.42 billion in 2005, 65 percent higher than in 1998 (table 8.5). In 2005, 7.1 percent of GDP was allocated to finance health services, a proportion that has grown over the years. Private health

**Table 8.5  Costa Rica: Health Expenditure Indicators 1998, 2000, and 2003**

| Sector | 1998 | 2000 | 2005 |
|---|---|---|---|
| Total health expenditures (US$ millions) | 859.85 | 1,004.62 | 1,415.00 |
| Health expenditures (% of GDP) | 6.1 | 6.3 | 7.1 |
| Private health expenditures (% of GDP) | 1.3 | 1.3 | 1.7 |
| Public health expenditures (% of GDP) | 4.8 | 5.0 | 5.4 |
| Per capita health expenditures (current US$) | 230 | 258 | 327 |
| Public health expenditures (% of total health expenditure) | 77.9 | 79 | 76 |
| Public health expenditure (% of total government expenditure) | 21 | 21.7 | 21 |
| Private health expenditures (% of total health expenditure) | 25 | 28 | 24 |
| Participation of hospitals in public health expenditures (%) | 51.1 | 49.6 | 51.6[a] |

*Sources:* World Development Indicators 2006; MOH-PAHO 2003a; CCSS 2005.

a. This figure is for 2003.

outlays increased and then decreased compared to public health spending, allowing private expenditures to fall from 25 percent to 24 percent of total health expenditures. Despite this upward trend in private health expenditures, Costa Rica has one of the lowest private participations and one of the lowest proportions of out-of-pocket expenditure—19 percent of total health spending in 2005—in Latin America (World Development Indicators). Per capita expenses also rose, by 42 percent between 1998 and 2005, from US$327 to US$305 ($684 in current international U.S. dollars). Per capita public health expenditures exceeded US$200 in 2003. Public health expenditures accounted for more than a fifth of all government spending, and 52 percent of it was allocated to finance hospital activities in 2003.

## Benefit-Incidence Analysis

In 2001, the distribution of public health spending by income category reflected a positive redistribution of resources in favor of poorer families (figure 8.3). For instance, regarding the CCSS spending, the poorest 20 percent of the population (receiving 4.7 percent of national income), got almost 30 percent of CCSS health-related expenditures. The wealthiest 20 percent of the families (representing 48 percent of the national income) received 11.1 percent of social security resources.

Trejos (2002) estimated the proportion of public health expenditures associated with the different income groups, by program. On average, the poorest 20 percent of families received 29 percent of public health spending, in contrast to the 11 percent received by the richest 20 percent. Individually, poor families (first quintile) benefited from nutritional programs (55 percent of the corresponding budget), primary care (37 percent), outpatient services (26.5 percent), and hospitalization (26.3 percent). In no case did the poorest quintile receive less than 22 percent of the budget.

**Figure 8.3   Costa Rica: National Distribution of Public Spending on Health, by Income Category, 2001**

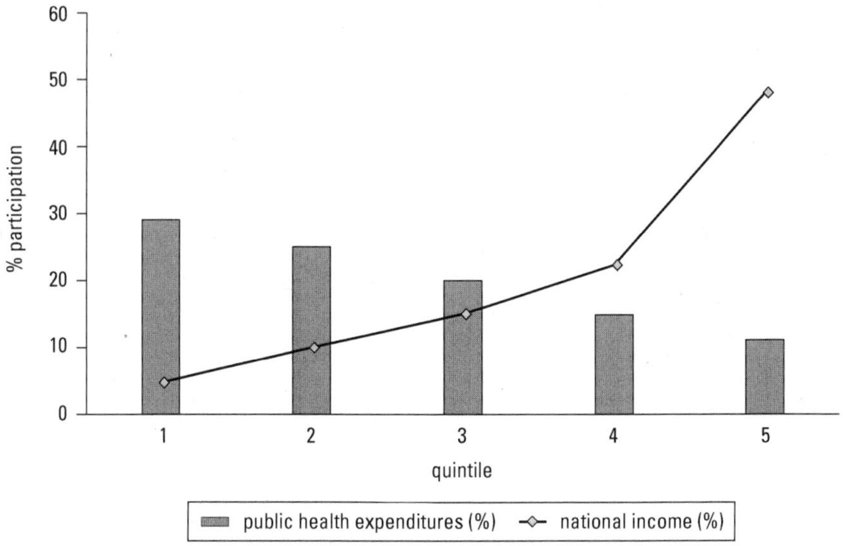

*Source:* INEC 2001.

## Benefits Package

The benefits package, defined and provided by the CCSS, includes: general medical assistance, specialized services, and surgery; hospital assistance; pharmacy services; dental services; a cash subsidy for direct affiliates; a funeral stipend in cash; and social provisions.

The benefits package is comprehensive; only a few interventions (e.g., some plastic surgeries) are excluded from the list. The Constitutive Law of the CCSS empowers the board of directors (BOD) to define the components of the package. However, recent resolutions of the Constitutional Court suggest that other entities (like the Court itself) are able to modify the package. The absence of a specific reference regarding the right to health in the Constitution has created a vacuum in Costa Rican legislation. Should conflicts arise, the Constitutional Court, at the last minute, will rule on the specific situation.

Rulings by the Constitutional Court are binding on the CCSS and create jurisdiction for future cases, which has an enormous impact on the definition of the package of services. Some rulings have been broad, such as the one establishing that the benefits package cannot explicitly restrict access to health services, and narrow, such as the recently issued resolution forcing the CCSS to provide a specific drug to a breast cancer patient. In practice, the BOD has only partial control over the definition of the package of services and drugs; it cannot exclude health services or drugs from the package because of a patient's contribution status or type of disease.

## Financing and Payment

This section describes the financing scheme that operated in the Costa Rican mandatory health insurance system. The section covers two issue: the sources of financing and the payment mechanisms as tools for resource allocation.

*Financing sources.* Revenues to finance health care and health-related activities come from three sources: taxes, as in the case of the Ministry of Health; contributions (especially payroll contributions) to finance health insurance (CCSS); and fees, as in the case of the water and sewage entity (the AyA). The CCSS is the most important health institution, handling 76 percent of public health expenditures.

The contributory base of the CCSS is the result of three parties: workers, employers, and the state (table 8.6). Legislation also regulates revenues collected from independent workers. The BOD determines premiums according to actuarial analyses, and under no circumstances are the premiums paid by the workers allowed to exceed the premiums paid by employers. The mandatory health insurance financing relies on a 15 percent payroll tax for formal employees, 10.25 percent of the income reported by independent workers, and 14 percent of the pension received by a retiree.

As expected, the largest source of financing for the CCSS—88 percent of total revenues—is contributions from employers, workers, and the state contributions. Contributions from workers and employers increased from 83 percent in 1990 to 87 percent in 2004, and revenues collected from workers grew faster than revenues from employers.

Poor households are covered by the state. The Ministry of Finance (MOF) collects revenues for this purpose through taxes on luxury goods, liquors, beer, colas, and other similar imports. The procedure is complex for allocating budget to cover expenditures by poor households. Based on the Household Survey, the MOF estimates the number of poor people. Then, the average "contribution" per poor person is calculated by applying a 14 percent rate to the average premium paid by the

**Table 8.6   Costa Rica: Payroll Fees, by Insurance Scheme**

| Health insurance type | Contribution by source (%) | | | | |
|---|---|---|---|---|---|
| | Employee | Employer | State | Pension regime | Total |
| Salaried | 5.50 | 9.25 | 0.25 | n.a. | 15.00 |
| Independent | 4.75 | n.a. | 5.50 | n.a. | 10.25 |
| Voluntary | 4.65 | n.a. | 5.50 | n.a. | 10.15 |
| Contributory pensioner | 5.00 | n.a. | 0.25 | 8.75 | 14.00 |
| Noncontributory pensioner | n.a. | n.a. | 0.25 | 13.75 | 14.00 |
| Insured by state | n.a. | n.a. | 14.00 | n.a. | 14.00 |

*Source:* CCSS.

*Note:* n.a. = not applicable.

other contributors at the national level. The projected number of poor people, multiplied by the average contribution, is the budget the MOF plans to transfer to the CCSS.

In practice, however, the budget figures diverge significantly from the actual numbers. The CCSS does not have a program for identifying and registering poor households as health service beneficiaries, which means that affiliation of poor families mostly follows an *as-you-go basis*. Although no person can be denied health care in a public facility in Costa Rica, current regulation establishes that unaffiliated persons must pay for health care at subsidized rates. To avoid paying for care, poor persons must register at the CCSS or at the facility when services are provided. Exemption is effective when the CCSS validates the socioeconomic conditions of the person. However, due to shortages of staff and resources to track all the requests, the CCSS has problems detecting fraudulent cases of nonpoor people registering as state beneficiaries.

*Payment mechanisms.* In the mid-1990s, the CCSS board introduced the management agreement (*Compromisos de Gestión*), a legal and managerial tool for planning and improving resource allocation. Basically, the agreement is a means of regulating relations between the CCSS and health service providers, involving both primary care facilities and hospitals. These contract-type agreements include key indicators for assessing quality (e.g., intra-hospital infection, mortality, and readmission rates) and utilization (waiting lists and the average length of stay, ALOS). The agreements are also intended to improve coverage and health service quality by linking resource allocation with the achievement of prenegotiated health outcomes. Cost containment is an implicit objective.

The management agreement is also a regulatory instrument for the CCSS. It defines, for instance, the health services to be supplied by providers throughout the country. Services included are integral care for children under 10 years old, teenagers 10 to 19 years old, women 20 to 64 years old,[1] adults 20 to 64 years old, and the elderly (over 65 years old). For each area, the management agreement also incorporates prenegotiated health goals in terms of accreditation, quality, efficiency, and coverage.

Hospital performance contracts were implemented in 1997 and, by 2005, 29 hospitals and 104 health regions had signed one with the CCSS. The CCSS has also signed agreements with nonprofit associations, universities, and cooperatives that provide services to more than 400,000 persons, one of the mechanisms used to increase coverage starting in the 1990s.

Finally, payment mechanisms differ for primary and tertiary care facilities. Primary care services are paid on a historical capitation basis. For hospitals, a payment unit was defined, known as the "hospital production unit" (UPH in Spanish), for setting rates for hospital activities—in "patient days," "consultations," or "emergencies." The original payment scheme considered a variable component, generally 10 percent of total budget, as an incentive to reward the achievement of objectives and to cover unexpected events. The entire hospital payment system was originally expected to evolve into a results-based payment model similar to the related diagnostic groups. However, despite some significant progress on this issue, resource allocation has not yet been fully linked to performance. In fact, the incentives fund has not been activated.

## Equity: Health Indicators, Outcomes, and Their Distribution

This section presents the most important health outcomes achieved by the Costa Rican health system between 1990 and 2004. Then, the section assesses the existing gaps in terms of access and health outcomes by income quintile.

*Health Outcomes.* Table 8.7 presents a list of key health indicators related to health processes and health outcomes; the information is presented on an averaged biennial basis from 1990 to 2004. In general terms, health outcomes improved in mortality-related indicators and life expectancy; the balance in morbidity diseases and immunization is not fully satisfactory. Life expectancy, for instance, increased by almost two years, one of the highest jumps in Latin America, while infant mortality rates fell 32 percent during the assessed period. Universal access to potable water was nearly achieved, and measles disappeared. However, maternal mortality increased (mostly attributable to improvements in recording systems), vaccination rates remained the same or decreased slightly, and the incidence of some diseases like dengue and HIV rose significantly.

**Table 8.7   Costa Rica: Health Indicators, 1990–2004**

| Indicator | 1990–91 | 1995–96 | 2003–04 | Situation 1990–2004 |
|---|---|---|---|---|
| Gross birth rate | 26.4 | 22.7 | 17.3 | Decrease |
| Infant mortality rate (per 1,000 live births) | 14.3 | 12.5 | 9.7 | Decrease |
| Life expectancy at birth | 76.7 | 76.5 | 78.6 | Increase |
| Men | 74.7 | 74.3 | 76.4 | Increase |
| Women | 78.9 | 78.8 | 80.9 | Increase |
| Maternal mortality rate (per 100,000 live births) | 19.8 | 22.0 | 25.3 | Increase |
| Children with low birth weight (%) | 6.3 | 7.0 | 6.5 | Increase |
| Dengue per 100,000 inhabitants | 9.5[a] | 109.7 | 347.0 | Increase |
| Measles per 100,000 inhabitants | 103.2 | 1.4 | 0.0 | Decrease |
| AIDS per 100,000 inhabitants | 2.9 | 4.7 | 3.7 | Increase |
| Vaccination SRP-measles (% 1 year) | 91.0 | 88.0 | 89.0 | Decrease |
| Vaccination VOP3-poliomyelitis (% 1 year) | 92.0 | 86.0 | 89.0 | Decrease |
| Total population served by water system | n.a. | 95.8% | 99.0% | Increase |

*Sources:* Based on Ministry of Planning data; Proyecto Estado de La Nación 2005; and OPS data.

*Note:* n.a. = not available.

a. This rate corresponds to 1992–93.

*Equity problems: gaps.* As mentioned, Costa Rica's outcomes were mixed during 1990 to 2004. Some major gains were in line with the health reform objectives. The new delivery model emphasized primary care and prevention at community level. The significant decline in infant mortality and even the improvements in recording and registering maternal mortality can be explained, at least partially, by the new policies accompanying the reform. In other areas, the outcomes are not satisfactory. For example, the outcomes for morbidity-related conditions and vaccination coverage are not the best, despite the fact that vaccination is part of the management agreements between primary care providers and the CCSS. On balance, however, there is a perception that overall living conditions have improved in Costa Rica.

One of the main achievements of the reform was improvements in health outcomes, though not uniform, for practically every population group, income group, and region. In some cases, poorer regions got most of the benefits, but in others the gap between the best performer and the rest of the regions or groups widened. This section evaluates equity gaps in four areas: health insurance coverage, health service utilization, infant mortality rates, and per capita budget allocation.

Concerning *coverage,* by 2004, 88 percent of the Costa Rican population was covered by social health insurance (table 8.8). Significant differences persist, however, by income quintiles (table 8.8). For instance, while 85 percent of the Q-5 population was covered by health insurance, 70 percent of the Q-1 population was in the same condition. More important, only 10 percent of the poorest 20 percent group was a direct contributor, a number that increased to 49 percent among Q-5. Gaps by region existed, but differences were small, in the range of 2 to 4 percentage points. This can be considered a major strength of the health system: disparities by region have been narrower than in other countries. Additionally, the contribution results reveal the existence of a cross-subsidy from richer groups to poorer families. This situation is clearer from the different use patterns by income group.

Regarding *health service utilization,* poorer groups generally use public facilities more than richer groups (figure 8.4). The better-off tend to use private services instead of public ones, although richer groups presented higher rates of affiliation. Only hospital services showed similar rates of utilization between poorer and richer groups.

*Health outcomes* have improved for almost the entire population regardless of place of residence. Regionally, except in Chorotega, child mortality rates and the under-five (U-5) mortality rates have decreased, and the gaps between the highest and the lowest rates have narrowed (table 8.9). At the canton level, differences in infant mortality rates were up to 5.5 times higher between Talamanca (17.8 deaths per 1,000 live births), with the highest rate, and Turrubares (3.2 deaths), with the lowest; however, dispersion is falling. In total, 95 percent of the cantons had infant mortality rates below 20 deaths per 1,000 live births.

*Per capita budget allocation,* the last equity issue, deals with the distributional problems arising from the payment schemes. Although the reform has modified the way health services are paid and goes a step farther toward a performance-based

**Table 8.8    Costa Rica: Health Insurance Coverage, by Income Quintile, 2005 (percent of total population)**

| Indicator | Q-1 | Q-2 | Q-3 | Q-4 | Q-5 |
|---|---|---|---|---|---|
| **National** | | | | | |
| Insured | 70.7 | 77.6 | 82.5 | 86.3 | 84.7 |
| Direct contributors | 10.6 | 21.3 | 31.1 | 39.5 | 49.2 |
| Insured as family dependents | 34.4 | 46.1 | 45.2 | 44.0 | 33.5 |
| Insured by the state | 19.3 | 6.2 | 3.7 | 1.9 | 0.7 |
| Insured by other plans | 6.4 | 3.9 | 2.5 | 1.0 | 1.4 |
| **Urban** | | | | | |
| Insured | 72.0 | 77.9 | 83.8 | 86.5 | 87.8 |
| Direct contributors | 13.2 | 26.1 | 34.5 | 42.1 | 54.0 |
| Insured as family dependents | 35.0 | 42.6 | 45.6 | 41.5 | 35.6 |
| Insured by the state | 16.2 | 4.3 | 1.8 | 1.9 | 0.3 |
| Insured by other plans | 7.6 | 5.0 | 1.9 | 0.9 | 1.0 |
| **Rural** | | | | | |
| Insured | 68.2 | 75.3 | 81.1 | 85.5 | 82.4 |
| Direct contributors | 8.0 | 16.6 | 23.8 | 33.8 | 39.0 |
| Insured as family dependents | 30.2 | 47.4 | 49.2 | 46.1 | 40.6 |
| Insured by the state | 25.0 | 8.4 | 4.9 | 4.5 | 1.5 |
| Insured by other plans | 5.0 | 2.9 | 3.2 | 1.0 | 1.3 |

*Source:* Authors' estimations based on the INEC 2005 Household Survey.

**Figure 8.4  Costa Rica: Outpatient Consultations per Inhabitant, by Income Decile, 1998 and 2001**

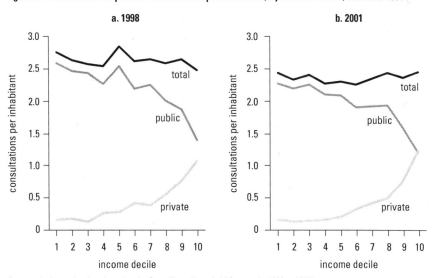

*Sources:* Author estimations based on the Costa Rican Household Surveys for 1998 and 2001.

*Note:* Income deciles (Ds) are defined using the 1998 and 2001 Household Surveys.

**Table 8.9   Costa Rica: Child and Infant Mortality, by Health Region**

| | 2001 | | 2004 | |
|---|---|---|---|---|
| **Region** | **Under five years of age** | **Under one year of age** | **Under five years of age** | **Under one year of age** |
| Chorotega | 9.5 | 8.2 | 12.8 | 10.7 |
| Central | 11.5 | 9.7 | 9.4 | 7.8 |
| Central Pacific | 12.0 | 9.8 | 8.8 | 8.2 |
| Brunca | 16.9 | 12.2 | 12.0 | 10.0 |
| Atlantic Huetar | 16.7 | 12.7 | 13.1 | 10.0 |
| North Huetar | 14.6 | 9.7 | 10.7 | 9.1 |

*Source:* Authors' estimates, based on Centro Centroamericano de Población database.

system, the allocation of funds is creating enormous gaps between regions. The MOH-PAHO-CCSS (2004) reported that some regions receive up to 60 times more funds (per capita) than others for no particular reason (i.e., no significantly different health profiles). This situation is especially true under the capitation formula used in primary care, which still bases allocations of funds on historical trends, not needs. Thus, because the formula does not fully take into account differences between regions (such as demographic profiles, distance, higher administrative costs), the mechanism perpetuates the perverse incentives generated by input-based models.

## Efficiency

This section on efficiency deals with four main topics: the structure of health spending by use; the structure of health financing by source; an equity analysis of the distribution of public health expenditures. It also briefly assesses health care financial sustainability.

*Spending by Source and Use.* The CCSS, Costa Rica's biggest health institution, contributes two out of three every colones spent in the health sector.[2] Households are the second most important source of financing, almost one-fourth of total spending. Most family expenditures on health go to drug purchases and outpatient visits. Families use public hospitals in preference to the more costly private hospitals. Nongovernmental organizations (NGOs) and private insurance represent a very low share of total health expenditures (less than 1 percent each).

The composition of public health expenditures, by level of care, has two main features. First, the share of hospital spending was practically unchanged between 1997 and 2004 (table 8.10). About half of public health outlays goes to hospital services, the most dynamic of the three levels of care. In the postreform period, hospital expenditures have been growing 5 percent a year in real terms. Arce (2001) estimates that, if this trend continues, in 20 years the system will be forced

Table 8.10    Costa Rica: Health Spending, by Level of Care (percentage)

| Level of care | 1997 | 2000 | 2004 |
|---|---|---|---|
| Primary | 18.8 | 22.4 | 21.8 |
| Outpatient | 30.1 | 28.0 | 26.6 |
| Tertiary | 51.1 | 49.6 | 51.6 |
| Total | 100.0 | 100.0 | 100.0 |

*Source:* CCSS 2005.

to allocate three times more resources to cover all the expenses generated by the hospital sector. For Arce and Saenz (2002), this behavior reflects the failure of the current hospital payment mechanism to control costs because the model incentives extended lengths of stay, and the reform has not been able to tighten the link between hospitals and primary care centers. The second relevant feature is the increasing share of primary care services in total public expenditures, a good sign that the system is moving in the right direction. However, if hospital reforms are not completed, the full benefits of incorporating more primary care services in the health sector will be hard to realize.

*Sources of Financing.* Social security contributions are the most important source of financing, almost 60 percent of all health sector revenues (table 8.11). The second source, sales of goods and services, corresponds to out-of-pocket expenditures by households. If out-of-pocket expenditures and social security contributions are considered together, households contribute half of total revenues. The government contributes 7.3 percent of total revenues (5 percent in the form of taxes and 2.7 percent in the form of contributions to the CCSS). This figure does not, however, include government contributions to pay for health insurance for poor households. The role of external funds is minimal, not more than 4 percent of total health revenues. External grants and donations mainly finance purchases of medical equipment and salaries of staff working in the reform program.

Table 8.11    Costa Rica: Sources of Health Financing (percentage)

| Source | Participation |
|---|---|
| Taxes | 5.0 |
| Contributions to Social Security | 59.7 |
| Contributions to INS | 4.8 |
| Grants and Donations | 3.4 |
| Sales of Goods and Services | 27.1 |

*Source:* MOH-PAHO-CCSS 2004.

**Figure 8.5   Costa Rica: Income and Social Expense Distribution by Function, 2000**

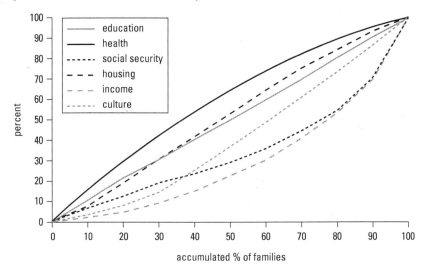

legend:
- education
- health
- social security
- housing
- income
- culture

y-axis: percent

x-axis: accumulated % of families

*Source:* Trejos 2004.

*Health Spending, Equity, and Sustainability.* In Costa Rica, public health spending is the most progressive social spending component: the poorest families receive more resources than proportionate to their weight in the population. Because health expenditures favor poorer families more than nonpoor families; health spending is a key factor in improving living conditions of the poorest and reducing income inequality (Trejos 2004). The Lorenz Curve in figure 8.5 illustrates this conclusion.[3] Curves above the 45° line are said to be progressive. In these circumstances, only two sectors, health and housing, appear above the income line. Because health is above housing, it is evident that the health sector is, of all the expenses evaluated, the most progressive within the social area.

The same pattern is also observed among regions. In all but the Central region, the poorest 20 percent of families receive at least 29 percent of the public resources invested in health (figure 8.6). In some cases, like the Brunca and the Chorotega regions (the two poorest regions of the country), the families in the first quintile receive between 38 percent and 42 percent of the health expenditures.

The Lorenz Curve in figure 8.7 shows the distribution of health insurance contributions and the associated level of spending by income level. The principles of solidarity and equity in access are clearly presented. First, the expenditure curve is similar to the 45° line representing high equity in access by all income groups. Solidarity is seen in the differences in expenditure and contribution participation. D-1, for instance, absorbs 12 percent of health insurance expenditures, but its contributions represent just 0.6 percent of total contributions. On the other hand, D-10

**Figure 8.6  Costa Rica: Distribution of Public Spending on Health Nationally and Regionally, by Income Group, 2001**

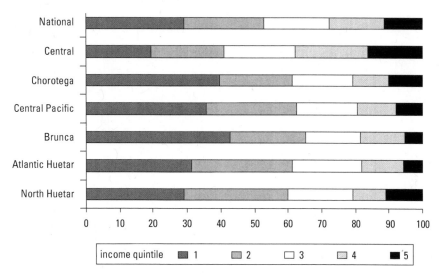

*Sources:* Based on data from INEC2001.

**Figure 8.7  Costa Rica: Health Expenditures and Contributions to CCSS, by Income Decile**

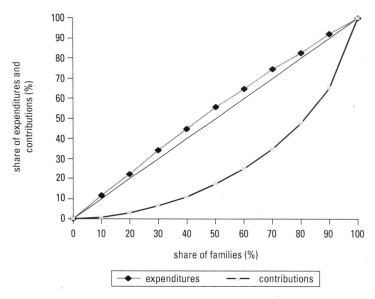

*Source:* Duran 2005.

families (richest 10 percent of all families) make 35 percent of the contributions but account for only 8 percent of the expenditures.

A final element that deserves special attention is the financial sustainability of the health sector. At the present time, an important list of factors jeopardizes its financial sustainability:

- *Progressive aging of the population.* People over 60 years of age represent a significant financial burden for the population. In 2002, health care for a person in this group was 3.4 times more expensive than a person aged 15 to 59 years and 4.4 times more expensive than a person 0 to 14 years old.

- *Low rates of affiliation among economically active population (EAP).* Only 52 percent of total EAP (61 percent of the salaried EAP and 38 percent of the non-salaried EAP) are affiliated with the system.

- *Evasion and default revenues are still high.* Despite recent measures to control these two problems, evasion and default are still high. According to the CCSS, evasion in the service sector is 35 percent of potential revenues; 27 percent in commerce; and 12 percent in agriculture (CCSS 2007). In total, 29 percent of potential revenues are evaded by employers. An estimated 40 percent of salaried workers and 60 percent of nonsalaried workers under-report their wages.

- *Government continuing default conditions.* The government usually pays a fraction of mandatory contributions for public employees and contributions to protect poor families. A growing backlog of debt owed by the state is one of the financial limitations faced by the CCSS. By 2005, 45 percent of the total debt to CCSS had a public origin (SUPEN 2006).

- *Incentives for evasion and inconsistencies between contributions and costs.* Differential rates favoring independent workers are an incentive for evasion. Lower contributory rates are also dissociated from the real costs of carrying these contributors, creating a permanent "deficit" in special groups like pensioners, independent workers, and others.

- *Poor mechanisms to verify the socioeconomic conditions of state-subsidized families.* For want of resources to check the veracity of statements filed by state-subsidized beneficiaries, the CCSS usually approves payments without further ado.

- *Increasing hospital costs.* Hospital costs (in real terms) are growing faster than any other spending component, as seen above.

Duran (2005) presented the expected financial balance of the CCSS by 2050, based on the occurrence of certain revenue and expenditure conditions. The main lesson to be learned, in spite of the assumptions about future expenditure behavior, is that the financial sustainability of the CCSS depends on how well the institute manages to increase revenues. Even under an optimistic expenditure scenario (table 8.12), if revenue collections do not grow appropriately, the expected deficit would be 8.1 percent of total expenditures.

**Table 8.12    Costa Rica: Estimated Health Insurance Financial Balance in 2050 under Different Scenarios (percent of total expenditures)**

| Expenditures | Revenues | | |
| --- | --- | --- | --- |
| | Pessimistic | Base | Optimistic |
| Pessimistic | −31.8 | −6.1 | 2.3 |
| Base | −21.4 | 8.0 | 17.8 |
| Optimistic | −8.1 | 26.6 | 37.8 |

*Source:* Duran 2005.

## Other Issues

This section discusses a wide range of complementary issues about the health system in Costa Rica. The topic ranges from risk-sharing mechanisms to the role of labor within the sector and relationships with other entities.

*Risk sharing and cross-subsidization.* The health system in Costa Rica is based on solidarity. No matter what a person contributes to the system, he or she will have equal access to health care services. This condition where risks, benefits, and contributions are not aligned one-to-one with contribution size allows cross-subsidization in favor of lower-income or higher-risk individuals. Poor people, an estimated 620,000 individuals, are covered by the "noncontributory" and the "insured by state" regimes. Cross-subsidization goes from contributors (formal employees) to the other groups. According to actuarial studies of the CCSS, about 50 percent of the contributions from formal employees are used to cover health expenditures of pensioners, independent workers, and poorer households.

*Insurance regulation.* The system is not overseen by a formal health insurance regulator. In effect, regulatory tasks are undertaken by the Ministry of Health (health issues) and the Office of the Controller General (budgetary and financial management). The controller, the most powerful supervisory entity in Costa Rica, has extensive power to force changes or refuse decisions and uses it frequently. The controller can, for instance, approve or reject the institutional budget or recommend modifications in contracts the CCSS signs with private firms. Additionally, the controller is the final approver of any investment project (especially those involving private firms), drug purchasing, and acquisition of medical equipment. Last but not least, the controller is empowered to recommend changes in the internal processes of the CCSS (e.g., contracting, purchasing, planning). Although most of this agency's resolutions are "suggestions" to the CCSS, in the final analysis the incentive to obey is implicit because approvals are generally linked to compliance.

*Centralization and decentralization.* In 1998, the MOH launched a decentralization process to improve its stewardship functions at local level. The structure consisted of one ministerial office, one general directorate, six central directorates, nine health regions, and 81 individual health stewardship areas.

The CCSS also led a decentralization process, because excessive centralization was one of Costa Rica's key problems before the health care reform. Several measures were undertaken in the last decade to dilute CCSS centralization. For example in 1998, the Congress approved Law 7852 on Decentralization, which enhanced the autonomy of hospital directors in budgetary procurement and administrative and human resource management. The act also set up local health boards to enhance community participation in local decisions. Some administrative changes were also made, such as collecting revenues at regional centers so that contributors pay in local CCSS headquarters. Currently, the CCSS is organized around six management centers, seven sanitation regions, and 103 health care areas.

*Cost-sharing mechanisms.* Costa Rica does not have a copayments system or any other cost-sharing mechanism. Informal copayments, however, are known to be common, especially in areas with long waiting lists or in cases of urgently needed care.

*Unions in the health sector.* Medical labor unions are strong. Six labor unions have a direct relationship with the CCSS. The Sindicato de Profesionales en Ciencias Medicas (SIPROCIMECA) and the Unión Medica Nacional are the most representative of the six. The influence of medical unions can be seen in many areas. For instance, doctors have a seat on the CCSS Board of Directors and a quite different monetary incentives structure from the payment scheme applicable to all other public employees.

*Freedom of choice.* In Costa Rica, users have no freedom to choose their health care providers within the mandatory health insurance (MHI) system. The CCSS assigns a provider by a person's geographic location (residence). However, Arce and Muñoz (2001) established that there is a "de facto, unregulated freedom of choice," allowing some socially prominent or wealthy individuals to get health services in a public facility where they are not registered. This system has some characteristics of a black market. In 1992, the CCSS introduced a program that offers its affiliates a chance to choose—and pay—a private provider while the institution partially covers selected services. Services may range from surgeries to childbirth, but the final approval of the service and the economic subsidy is in the hands of the Medical Division.

*Interaction with other programs.* The Costa Rican health sector should be viewed as a health system in the sense that it is composed of many other institutions with health-related functions. One of these institutions is the National Insurance Institute, which administers the state private insurance monopoly. The institute participates in the health sector by protecting workers against the risks of labor accidents and traffic accidents, for instance.

The Costa Rican Institute of Water and Sewer Systems provides potable water supply services, collects and treats sewage and industrial liquid waste, and sets the operating norms for rainwater systems in urban areas. To finance its activities, the institute charges user fees.

Finally, the University of Costa Rica contributes to the improvement of the health sector in three ways: by educating and training health professionals, by hosting and participating in research and social action projects in the health setting, and by providing health services to the CCSS under management agreements between the two institutions. The university's health professional teaching and training actions are financed from the general budget, in turn financed through direct annual transfers from the national budget.

In addition, the CCSS is in charge of administering one of Costa Rica's pension regimes (Invalidez, Vejez y Muerte). For many years, the institution managed the health insurance system and the pension system in a single administrative body, and revenues collected from both systems were commingled. There was no transparency in the use of these resources, and how much each system collected individually was not clear. The health reform separated the two systems and created the a Pension Division, to deal exclusively with this issue. Revenue collection is still in the hands of one entity, the Financial Division, which collects funds through the Centralized System of Revenue Collection (Sistema Centralizado de Recaudación, SICERE).

## Overview of the Health Delivery System

This section presents a brief characterization of the network of providers involved in the Costa Rican health system. It describes the availability of health-related inputs, the regulatory framework governing providers and the insurance market, and the role of other components of the delivery system. The most important weaknesses and strengths of the system are also assessed.

### Supply and Organization of Hospitals, Physicians, and Public Health Programs

For the understanding of the supply-side structure, this section discussed a series of critical elements regarding the organization of the network of providers and the availability of resources.

*Organization of the health sector and the network of providers.* Institutionally speaking, the Costa Rican health system is organized around the MOH (the health policy governing, regulating, formulating, oversight, and regulatory body) and the CCSS, in charge of administering health insurance. Health insurance, as a vehicle for attending to people's health, is complemented by occupational health risk insurance and by compulsory automobile liability insurance, administered by the INS, the second institution that finances, contracts and provides health services in

Costa Rica. The private sector,[4] though relatively small, has been growing. Its services are primarily concentrated on delivering ambulatory care and marketing pharmaceuticals. System oversight and regulation have been assigned to the MOH, currently reorganizing to take on these tasks. According to García G. (2004: 2) the health sector in Costa Rica ". . . is made up of a group of institutions and organizations that are part of the public and private sectors whose direct or indirect purpose is to contribute to improving the health of people, families, and communities, whether the institutions are from the health or other sectors." The proposed distinction is founded in two executive decrees: Executive Decree No. 14313 SPPS-PLAN, dubbed "health sector constitution," which formally created the health sector in Costa Rica and which regulates its structure and organization; and Executive Decree No. 19276-S of November 9, 1989, which created the NHS and establishes the General System By-laws, in which the MOH became the governing institution. The NHS groups together the health sector institutions and four additional types of organizations, such as municipalities, communities, and institutions in charge of training health staff, and the public or private institutions providing health services.

The Costa Rican provider network is mainly publicly owned. With the health sector reform that began in the mid-1990s, the MOH became the sectoral oversight and regulatory institution, while the CCSS gained control of administering the three levels of care. The network was consolidated in one institution after many years of effort. Until the CCSS took over in 1977, hospitals and secondary-level facilities had been run by the MOH or charitable organizations. Then, the reform completed the process by integrating primary care centers under the CCSS umbrella.

The public provider network is organized around three levels of care. The first level of care, the gateway of the system, is organized around 103 health areas that provide primary care services in five programs of integral care to children, teenagers, women, other adults, and elderly people. Primary care services are provided in health centers and clinics where 895 Basic Teams for Integral Health Care (Equipos Básicos de Atención Integral en Salud, EBAIS) work, delivering health services to an average 4,705 persons per EBAIS.[5] According to the CCSS, 99 percent of the population was covered by primary care services in 2005, making the establishment of the EBAIS one of the most successful coverage-oriented policies of the reform process.

The second level of care supplies outpatient services, medical treatments, surgeries, and hospitalization in a broad range of areas including internal medicine, pediatrics, gynecology and obstetrics, and surgery in a network of 10 major clinics, 14 peripheral hospitals, and six regional hospitals.

Finally, the third level is in charge of delivering complex health services and surgeries and highly specialized treatments in a network of three general hospitals and six specialized hospitals (children, women, geriatrics, psychiatry, and rehabilitation).

**Table 8.13   Costa Rica: Health System Inputs, 1995–2002 (per 1,000 inhabitants)**

| Input | 1995 | 2000 | 2002 |
|---|---|---|---|
| Hospital beds | 1.78 | 1.50 | 1.40[a] |
| Physicians | 0.85 | 1.32 | 1.75 |
| Dentists | 0.39 | 0.43 | 0.52 |
| Pharmacists | 0.35 | 0.45 | 0.55 |
| Microbiologists | 0.28 | 0.29 | 0.31 |
| Nurses[b] | 0.56 | 0.32 | n.a. |
| Total workforce | 8.21 | 8.18 | 8.77[c] |

*Sources:* Information on hospital beds and physicians was taken from WDI 2006; information on dentists, pharmacists, microbiologists, nurses and total workforce comes from MIDEPLAN (http://www.mideplan.go.cr/sides/social/index.html).

a. Last value corresponds to 2003.

b. Figures refer to nurses employed by the CCSS only.

c. Last figure corresponds to 2004.

*Supply of resources.* The availability of health-related inputs has improved in the last decade (table 8.13). The number of physicians and pharmacists (per 1,000 habitants) increased more than 50 percent between 1995 and 2002; the number of dentists, by one third. Only nurses seemed to decline over time, but this situation is explained by three factors. First, the figure represents only nurses hired by the CCSS, an entity that has been representing a lower share of the total health workforce (though still the biggest). Second, in the same line, many nurses work independently or for the private sector. Third, there has been a brain drain of nurses migrating to other markets (especially to the United States) for better working opportunities. Despite this, the MOH-PAHO-CCSS 2004) estimated there were 1.1 nurses per 1,000 inhabitants in Costa Rica, a higher figure than in similar countries like Chile (1.0 nurses), Argentina (0.52 nurses), and Uruguay (0.7 nurses).

Total staff working for the CCSS (still the most important health-related employer and the second biggest employer in Costa Rica) increased 27 percent (1995 to 2004) due to the significant growth among health professionals (3.2 percent per year). Policies to increase primary care coverage are a critical factor for understanding these accelerated dynamics. As part of the consolidation of the EBAIS, the CCSS hired many general practitioners and primary care technicians early in project implementation. Between 1995 and 1997, the CCSS created 1,180 positions to launch the first EBAIS, and in 2005 more than 3,000 employees worked for EBAISs.

In contrast, hospital beds have been declining in the last years. Between 1995 and 2005, the number of beds (in CCSS hospitals) fell from 6,035 to 5,823 beds. This situation is in line with the reform objectives of improving efficiency by limiting the capacity of general and specialized hospitals, ultimately giving primary care more predominance.

## Regulatory Framework

The General Act on Health empowered the MOH to regulate the health sector through the Central Directorate of Health Services, the Directorate for Protection of the Human Environment, and the Directorate of Records and Controls. The MOH has the right to control benefits, set up tariffs, and define which providers can participate in the market.

The MOH has organized a health regulation system in three subsystems: regulation of health services, regulation of health inputs, and regulation of the environment. The first subsystem regulates providers by establishing a minimum set of standards to be met by providers for licensure and accreditation. This regulation applies to both public and private providers and is oriented mainly to defining standards in terms of infrastructure and health service quality. The MOH is also in charge of regulating pharmaceuticals (regulation of health inputs), and was therefore the institution that approved a drug-registration regulation for the distribution of new pharmaceuticals in the country. Jointly with the laboratories of the University of Costa Rica and the CCSS, the MOH controls the quality of medications.

In terms of environmental regulation, serious conservation problems were observed in the last decade regarding water pollution (explained by inappropriate waste management in coffee factories), soil erosion, and progressive deterioration of the forests. The MOH with the Ministry of Environment implemented some specific measures to reduce environmental problems, and some improvements have been observed. For instance, the coffee-related pollution, once responsible for 21 percent of industrial pollution, has fallen to 5 percent in recent years.

Despite significant progress in the field, regulation is still incomplete. First, the regulation of private providers is weak, unclear, and does not adequately protect patients. Minimum standards in terms of equipment, infrastructure, staff, health service quality, protocols, monopolistic competition, and market control are not sufficient to regulate private providers effectively. Similarly, the management agreement, the key CCSS tool for regulating its public and nonprofit providers, is a good instrument but incomplete due to the absence of sanctions for noncompliance with the negotiated terms.

## Other Components

This section presents the main features of four elements that complement the Costa Rican health system: medical education, the supply and distribution of drugs, medical technology, and information systems.

*Medical education.* Medical education has a long tradition in Costa Rica. The School of Medicine of the University of Costa Rica is one of the oldest faculties in the nation. Traditionally, a medical degree has conferred high status and is very attractive to high school students and to private universities[6] as well. Beginning with two medical schools, the number started growing after 1985. By 2005, Costa Rica had 11 teaching faculties for medicine and other health-related disciplines (like physiotherapy). The number of graduates increased even faster. Between 1990 and 1995, the number of new doctors more than doubled, while the general population grew just 10 percent. The system has been unable to absorb the new doctors, especially because the CCSS (which used to hire more than 80 percent of the national doctors) now hires around 50 percent. The proliferation of new schools reflects the absence of a needs-based national plan for human resources and the paucity of regulations on the issue. Accreditation of new schools (in the hands of two national councils where the MOH has no participation) is done according to administrative criteria (e.g., fulfillment of faculty conditions, laboratory standards) and not according to real needs. This situation also creates problems in the market. The CENDEISS (the center in charge of planning human resource needs and training requirements within the CCSS) cannot provide slots for every new doctor. The graduates without a post usually start practicing on their own, pushing down the consultation costs.

*Pharmaceutical supply and distribution.* Drug spending in Costa Rica exceeded US$200 million in 2005, and the CCSS is the most important single purchaser (38 percent of total drug expenditures). Both supply and distribution are concentrated in a few companies (oligopolistic markets), and the top seven CCSS suppliers furnish 50 percent of the institutional drug purchases. In the private market, competition is greater, and the top five laboratories handle 28 percent of private drug purchases. Such high concentration has a negative impact on medicine costs. To improve access to some key medicines, the MOH has exerted partial control over some drugs. During 2000, the ministry made available a free phone service to orient users about the price of certain drugs and to provide therapeutic information.

Distribution is even more concentrated in a few companies. Although the market has more than 40 drug distributors, the top two firms account for 42 percent of drug sales, and the top four companies handle 61 percent of all sales. The College of Pharmacists lists about 850 pharmacies in the entire country. The CCSS has defined a list of official drugs (399 active principles classified in 54 therapeutic groups) that all the pharmacies must stock. In addition, every pharmacy must have a graduate pharmacist to provide free client services.

*Medical technology.* Research and innovation practice is regulated by the MOH. Public health experts generally believe that the system devotes too few resources to improving research and innovation. Costa Rica has a wide range of institutions in charge of different health sector tasks. For example, public health research is developed by the Institute of Health Research and by the Clodomiro Picado Institute (University of Costa Rica). There are three more public entities with very different profiles: a research institute on nutrition, a national drug center, and an institute on alcoholism and pharmacodependency.

*Information systems.* Despite the existence of many heath information systems (HIS) in the CCSS, they play a minor role in policy making. Strategic planning, critically lacking before the reform, has been weakly incorporated into the daily tasks of the CCSS. The information collected by the HIS is used mostly for following up the contract performance but rarely for estimating population needs. The high rates of evasion and default force the CCSS to improve collection using modern tools. In 2001, the CCSS installed the Sistema Centralizado de Recaudación (Centralized Collection System, SICERE) to ease management procedures for billing and contribution collection.

## Strengths and Weaknesses of the System

Table 8.14 summarizes the major strengths and weaknesses of the Costa Rican health system. The list includes mainly the aspects assessed above and some other issues derived from the analysis.

**Table 8.14   Costa Rica: Major Strengths and Weaknesses of the Health Sector**

| Strengths | Weaknesses |
|---|---|
| Solid institutions with more than 50 years of operations; strong national health system | Falling rates of contributory coverage among economically active population |
| Strong political support from all sectors | Weak regulation in key areas like medical education |
| Functional solidarity principle | Increasing hospital costs |
| Universal access to primary care centers and wide access to public hospitals | Problems with service quality, especially in hospitals |
| Positive incidence of benefits among poorer income groups, whose benefits exceed their financial contributions to the system | Persistent gaps in equity and health outcome by gender and between regions |
| High financial protection, especially for poorer households; low out-of-pocket expenditures and no cost sharing mechanisms (formal) | Lack of adequate long-term strategic planning |
| Extensive benefits package | Slow transition to full performance-based system |
| High levels of equity between rural and urban areas | Weak internal organization of CCSS |
| Stable public financing over the years | High rates of evasion and default |
| Strong external control from other public institutions to avoid corruptive practices | No freedom of choice |
| Adequate number of health professionals | Lack of consolidated medical technology program |
| Low dependence on external funds | Excessive number of medical schools |
| Cumulative experience transformed into concrete outcomes | Not a patient-centered system |

*Source:* Author elaboration based on previous sections.

## Health Coverage Reforms

Between 1943 and 1990, policies to increase health insurance coverage were oriented mainly to increase the *breadth of coverage* (that is, the number of individuals covered by health insurance). The health reform of 1994 shifted emphasis to *depth of coverage* (that is, the increasing of the share of the population with access to primary care services).

### Policies Oriented to Increase Health Coverage

Since the 1940s, with the creation of the CCSS, efforts were made to make social security coverage in Costa Rica universal and to maintain what had already been achieved in health. As first conceived, the health insurance scheme covered only public employees and manufacturing workers. Later, CCSS expanded the breadth of coverage to include farmers, independent workers, and unemployed/poor people.

In 1961, the Congress approved Act 2,738 and established universal health insurance for workers and their families. This reform represents the turning point in health insurance coverage by including family dependents as insurance beneficiaries. This reform became the most important step toward universalization of health insurance in Costa Rica.

In 1973, Act 5,349 transferred to the CCSS all public hospitals previously controlled by the Ministry of Health. The act defined the first bases of a social assistance program in which the government engaged to pay for health services for poor people. Although this effort was not a formal health insurance program for the poor, it at least guaranteed poorer families greater access to health services.

Later, in 1975, the CCSS expanded health insurance coverage to farmers and independent workers. A year later, the Board of Directors (BOD) established the obligation of all inactive pensioners to be insured under the sickness and maternity scheme. In 1978, the CCSS created and regulated the voluntary health insurance scheme for independent workers. Then in 1984, the government of President Monge created the state-subsidized insurance plan for covering poorer families and unemployed persons. Unlike the program established in 1973, this was a permanent insurance program with all the characteristics of a health insurance plan. The last two milestones in the long history of coverage-related policies occurred in 2000 and 2006. In 2000, the Act of Worker Protection declared all independent workers' obligation to join the health insurance program. More recently, the CCSS reformed the health insurance regulations for the first time in 10 years. The reform allows affiliated workers to cover handicapped brothers or sisters who cannot work. Also, the affiliated can insure brothers or sisters taking care of their parents if the parents are handicapped and over 65 years old. Finally, the reform expands health insurance protection to students younger than 25 and registered in nonuniversity tertiary education centers (like university colleges and parauniversity institutes). Formerly, only students below 25 years of age and studying at universities were protected by the legislation.

The economic crisis at the end of the 1970s and the beginning of the 1980s caused a major upheaval in Costa Rica's public finances. Health sector investments abruptly ceased, and service coverage could not be broadened. In addition, within the context of state reform at the beginning of the 1990s, a health sector assessment identified the most relevant problems to be solved to improve health system efficiency and effectiveness. These included: structural, organizational, and functional fragmentation; deficiencies in the regulatory framework; inefficiency and inequity in resource allocation; service-scheduling deficiencies arising from excessive centralization; nonexistence of demand self-regulation mechanism as a result of the privileged position given to tertiary care at the expense of integral individual care; lack of continuity in user care, caused by the nonexistence of a referral and counter-referral framework and by overspecialization in medical practice; dissatisfaction among service users and providers; and inadequate training in human resource management.

A critical problem in the sector before 1990 was low coverage for primary care services. before 1990, around 82 percent of the population was covered by health insurance. Nonetheless, the traditional PHC model was dilapidated, people did not have access to a nearby PHC facility (within 30 minutes of their residence). PHC coverage dropped from 46 percent in 1990 to 25 percent in 1995. Thus, the main challenge was not to increase *breadth of coverage* but *depth of coverage.*

## The Health Sector Reform: Policies and Evaluation

To deal with these problems, the health sector reform was organized into three broad areas for action: the financing model, institutional reorganization, and modernizing management of the service provider network.

*Financing model.* For almost 40 years, social security financing had experienced legal constraints on enforcing mandatory affiliation. The reform sought to reduce this problem by promoting two critical elements: (1) increasing contribution coverage by designing means of enforcing compulsory contributions, setting up systems for tracking evasion, and extending contribution coverage to the independent workers; and (2) redesigning the financing model, redefining contribution rates for independent workers and pensioners, and modifying the system for calculating state contributions to the CCSS to cover the poor and the uninsured.

Efforts to reform the financing model were not entirely successful, partly due to unforeseen events. The main results from the reform period may be summarized as follows:

*The gap between contributions and real expenses per insured began to narrow.* As a percentage of GDP, health insurance contributions were stable at around 5 percent between 1990 and 2004. The differential between real income and real expense per direct insured has been falling. Between 1990 and 1999, the "surplus" per direct insured was 21 colones. After 2000, it declined to 10 colones, indicating that the subsidy to noncontributors had fallen to less than half. In 2003, the real contribution was insufficient to cover the real expense incurred in meeting the insured parties' demand for health services.

The Costa Rica's ongoing demographic transition partly explains this spending behavior. Arias (2004) points out other factors affecting the trend toward financial imbalance. These include evasion, late contributions, deficiencies in insurance administration, and inappropriate use of medical insurance by insured family members. Arias, for 2003, estimated evasion in the noncontributing, independent, and retired regimens at C 143,179 billion (US$359 million), equivalent to 51 percent of collections from the salaried worker regimen.

*Increases in the contributions have relieved the funding shortfall.* Modifications in premiums are always a big change, because more than 90 percent of health insurance income comes from member contributions. Contributions began to increase, beginning in 2000, but other unsolved financing problems appeared:

- State contributions for financing the regimens cover only 14 percent of the effective costs.
- Contribution evasion is estimated at around 30 percent of the regulatory health insurance income.
- High defaults on payments by employers and even the state (as an employer) also weaken the financial structure of the CCSS. In 2005, the state and employers owed the CCSS C 50.2 billion (US$106 million), 86 percent of it owed by the state.[7]

*The CCSS contribution coverage has been decreasing.* Both salaried and non-salaried worker coverage has decreased in the last decade (figure 8.8). Between 2000 to 2004 the share of independent workers, contributing to the CCSS declined from above 80 percent to just under 40 percent—although a significant part of this decline is due to the introduction of a new method for estimating the size of the independent workers labor market. For salaried workers the declining trend implied a fall of the coverage rate from 75.3 percent in 1990 to 61.8 percent in 2004 in that group. In the last two years, the CCSS added 114,000 workers contributing to health insurance. Thus, for example, in September 2004, 1,076,028 workers were contributing to insurance, as compared with 961,266 in 2003, a 12 percent increase in coverage.

*Financial protection for the population, especially the poorer groups, is good, judging by evidence from national surveys.* According to estimates in the Survey on Household Revenues and Expenditures (SHRE 2006), Costa Rican households allocate 2.6 percent of their income to health spending, 4.1 percent of current, noncapital spending. Most household health expenditures go to specialist/hospital services and drugs, and such expenses affect urban households (5.1 percent of their income) more than rural families (3.6 percent). The share of health expenditures in the fifth quintile is approximately 6.6 percent of their income, 3.7 times higher than the share of health expenses in poorer households (first quintile). In other

Figure 8.8    Costa Rica: Health Insurance Coverage, of Economically Active Population 1990–2004

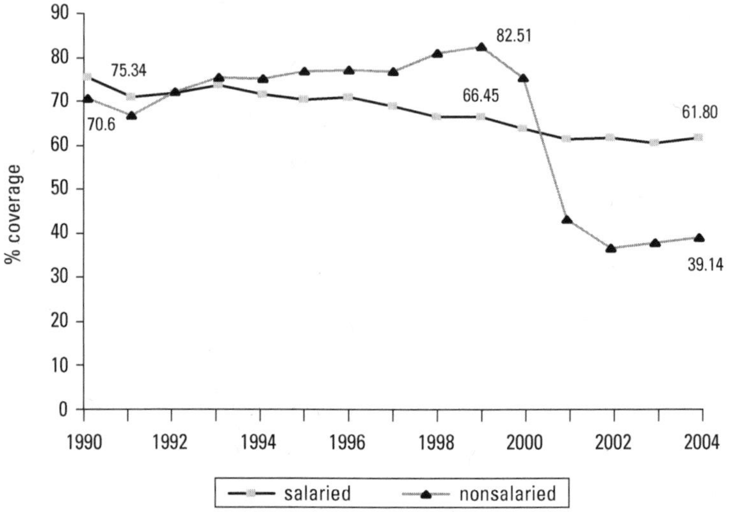

*Source:* Proyecto Estado de la Nación 2005.

words, wealthier families are responsible for most of the out-of-pocket spending. Poorer households are not only less encumbered by health spending, but their burden also decreased between 1998 and 2004. In 1988, the SHRE reported that poor households allocated 2.1 percent of their income to cover health expenditures. By 2004, that share declined by 15 percent to 1.8 percent of their spending.

***Institutional reorganization.*** The institutional reorganization entailed strengthening CCSS and MOH by establishing four strategic functions, separating management and financing of health and pension benefits, and modernizing provider network management. The Law on Decentralization of 1998 was a key instrument in this reorganization.

*A key element of the sector-wide reforms was to clearly separate the stewardship functions, assumed fully by the MOH, from the financing, purchasing and provision functions which were managed by the CCSS.* The MOH assumed the tasks related to oversight, coordination, and regulation of the system. The CCSS took over the insurer and health service provider functions at the three traditional levels, including health promotion and preventive services previously carried out by the MOH. This process went into operation beginning in 1998. One of the more important actions was the establishment of the Sector Council as a coordination body, under the supervision of the MOH, to be used to manage and lead sector policies. This was done despite the fact that its autonomy allowed the CCSS a fair amount of discretion in its own governance and policy formulation and planning.

*Four strategic functions were established within the MOH*: political direction and leadership, health oversight, technological research and development, and health development regulation (MOH 2002). Some major progress in the ministry's oversight and regulatory function included the formulation of the National Health Policy 2002 to 2006, the publication of the joint health sector agenda for 2002 to 2006, implementation of the Institutional Evaluation and Development System (SEDI in Spanish), design and implementation of the national health account system, and evaluation of integral first-level care.

*The administrative separation of financing from purchasing and provision in health services, and separation of pensions from health, were the most prominent features of the CCSS institutional reforms in the past decade.* Within the new health insurance structure, three basic functions were defined: health service financing, health service purchasing, and health service provision. Carrying out these new functions required certain changes, such as the creation in 1999 of the health service purchasing management area, responsible for service planning and purchasing activities and the approval of the Law on Decentralization of the CCSS Hospitals and Clinics in 1998. As a result of this process, overlapping subsidies between the two types of insurance (health and pensions) were eliminated, and administrative costs were efficiently allocated between the two insurers. The process, however, has run into some difficulties, and some challenges still lay ahead. They include:

- Some interest groups within the CCSS are opposed to the reorganization.
- The health service purchasing management area was assigned to the CCSS administrative division without any clear, direct link to the financial division. Therefore, the planning and purchasing processes lack an appropriate interrelationship to facilitate financial and budget scheduling, resource allocation, and service provision.
- The institutional reorganization needs to be redefined in terms of processes instead of structures. This means moving from the prevailing activity-oriented approach (enrollment, administration, statistics) to a more integrated approach (the health service purchasing cycle, for instance). This situation is equally required in both the MOH and the CCSS. In any case, the new institutional structure should be defined according to the new approach that favors increased decentralization, enhanced quality of care, improved health network management, and a performance-based orientation (Arce and Sáenz 2002).
- Although the MOH has made significant advances in strengthening the stewardship function in the sector, there is a large unfinished agenda with regard to how the MOH interacts with the CCSS in terms of oversight of the financing and provision of care and in terms of the development of public health activities in the sector. Furthermore, MOH activities in the environmental, food and drug safety and technology assessment have lagged considerably behind.

- The regionalization system used needs to be brought back to the table because the CCSS and the MOH use two different systems. Staff, financial resources, and materials are unnecessarily duplicated, and efficiency suffers when attempting to coordinate sector policies.

*Law 7852 on Decentralization of 1998 contributed to the regulation process in three essential aspects of the health reform process.* First, it promoted administrative decentralization in the CCSS. Second, it created Health Boards as community groups that promote the involvement of community leaders, democratically elected, to supervise the delivery of services from the perspective of responsiveness to the population's needs and expectations. Finally, the law introduced the possibility of eliminating the life-time tenure enjoyed by hospital directors and promoted additional measures to improve incentives for hospital management.

*Service provider network management modernization.* In provider network management, the modernization reform was intended to replace the traditional financing plan, based on the historic budget, with a more prospective arrangement, in which service production and compliance with quality standards were indicators that would define budget allocation. A first attempt was made at the end of the 1980s with the introduction of cooperatives and single payments that predefined a coverage region. Later, in 1997, management agreements were introduced, which generated major changes.

*Primary care has become more prominent in total expenses.* Between 1997 and 2004, the proportion or resources allocated to primary care increased from 19 to 22 percent. This increase was financed by reducing the rate of growth of hospital expenditures, thereby reducing the overall allocation to hospital services in favor of increasing funds for primary care. The real expenses incurred over this period illustrate the impact that resource allocation has had on primary care. For ambulatory services, actual expenses increased 78 percent, versus a 55 percent increase in hospital expenses.

*The targeting of health reform to the poorest areas, with the greater socioeconomic needs, produced significant gains in access to care and health outcomes.* Rosero-Bixby (2004) has shown that key indicators, such as infant mortality, decreased more rapidly in these areas because they were targeted in the first phase of the reforms.[9]

*Primary care coverage results.* Readjusting the health care model favored an integral and social health promotion approach. The pivotal point of the readjustment was the creation of the health areas (103 areas in 2005) based on geographic-population criteria and criteria pertaining to accessibility, population distribution, and the country's political-administrative divisions. Each health area was subdivided into segments that were assigned at least one EBAIS. The number of primary care establishments with an EBAIS team has grown constantly since

**Figure 8.9   Costa Rica: Primary Health Care Program Coverage, 1990–2003**

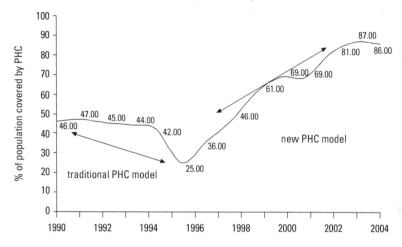

*Source:* CCSS.

1995. Thus, for example, 232 establishments were founded in 1995, and by 2004 there were 855 EBAIS, (i.e., 3.7 times more that at the beginning of the program). Priorities were determined for each region, based on the population's epidemiological profile, which was a major step in defining needs-based plans. The new model that accompanied the health reform in 1994 strengthened the role of primary care through the EBAIS. In terms of coverage, the rate jumped from 36 percent of the population in 1995 to 69 percent in 2000, and to 86 percent in 2003 (figure 8.9). According to the presidency of the Republic, practically everyone in Costa Rica was covered by the primary health care (PHC) program in 2005. As a result of the Reform, the percentage of people without equitable access to primary health services dropped by 15% between 1994 and 2000 in areas where health sector reform was implemented in 1995–1996, whereas areas that had not yet initiated health sector reform in 2000 experienced only a 3% reduction.

In addition to the reorganization of the network by health areas and the creation of the EBAIS, another strategy developed by the CCSS to increase PHC delivery entailed the introduction of special partnership models between the CCSS and nonprofit institutions. The first attempts to resolve shortcomings in primary care coverage started in 1988 when the CCSS broke the traditional public-based delivery model and began purchasing health services from health cooperatives. Because the early experiences were successful in terms of quality and cost, the CCSS decided to expand the program during the reform period. By 2004, the CCSS had established management agreements with four cooperatives and one foundation (belonging to the University of Costa Rica), covering more than 10 percent of the Costa Rican population.

## Key Conditions for Success

In both breadth and depth of coverage, Costa Rica is a high performer but not problem-free. In terms of breadth, coverage is close to universal, with almost 90 percent of the population affiliated to the CCSS. By 2006, 3.9 million people (89.2% of the population) were affiliated to CCSS in any of the health insurance programs that exist for that purpose (direct, self-insured, State, pensioners). Important internal problems regarding financing and administration persist, but over the years the CCSS has been transformed into one of the most solid institutions in Costa Rica. In terms of *depth of coverage*, the reform has also been successful. In less than 12 years, the system moved from a 25 percent coverage rate (primary care services) to 99 percent in 2005. Again, the EBAIS model improved access and the role of primary care in the system, although some problems persist in service quality and immunization coverage.

The reform results suggest a net positive balance overall. Among the main factors explaining the success of the reform are:

*Political commitment: the two most important political parties agreed change was needed, the new government in 1994 followed through, and stakeholders were involved in the process.* Although the *Partido Liberación Nacional* and the *Partido Unidad Social Cristiana* did not agree on every detail, they did agree on the need for health care reform and strongly backed the process, allowing the Reform to continue despite alternation of the presidency in 1994. The rapid approval of the reform loans in the Congress was a signal of such political support. The Ministry of Planning and the CCSS itself were heavily involved in the design and implementation of the reform.

Opposition to the reform existed, but it was more the result of sporadic groups than the collective opposition of key stakeholders. Transparency and continuous communication were critical to facilitate the implementation. *Mixed commissions* were created to involve unions and hospitals in the discussion and the understanding of the process. This support took unusual dimensions. The pilot test of the new resource allocation model was, for instance, publicly supported by the hospitals included in the sample. In short, one of the main advantages of the Costa Rican case was the relatively general consensus among the main stakeholders: government/CCSS, opposition, unions, and providers.

*Origin of the reform: the idea for health reform came from within the health sector, not from outside.* This special feature has allowed the reform process to unfold smoothly without confrontations between key institutions like the CCSS and the MOH.

*Availability of funds: political support was expressed in economic support.* The reform program was financed with external loans and local contributions. The first loan amounted to US$22 million from the World Bank, and it was part of a US$32 million project for financing the core component of the reform agenda. A second loan was approved by the Inter-American Development Bank, for US$42 million. The total cost of the second project amounted to US$60 million.

**BOX 8.1** *Costa Rica: Cooperatives as Health Care Providers*

The introduction of market-like mechanisms began in 1988 with the introduction of the first health care cooperatives. Each cooperative was founded by the employees of a primary health care clinic. They formed autonomous, legal entities that assumed responsibility for managing the facility. The facilities were leased from the CCSS to the cooperative for a yearly fee of US$1, and all equipment and infrastructure were transferred to the cooperative. From this point on, the cooperative assumed full responsibility for maintaining the transferred equipment and buying new equipment (unless cooperatives could prove that damage or deterioration of the transferred equipment were due to faulty construction or quality). The cooperatives bought drugs, medical supplies, and other inputs from CCSS centers at cost plus 15 percent for administrative and shipping expenses, or directly from the market. The same services as in public clinics were provided, and the catchment population continued to be the residents of the geographic area served by the cooperative. The cooperatives received a yearly capitation fee based on the estimated number of members in the geographic area. No additional services were provided or fees charged by the cooperatives, because the new model was supposed to maintain an identical package of services with only a change in management responsibility. The cooperatives were, however, allowed to charge uninsured individuals seeking care on equal terms with the CCSS clinics. Several groups had strongly opposed the introduction of cooperatives because they suspected that it was effectively a privatization. This, they viewed as a renunciation by the state of its responsibility to provide free or low-cost health services.

In 1988, a self-managing cooperative, COOPESALUD R.L., was named service administrator and put in charge of the CCSS Pavas Clinic. Cooperative management was selected by an administrative council, elected every two years by the general assembly of all cooperative members. Legally, all workers in the cooperatives became shareholders and periodically received earnings generated by the cooperative. The cooperatives operated under private law, without public encumbrances related to contracting, firing, and management of personnel and resources. The cooperatives enjoyed income tax exemptions and considerable political support. They had full autonomy to manage the capitated payments from the CCS, but were obliged to present annual financial statements to the CCSS for external audit. All profits were either reinvested in new equipment or infrastructure or distributed to cooperative members. In return, the cooperatives were required to follow the guidelines and policy objectives set by the CCSS and the Ministry of Health. The contracts signed with the CCSS obliged cooperatives to provide the following services: general and specialized medicine, emergency care, minor surgery, dental care, pharmaceuticals, laboratory and radiology services, biopsies, laboratory smear tests, social work services, services related to rights and benefits verification, transportation for patients, and support services.

Gauri, Cercone, and Briceno (2004) showed that cooperatives conducted an average of 9.7 to 33.8 percent more general visits, 27.9 to 56.6 percent more dental visits, and 28.9 to 100 percent fewer specialist visits than CCSS clinics. The number of nonmedical, emergency, and first-time visits per capita were no different from the traditional public clinics. These results suggest that the cooperatives substituted generalist for specialist services and offered additional dental services, but did not turn away new patients, refuse emergency cases, or substitute nurses for doctors as care providers.

*Source:* Gauri, Cercone, and Briceno 2004.

Most of the funds were allocated for modernization of the primary care network. In total, US$17 million from Project 1 and US$19 million from Project 2 were assigned to primary care transformation.

*Wide participation of main stakeholders: CCSS workers (especially medical staff), MOH staff, medical doctors, and communities all participated in the reform process.* The information given the stakeholders was transparent. Although several groups opposed the reforms, as was to be expected, continuous negotiation and consensus building allowed the main part of the reform to go forward. Nonetheless, the original reform agenda has still not been fully implemented, and some elements are missing. For instance, the issue of allowing patients the right to choose their provider has not yet been considered.

*Priority to rural and poor areas: the first EBAIS were launched in rural areas, particularly in poor regions.* Almost all of the first 229 EBAIS were opened in poor, rural areas, following social equity principles. This has allowed the system to gain quick benefits and to create a solid basis of support for further changes. This is a distinctive characteristic of the health coverage reform.

*Strong technical team: all members of the team were highly qualified.* The group of professionals that designed and implemented the reform and the "political team" (the BOD and the executive president of the CCSS) had a solid background in similar tasks, an understanding of the national problems, and experience in negotiating key changes.

*Clear reform objectives: The CCSS was clear about its objectives.* Although there were many problems at the time of the assessment, technical and political efforts had to be concentrated on just some of them. Putting too many objectives and "components" in the reform agenda may dilute the strength of the reform.

*Transformation of the CCSS for a sustained reform process.* Changes in the model meant that some internal reorganization had to be made in the way the CCSS functions. Some measures were implemented, like the creation of a Purchasing Unit and the establishment of the CENDEISS, the department in charge of training CCSS staff.

*Continuous monitoring and evaluation.* The reform was constantly monitored to verify that different measures had been adopted and observe the outcomes.

*Focus on access to primary care.* The health sector reform greatly benefited from expanding PHC services rather than concentrating on hospital care. The new strategy moved to a PHC-centered delivery model that increased coverage in rural areas and improved physical access to basic health services throughout the country. This strategy yielded concrete benefits during the first two years of implementation. In about a decade, the new PHC model achieved nearly full coverage. The outcomes of the new strategy were the result of multiple concurrent factors: institutional transformations, community participation in decision making, increased budgets, enhanced participation by the for-profit and nonprofit sectors, adequate planning, and incorporation of quality standards.

## The Outlook for Further Reform

Perhaps corruption is the most important enemy of the reform process at this moment. A critical case of corruption, known as "the Finnish scandal," hit the CCSS in 2004 when the general prosecutor of the republic brought charges for misappropriation of funds against the CEO of the institution, together with a former president of the republic, members of the BOD and staff of Corporación Fischel.[10] According to the brief, the CCSS had been granted a US$39 million loan from the government of Finland for modernizing the hospital network. At least half of the loan was tied to purchases of Finnish products. The contract was awarded to the Finnish consortium Instrumentarium Corporation Medko Medical, and a commission of US$8.8 million (20 percent of the value of the loan) was paid to Corporación Fischel (the consortium's Costa Rican representative). Part of this commission was paid to bank accounts of CCSS board members and former president. The scandal severely damaged citizens' confidence in the efficiency of the institution. The common perception of the effects of corruption scandals in the CCSS is that they greatly affect the health services.

The 2004 scandals severely curtailed any effort to implement further changes in the organizational, financing, and delivery model. Many consulted experts believe that any attempt to change the status quo is now associated with corruption and is under strict public scrutiny. As a result, reforms have slowed down and are more difficult to put into action.

Despite substantial progress in the overall health model, the reform still lags in several areas. Some of those topics will definitely be "points of disagreement" between the CCSS and other stakeholders or within the CCSS. Among the most important issues are

- The monopoly of the CCSS in the administration of health insurance schemes in Costa Rica. Should the market open to new insurers? Privatization has no room in Costa Rica at this moment (the CCSS is the public institution with the greatest support from the citizenship), but market openness should be discussed in more detail.

- Free choice of providers, especially of hospital services.

- Implementation of new financing mechanisms beyond the current tripartite model.

- The definition of a modern institutional organization. This was discussed in the early reform years but never appear in the final agenda. Moreover, the 2004 scandal was facilitated by the "restructuring process" implemented by the new CCSS authorities, which gave managers more power and decision-making autonomy. Thus, any plan to further change the administrative structure usually arouses suspicion and encounters obstacles to its full implementation.

## Lessons for Policy Makers

The enabling factors (financial, institutional, others) that create adequate conditions for success in the field of health coverage are analyzed in this last section. Some elements of the Costa Rican political economy are evaluated, and some lessons are derived for possible use by policy makers in low- and middle-income countries.

### Enabling Technical and Political Factors

From the Costa Rican experience, the key enabling factors for the success of a coverage-oriented reform are

*The political actors must compromise to reach a consensus and follow through.* In Costa Rica, the reform was designed by one government but implemented by the opposition in the next presidential term. Achieving commitment implies constant dialog, negotiation, and consensus building with the main stakeholders.

*Designing a health reform is a complex exercise that demands technically sound strategies.* It requires adequate diagnosis of the sector, an economic and political strategy for implementation, and incorporation of country-specific conditions. When designing a reform, it is important to single out some key aspects on which most of the effort will be concentrated, instead of trying to solve every problem at the same time. Appropriate phases of the reform should also be discussed.

*Sustainability of the reform depends on the financial support throughout implementation.* This implies two things. First, there must be a "short-term" budget to launch the program, such as the two loans Costa Rica had. Second, it is critical to commit to investing resources for the long haul. The example of Costa Rica shows that, if sustained over time, health investments pay off. Since 1950, Costa Rica has allocated ever-increasing amounts of money to the health sector. As a result, life expectancy increased from 45 years in the mid-1940s to almost 80 years in the mid-2000s.

*Active participation by local communities in decision making is an important part of reform design.* Final users who help shape the reform will understand the scope of the changes. Opposition (usually heated in health-related issues) will cool off.

*Ask which measures will yield positive benefits in the short term.* It is hard for people to accept change if they cannot quickly see some benefits. In Costa Rica, the first steps were oriented to increasing coverage in rural and poor communities.

*Private participation is important.* Anything but public service delivery invites opposition in many countries. However, in countries where the network of providers is thin and the needs urgent, the contribution of the private sector may be critical to avoid bureaucratic regulations that can delay infrastructure projects, for instance.

## Institutional Financing Arrangements

Parallel to changes in the health sector, some internal administrative and organizational transformation should be implemented:

*Creation of the Purchasing Unit was the most important organizational change introduced in the CCSS during the reform period.* Separating purchasing from provision functions has allowed a single department to concentrate fully on planning, negotiating, monitoring, and evaluating the performance of health care providers. At the same time, this separation has permitted the Purchasing Unit to focus on coverage issues.

*Both clinical and nonclinical staff were trained on the new orientations of the model.* During reform implementation, the CENDEISS did the training CCSS staff. Giving a training program permanent status, with its own budget and clear long-term objectives, might be a good idea.

*Adequate information goes hand in hand with the sectoral transformation.* Good information systems allow an institution to improve its capacity to track contributions, evasions, consultancies, costs, and reporting and to improve the planning cycle. The SICERE system, for example, enables the CCSS financial management to track revenue flows daily instead of only 30 days after the fact, as before.

*Restructuring payment mechanisms could be a powerful tool to increase coverage.* In Costa Rica, the management agreements between the CCSS and primary care providers explicitly define coverage (e.g., immunization, smear) as a target to which payments will be linked.

*Clear incentives to promote administrative staff efficiency should be set up.*

## Lessons for Low- and Middle-Income Countries

The reform experience of Costa Rica suggests eight sets of lessons for low- and middle-income countries.

*Reforms can be applied even if the context is far from ideal.* Almost everyone, including workers, opposed the creation of mandatory health insurance in Costa Rica in the early 1940s. Nonetheless, the president insisted that the people needed a health insurance system for financial protection. After intensive negotiations, the project was approved in the Congress with the support of the Roman Catholic

Church, the governing party, and the Communist Party. Completely opposite forces, like the Church and the Communist Party, strongly supported the initiative.

*Health reforms take time for implementation—and results.* Changing a health service delivery model takes time. A new model demands not only new staff and equipment, but also changes in perceptions and behavior of the professionals and their prospective patients. In Costa Rica, one change was the switch in orientation from cure to prevention. Achieving full primary care coverage with services took Costa Rica less than 15 years; fully universal health insurance coverage is still a goal, after more than a half-century. Experiences will vary from country to country and from topic to topic.

*Expand primary care to reach universal coverage.* The main focus of the health sector reform in Costa Rica was the expansion of primary care services as the main channel to provide universal access to the whole population. The new strategic orientation yielded important health outcomes. The success of the PHC-oriented strategy resulted from the convergence of multiple factors. They included

- The top CCSS authorities knew a new model was needed.
- Budget increases concentrated on PHC activities.
- Cooperatives and the private sector were intelligently incorporated in health service delivery and regulated by management agreements that include specific coverage and quality targets.
- Adequate planning of the new model favored division of the country into small catchment areas, each with at least one EBAIS.
- Costa Rica is a small country with easy access to rural areas.
- Heavy investments were made in infrastructure in the first stages of reform.
- PHC coverage prereform was low, and all stakeholders recognized the need for a new model and came to support it.

*Money counts.* Without enough money, good results cannot be sustained. Budgets must be adequate to trigger the reforms and to consolidate a base for further transformations. In Costa Rica, strengthening primary care was one of the pillars of the strategy to expand coverage. The share of PHC in the total health budget of Costa Rica increased 22 percent in 10 years. With the additional money, the CCSS to set up more than 855 EBAIS, each taking care of 1,000 households (4,000 persons) throughout the country by 2006.

*The public and the private sectors, working together, can do more to improve health conditions than either sector can achieve on its own.* Costa Rica, breaking with the traditional public-centered delivery model, incorporated new provision models in which the private sector was given an important role. Both international experience and the Costa Rican case show that the private sector can be an extraordinary means of increasing coverage, especially service coverage. Participation of nonpublic entities should be limited to private firms, and to delivery, not financing. In Costa Rica, the spectrum of potential providers ranges from cooperatives to universities to nonprofit associations and NGOs. The incorporation of cooperatives and private foundations complemented CCSS efforts to extend primary care throughout the country. By incorporating the management agreements and creating an adequate regulatory framework to normalize relations between the CCSS and private providers, the model was able to launch the EBAIS in poor districts.

*Think about the needs of the disadvantaged first.* The decision to site the first EBAIS in rural and poor regions yielded multiple benefits to the reform process (see endnote 9). First, it increased equity and access in traditionally underserved communities. Second, starting with poor regions is likely to generate quick benefits. Quick benefits win recognition from different social groups, creating a solid base for further reforms.

*Be open and above board.* Transparency and accountability mechanisms should be activated at the outset to enhance communication with all interested parties and build their trust.

*Pay attention to the financial health of the system.* Costa Rica is good example of financial sustainability—but not cost containment. Contributions per insured person have been increasing, but so have costs. Real expenditure per direct contributor increased 5 percent during the 1990s, while the real contributions per direct contributor increased 11 percent (World Bank 2003). The difference has been enough to finance the deficit generated by other groups like pensioners, voluntary affiliates, and state beneficiaries. Several issues explain the dynamic behavior of contributions vis-à-vis the decelerated growth in expenditures:

- The CCSS implemented specific plans to reduce evasion and defaults.
- Waiting lists were used as cost-containment mechanisms.
- Channeling funds to PHC activities resulted in highly cost-effective interventions that allowed the system to achieve good results and helped in part to control expenditures.
- The existence of the Office of the Controller General (outside the organizational framework of the CCSS) is important to forestall irrational spending by health authorities.

The Costa Rican reform experience has shown that complex reforms in the health sector are possible if technical and political factors are considered and clear objectives are established and agreed by all stakeholders. While there is clearly an unfinished agenda to meet the challenges of quality, efficiency and user access, extensive analysis and consensus building will need to take place to ensure that the reforms continue.

## Endnotes

1. Mostly pre- and postnatal care and screening activities.

2. The colon (C) is the Costa Rican currency. The average reference exchange rate for 2003 by the BCCR US$1 = C 398.6.

3. The Lorenz Curve is a graphic representation generally used to show inequalities in the distribution of a determined variable (e.g., income, social spending, public subsidies, assets). On the x-axis, the graph shows the cumulative share of households/families. The y-axis presents the cumulative proportion of the assessed variable. Perfect equality is represented by a 45° line. If the final curve lies above 45°, the variable presents a progressive distribution. If the curve is below the 45° line, the variable is regressive.

4. Diverse estimates exist, each with a specific methodology offering different results. For example, Kleysen (1992) estimates that the relative weight of the private sector is 20 percent, while Sáenz and León (1992) calculated it at 23 percent, and Durán and Herrero (2001) at 31 percent.

5. Each EBAIS has a basic structure of one physician, one nurse, and one primary care technician.

6. In Costa Rica, there are four public universities and more than 40 private universities.

7. According to data published by *La Nación* newspaper (June 27, 2005), current debt could cover almost all the health needs for one year, including, among other items, buying medicine for all members, building new facilities, and social benefits for specific groups such as senior citizens.

8. The big reduction between 2000 (75 percent coverage) and 2001 (43 percent coverage) is partly explained by a purging of the CCSS databases. The Law for Worker Protection forced the CCSS to extend, for a five-year term, compulsory health insurance to independent workers, so only a fraction of the original group remained as voluntary affiliates.

9. The proportion of the population with poor access to health services went from 30 percent to 22 percent in the first four geographic areas (Buenos Aires, Pérez Zeledón, Golfito, Turrubares) where reform began in 1995 to 1996 (Rosero 2004).

10. The case is still pending in October 2007.

## References

Amenábar, Ana Victoria C. 2005. "Industria Farmacéutica en Costa Rica: El negocio de los medicamentos." *Revista Actualidad Económica* 18 (December 2004–January 2005): 308–9.

Arce, Claudio. 2001. *"El desempeño hospitalario: entre luces y sombras."* San José: CCSS (Unidad Coordinadora Proyecto de Reforma, Gerencia de Modernización y Desarrollo).

Arce, Claudio, and Carlos Muñoz. 2001. *La Reforma Pendiente: Introducción de Libre Elección en el Seguro de Salud.* San José: CCSS.

Arce, Claudio, and Luis Sáenz. 2002. *"Hallazgos preliminares, logros y desafíos de la reforma en el sector salud de Costa Rica durante los años noventa."* Report prepared for Proyecto Estado de la Nación [State of the Nation Project], San José.

Arias, Rodrigo. 2004. *Evasión, costos y financiamiento del seguro de salud.* San José: Departamento Actuarial, CCSS.

Gauri, Varun, James Cercone, and Rodrigo Briceno. 2004. "Separating Financing from Provision: Evidence from 10 Years of Partnership with Health Cooperatives in Costa Rica." *Health Policy and Planning* 19(5): 292–301.

CCSS (Caja Costarricense del Seguro Social). 2005. Anuario Estadístico 2004. www.ccss.sa.cr.

———. 2007. *Políticas prácticas en materia de cobertura contributiva en CCSS*. San José: CCSS.

Castro, Carlos, and Luis Sáenz. 1998. *"La Reforma del Sistema Nacional de Salud."* San José: Colección Tiempos de Cambio, MIDEPLAN.

CCP (Centro Centroamericano de Población). *Información Censal de los Cantones de Costa Rica (INFOCENSOS)*. San Jose: Universidad de Costa Rica. http://infocensos. ccp.ucr.ac.cr.

Duran, Fabio. 2005. "Hacia dónde va la Seguridad Social de Costa Rica?" In *Ensayos en Honor a Víctor Hugo Céspedes Solano*, ed. Grettel Lopez and Reinaldo Herrera. San Jose: Academia de Centroamérica.

Duran, Fabio, and Fernando Herrero. 2001. *El Sector Privado en el sistema de salud de Costa Rica*. In Serie Financiamiento del Desarrollo, Proyecto CEPAL/GTZ "Reformas de los sistemas de salud en América Latina," Economic Commission for Latin American and the Caribbean, Unit of Special Studies of the Executive Secretary, Santiago.

García G., Rossana. 2004. *Curso de Gestión Local de Salud para Técnicos del Primer Nivel. El Sistema Nacional de Salud de Costa Rica: Generalidades*. San José: Centro de Desarrollo Estratégico e Información en Salud y Seguridad Social (CENDEISSS), CCSS.

Gauri, Varum, James Cercone, and Rodrigo Briceno. 2004. "Separating Financing from Provision: Evidence from 10 Years of Partnership with Health Cooperatives in Costa Rica." *Health Policy and Planning* 19(5): 292–301.

INEC (Instituto Nacional de Estadística y Censos). 2006. *Survey on Revenues and Expenditures*. San José: INEC.

———. 2005. *Encuesta de Hogares de Propósitos Múltiples*. San José: INEC.

———. 2001. *Encuesta de Hogares de Propósitos Múltiples*. San José: INEC.

Kleysen, Brenda. 1992. *Los Gastos Privados en Salud en Costa Rica*. Working Paper No. 154, Instituto de Investigaciones Económicas, San José.

MIDEPLAN (Ministerio de Planificación y Política Económica). "Sistema de Indicadores sobre Desarrollo Sostenido, Variables e Indicadores Sociales." San José: MIDEPLAN. http://www.mideplan.go.cr/sides/social/index.html.

MOH-PAHO (Ministry of Health–Pan American Health Organization). 2003a. *Gasto y Financiamiento de la Salud en Costa Rica: Situación Actual, Tendencias y Retos*. San José: PAHO.

———. 2003b. *Las desigualdades de salud en Costa Rica: una aproximación geográfico— poblacional*. San José: PAHO.

MOH-PAHO-CCSS (Ministry of Health–Pan American Health Organization–Caja Costarricense del Seguro Social. 2004. *Perfil del Sistema de Servicios de Salud en Costa Rica*. http://www.cor.ops-oms.org.

OPS (Organización Panamerican de la Salud). *Iniciativa Regional de Datos Básicos en Salud. Sistema Generador de Tablas*. http://www.paho.org/Spanish/SHA/coredata/tabulator/ newTabulator.htm.

Proyecto Estado de la Nación [State of the Nation Project]. 2005. *11 Informe del Estado de la Nación, Anexo Estadístico*. San José: UNDP. http://www.estadonacion.or.cr/Compendio/ ind_compendio.html.

Rosero-Bixby, Luis 2004. "Supply and Access to Health Services in Costa Rica 2000: A GIS-Based Study." *Social Science and Medicine* 58: 1271–84.

Rosero-Bixby, Luis. Assessing the impact of health sector reform in Costa Rica through a quasi-experimental study. Pan American Journal of Public Health, Volume 15, Number 2, February 2004, pp. 94–103 (10).

Sáenz, Alberto. 2005. "The Role of Equity and Solidarity within Social Health Insurance: Chances and Risks of the Costa Rica Way towards Universal Coverage." Paper presented at the International Conference on Social Health Insurance in Developing Countries. http://www.shi-conference.de/contribut.html.

Sáenz, Luis B., and Miriam León. 1992. "Gastos de los hogares en servicios de salud privados en Costa Rica: 1987–1988." *Acta Médica* 35 (1) 1992: 30–38.

Superintendencia de Pensiones de Costa Rica (SUPEN). 2006. *Informe al Comité de Vigilancia del Réginen de Invalidez, Vejez y Muerte.* San José: SUPEN.

Trejos, Juan Diego. 2004. "La Equidad de la Inversión Social en el 2000." Paper presented at the Octavo Informe sobre el Estado de la Nación en Desarrollo Humano Sostenible, UNDP, San José. http://www.estadonacion.or.cr/info2002/nacion8/ ponencias.html.

United Nations Population Division. 2004. *World Population Prospects: The 2004 Revision Population Database.* New York: United Nations. http://esa.un.org/unpp/index.asp.

WHO (World Health Organization) 2004 *Global Burden of Disease Estimates.* Geneva: WHO, Department of Measurement and Health Information. http://www.who.int/ healthinfo/bodestimates/en/index.html.

World Bank. 2006. *World Development Indicators 2006.* Washington, DC: World Bank.

———. 2003. *Costa Rica: El Gasto Social y la Pobreza.* Washington, DC: Unidad Sectorial de Desarrollo Humano Departamento de América Central, Latin America and Caribbean Región, World Bank.

## Relevant Legislation

Act 17, Constitutive Law of the CCSS (1943)

Decentralization Act No. 7852 (1998)

Act 2,738 (1961), which established universal health insurance for workers and their families

Act 5,349 (1973), which transferred to the CCSS all public hospitals previously controlled by the Ministry of Health

Act 7,374 (1993), which split responsibilities between the MOH and the CCSS

Law 7,852 (1998) on Decentralization

Act of Worker Protection (2000), which declared all independent workers' obligation to join the health insurance program

Executive Decree No. 14,313 SPPS-PLAN, which formally created the health sector in Costa Rica and regulated its structure and organization

Executive Decree No. 19,276-S (1989), which created the National Health System and establishes the General System Bylaws, in which the Ministry of Health became the governing institution

# Estonia: "Good Practice" in Expanding Health Care Coverage

*Triin Habicht and Jarno Habicht*

## Background

*Estonia is a small (45,227 sq. km) upper-middle-income country in the Europe and Central Asia (ECA) Region of the World Bank, with a population of 1.4 million and a GDP per capita of US$5,328 in 2005.[1] Compared with similarly sized European countries, Estonia's population density is low, 30 inhabitants per square kilometer (km²).*

*Until regaining political independence in August 1991, Estonia's health system was that of the Soviet Union. Health care was centralized, universal, and provided nominally free of charge to everyone. The first Health Insurance Act was approved by the Parliament even before Estonia regained independence. The main rationale for health reform was to introduce a system that would ensure secure, sustainable financing for the health sector.*

*In the late 1980s and early 1990s, all Estonians were open to change and eager to move away from Soviet system to a market economy. However, it was understood that privatization and other market economy reforms would have to be balanced by a strong, sustainable social sector that included health insurance and pension systems.*

*The success of the health financing reform has been facilitated by strong economic growth, which has enabled the continuous expansion of health insurance revenues and has supported the restructuring and scaling up of the health system. These factors have guaranteed stability and continuity for the longer period, which Estonia has used to build up an institutionally sound health insurance system.*

*The health insurance system is mandatory. Contributions are related to being active in the workforce. Noncontributing individuals (children, pensioners) represent almost half (49 percent) of the insured population, and their expenses are implicitly subsidized by the others. State contributions cover only about 4 percent of the insured population. By the end of 2003, 94 percent of the population was covered. The uninsured 6 percent, working-age individuals outside the formal labor market, are ineligible for social insurance.*

## Introduction

Estonia began radical economic reforms in the late 1980s to restore a market economy modeled on the planned economy under Soviet Union.

### Economic Situation and Main Social Trends

Monetary reform was a first step toward economic modernization. A national currency (Estonian kroon, EEK) was introduced with a fixed exchange rate and a currency board arrangement, liberal external policies, and, most important, the immediate removal of most restrictions on capital account transactions. The main characteristics of Estonian reforms have been radical and rapid introduction of market-oriented institutions. Privatization of the economy has been completed, and only a few strategic companies (e.g., Estonian Energy Company) remain under the central government.

In the early years of independence (1991–94), Estonia's GDP contracted, but the recession ended by 1995. The economy recovered quickly, and GDP has grown every year since then. In 2004, the first year of full membership in the European Union (EU), the Estonian economy grew by 7.8 percent—5.6 percentage points higher than the EU average. Rapid growth assists the convergence process, and Estonia is witnessing a remarkable convergence in real terms to EU levels. Purchasing power parity per capita GDP increased to 51 percent of the EU level in 2004 from 35 percent in 1995. GDP per capita in 2004 rose to 14,555 international dollars from 6,289 in 1995.

Economic growth is expected to continue at around 6 percent, about three times faster than the EU average. However, vulnerability to external shocks is high because Estonia is small open economy, with a large, persistent current account deficit (US$1.4 billon in 2004) and rapidly expanding gross external debt (US$10 billion in 2004).

The purchasing power of the population increased by 30 percent between 1992 and 2002, but this growth was not evenly distributed among different socioeconomic groups. Income inequality, as measured by the Gini coefficient, widened substantially in the 1990s (to 0.38), but began a steady decline, reaching 0.36 in 2004. Nonetheless, large differences persist in average monthly income per household member among income groups: the income of the richest 20 percent of the population is 6.1 times larger than that of the poorest 20 percent. However, the proportion of people living below the national poverty line decreased tremendously from 36.1 percent 1997 to 17 percent in 2003. The groups at highest risk of poverty are the unemployed (especially the long-term unemployed), large families, and single-parent families. The poverty headcount ratio at $1 a day and $2 (international dollars) were respectively 2 and 8 percent of the population in 2003.

Estonia follows a conservative fiscal policy; a yearly balanced budget policy guarantees a favorable and stable environment for economic development. The government is committed to long-term fiscal sustainability and considers its aging population a macroeconomic policy priority. This conservative approach is also pursued in the health insurance budget, so far kept in balance.

The Estonian taxation system is simple and transparent, with few exceptions and differentiations. The Estonian flat-rate personal income tax system is one of the most liberal tax regimes in the world. The goal of taxation policy is to motivate entrepreneurship and initiative and to tax consumption rather than earnings. This has guaranteed economic growth, but some fundamental changes are planned because Estonian labor is heavily taxed compared with neighboring countries.[2] The high tax burden on labor stems mainly from the social insurance tax paid by employers on behalf of employees, 33 percent of each employee's salary. Of this revenue, 13 percent is earmarked for health insurance, and 20 percent funds pensions for current retirees. A reduction in the personal income tax rate is scheduled, from 26 percent in 2004 to 18 percent by 2011 with annual decrease by one percent point. This reform supports the government policy of low taxation of earnings.

## Demographic and Epidemiological Situation

Similarly to countries across Europe, the Estonian population is aging. Around 20 percent of the population was over 60 years of age in 2002, a group expected to grow to more than 25 percent by 2025 (figure 9.1). Among other similarities with Europe, aging urbanization has also increased. By 2005, 69.3 percent of the population lived in the cities.

Since 1991, Estonia's population has been declining, due mainly to negative natural growth and emigration, particularly to Russia. In 2005, Estonia had a crude birth rate of 10.7, a crude death rate of 12.9, and a fertility rate of 1.37, below the population maintenance rate. Hence, the overall population natural growth rate is negative, −3.8. The dependency ratio (the proportion of population aged 0 to 14 or over 65 years) is 48 percent, below than average EU rate. However, this is likely to increase in the future as the population continues to age.

These demographic trends will have serious consequences for Estonia's health sector because of the reduced tax base. Health expenditures are financed mainly through labor-related taxes (65 percent), and children and the elderly are insured, but no contributions are made on behalf of these groups. The epidemiological transition, as the population ages, also puts pressure on the health budget with the growing burden of chronic illnesses that are costly to treat.

The average age of mothers giving birth, including the average age at first birth, has continuously risen since 1995 from 23 years to 24.8 years in 2003.[3] Birth activity among women under 25 has also continuously decreased. Evidence of positive changes in family planning habits comes from the steady and continuing decrease in the absolute number of induced abortions and the number of abortions per

**Figure 9.1   Estonia: Population Pyramids, 2004 and 2025**

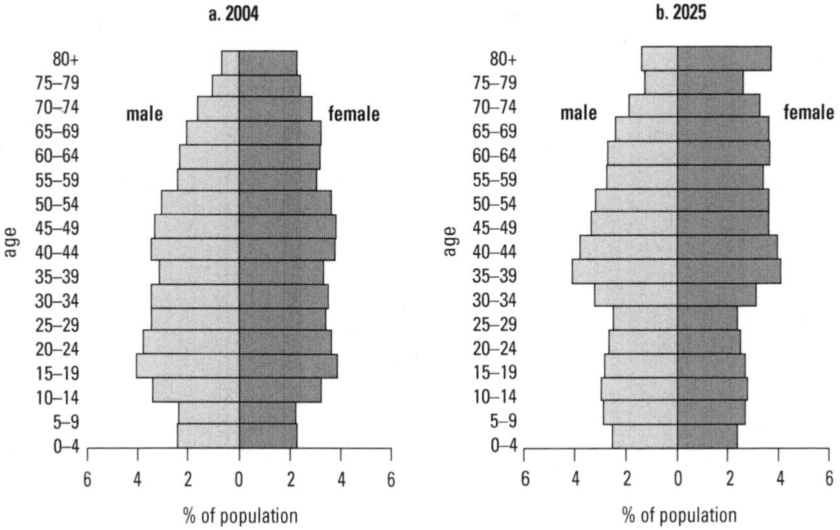

a. 2004

b. 2025

*Source:* Eurostat 2006 (http://europa.eu.int/comm/eurostat/).

1,000 women between the ages of 15 and 49, from 50.0 in 1995 to 31.0 in 2003.[4] In 2000, the number of induced abortions fell below the number of live births for the first time.

The number of deaths has been stable, only slightly crossing the 18,000 margins. More than half the deaths are caused by circulatory system diseases; cancer and accidents, poisonings, and acute injuries are the next most important causes. The causes of death differ by gender. In 2003, 63 percent of women's deaths were caused by diseases of the circulatory system (for men 47 percent), 17 percent by neoplasm (for men 20 percent), and less than 5 percent by accidents, poisonings, and acute injuries (for men 16 percent).

The mortality and morbidity patterns are similar to those of East European countries. According to the latest burden of disease study in Estonia (Ministry of Social Affairs and University of Tartu 2004) the main causes are cardiovascular diseases, neoplasm, and external causes. Still, due to the burden from disability or decrease in health status other disease groups rank high: joint and muscle diseases, pulmonary diseases, and mental health disorders (figure 9.2). More than half the burden of disease is concentrated in the working age population, among men 58 percent. Less of the burden is among over 65-year-olds (39 percent) and young people aged 0 to 19 years (8 percent). There is clear difference among men and women: only 2 of the top 10 causes are same, and among men external causes are much more prevalent, 11 percent of the total disease burden.

**Figure 9.2    Estonia: Burden of Disease**

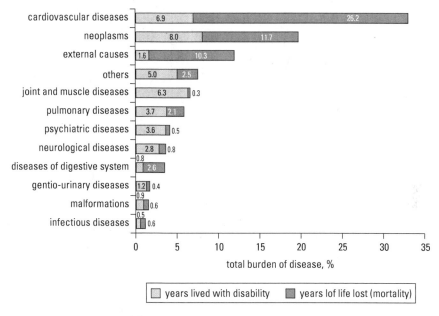

*Source:* Ministry of Social Affairs 2004.

Average life expectancy decreased in the first half of 1990s to a low turning point in 1994, 61 for men and 73 for women. This was the result of radical changes following independence, expressed in increases in mortality from external causes. Since 1995, life expectancy has slowly increased, to 66 for men and 77 for women in 2003, but remains among the lowest among EU countries (figure 9.3).

Over the years the infant mortality rate has fallen from 14.8 in 1995 to 5.7 in 2002. The maternal mortality rate of 23 per 100,000 live births (7.7 in 2002) is very low.

The five main risk factors creating the disease burden are smoking (8.3 percent), low physical activity (7.4 percent), high alcohol consumption (6.6 percent), overweight (5.1 percent), and low fruit and vegetable intake (3.8 percent). The smoking and alcohol consumption risk factors are concentrated among men, together causing more than 12 percent of the disease burden. Smoking alone causes 40 percent of cardiovascular diseases and 40 percent of cancers in Estonia.

## Political Environment

Estonia is a parliamentary republic. The Parliament (Riigikogu) consists of one chamber with 101 members elected to four-year terms. Since independent Estonia's first elections, in 1992, all governments have been coalitions of two or three

**Figure 9.3   Estonia: Average Life Expectancy at Birth Compared with EU Countries, 2003**

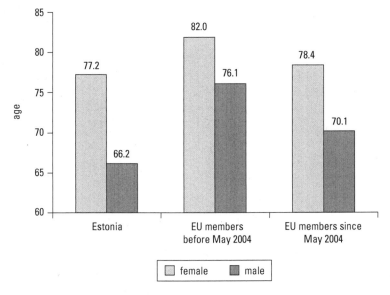

*Source:* Health for All Database 2006 (http://www.euro.who.int).

political parties. Although none of the coalitions have governed for a full term, they have been stable enough to launch and implement economic and social reforms.

Estonian political parties are at the center or to the right of the political spectrum. To date, governments have been on the right, although social democratic values and ideology have become more visible in recent years. In the early 1990s, health and social sector policies were driven by social values. The coalition that was in government between 2004 and 2007 has agreed to lower the proportional rate of personal income tax and to make a one-shot increase in state pensions. In health policy, the coalition agreement enables wide interpretation and is not clearly formulated. However, the priorities are prevention of HIV[5] and drug dependency, tackling the risk factors related to noncommunicable diseases (NCDs), remuneration policies (health services and pharmaceuticals), and improving access to care.

The second political layer in Estonia consists of 227 municipalities, which have budgetary autonomy and local tax-raising powers. Administratively, however, Estonia is divided into 15 counties, each run by a governor and administered by "the county government." Both the governor and the county government staff members are civil servants under the central administration. Many state agencies, including those engaged in health care administration and finance, operate not on a county basis, but through regional departments covering two to four counties. The role of the counties and municipalities in the health sector has varied. During the decentralization era in the early 1990s, a number of responsibilities were distributed to counties, as was the fragmented health insurance system. Counties, with specially recruited staff members, were responsible for planning and oversight of health care services. In the late 1990s, during centralization of planning and development, the role of planning primary health care and liaising with municipalities on behalf of government remained with the counties. The municipalities also have some role in the health sector, running local public health activities and supporting the health care sector (as well as owning some of the hospitals), but the practice varies across Estonia.

## Overview of Health Financing and Coverage

This section describes the Estonian health financing system: the collection of funds, pooling, benefits package, cost sharing, and purchasing of health care services. Finally, the performance of the current system is described as well as its impact on efficiency and equity.

### Collection of Funds

In 2004, total health expenditures were 5.1 percent of the Estonian gross domestic product (GDP). Among EU countries, this share ranges from similar to over 10 percent and averages 6.4 percent. The level of health expenditures in Estonia has been stable over time with small variations due to changes in the economic environment. In recent years, the health expenditure share of GDP has increased slightly because a good economic environment ensured stable tax collections and favored increases in out-of-pocket payments. The annual increase in total health expenditures in absolute terms was around 4 percent in the late 1990s and about 14 percent[6] more recently. In 2004, total health expenditures amounted to US$618 million.

The share of public expenditures in total health expenditures is relatively high, 76 percent, and 4.2 percent of GDP in 2004. In the total government budget, public health expenditures have been around 11 percent. Most public funding comes through the health insurance system—87 percent of health expenditure in the public sector and 66 percent of total health expenditure in 2004 (table 9.1).

Table 9.1    Estonia: Total Health Expenditure, by Source, 2004

| Source | Expenditure (US$ millions) | Share (%) |
|---|---|---|
| Central government | 52 | 8.5 |
| Municipalities | 8 | 1.3 |
| Social insurance | 406 | 65.7 |
| Out of pocket | 132 | 21.3 |
| Other private | 17 | 2.7 |
| External sources | 3 | 0.4 |
| Total | 618 | 100.0 |

*Source:* Ministry of Social Affairs 2006 (www.sm.ee).

**Figure 9.4   Estonia: Distribution of Funding Sources, 1999 and 2004**

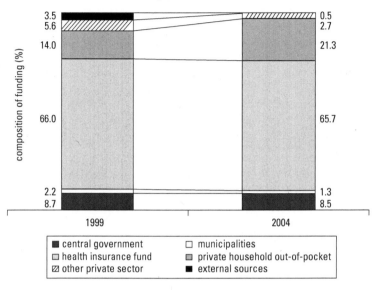

*Source:* Ministry of Social Affairs 2006.

When the health insurance system was introduced in 1992, municipal and central government financing was expected to grow in line with health insurance funding. Instead, their share has been decreasing, and the role of financing through health insurance is increasing (figure 9.4).

The main source of health insurance revenues (98 to 99 percent) is a social health insurance contribution paid by salaried workers and self-employed people. This is also known as a "social tax," which covers health and pension contributions, respectively 13 percent and 20 percent of employee wages and of self-employed individuals' earnings.

Health insurance contributions, related to the active workforce, cover about half the people. The health expenses of noncontributing individuals (49 percent of the insured population) are implicitly subsidized by the other categories, which shows great solidarity within the system. These noncontributing groups, including children, pensioners, disability pensioners, and students (during their nominal study time) are eligible for the same benefits package as everyone else in the insurance pool without any contribution from either themselves or the state. The state officially makes contributions for only a small proportion of the covered population (4 percent), including individuals on parental leave with children under three years of age, individuals registered as unemployed (eligible for up to nine months' coverage), and caregivers of disabled people. The state's contribution for these groups is defined annually when the state budget is approved and depends upon the number of eligible persons. However, the contribution rate is low, 15 times lower than the average contribution made by workers and the self-employed. In 2005, an increase the per person contribution rate is planned to make it equal to the health insurance tax paid on minimum salary. This cuts the difference in contribution rates from 15 to 2.5. Under Estonia's system, solidarity is high; half of the insured population contributes, and every insured person is entitled to the same benefits (cross-subsidization within the pool).

In 2004, central government funding accounted for 8.5 percent of total expenditures, and local municipalities accounted for 1.3 percent of total health expenditures. The central government finances ambulance services, emergency health care services[7] for uninsured people, and public health programs (e.g., HIV/AIDS; tuberculosis prevention; cardiovascular disease prevention). Local municipalities have no clear responsibility for covering health care expenditures and therefore financing practices vary widely.[8] Municipalities mainly cover health expenditures of the uninsured (some extra care in addition to central government–covered emergency care), and support for travel to health care facilities, for selected public health programs, and for out-of-pocket payments by people facing high health expenditures. Other municipalities cover some costs of family physician (FP) services in their region, but in-kind contributions for FPs are also common (e.g., office space to set up practices). Municipalities that own hospitals pay for some of their capital costs.

Out-of-pocket payments comprise statutory cost-sharing for Estonian Health Insurance Fund (EHIF) benefits, direct payments to providers for services outside the EHIF benefits package or from non-EHIF-contracted providers and informal payments. Out-of-pocket payments constituted about 21 percent of total health expenditures in 2004. Most out-of-pocket payments go for pharmaceuticals (53 percent) and dental care (23 percent). According to the National Health Accounts, households paid out of pocket for 45 percent of total pharmaceutical expenditure and 61 percent of dental care in 2004. Both shares have been increasing due to introduction of new drug reimbursement rules (introduction of reference prices) and exclusion of adult dental care from the EHIF benefits package. The share of out-of-pocket payments for total health expenditures has been increasing in Estonia (figure 9.4) and is expected to increase further. Still, the share of out-of-pocket payments is relatively low (21.3 percent) compared with similar countries in Eastern Europe (e.g., 45.9 percent in Latvia and 24.2 percent in Lithuania), but higher than in most of EU member countries, but about the same as for the EU as a whole after its May 2004 expansion (figure 9.5).

Other private expenditure includes employer-paid health care travel insurance, employer-paid health checkups and pharmaceuticals (bought mainly by foreign visitors but also by corporations). However, the share of these expenditures is low, less than 3 percent of total health expenditures. Informal payments are not common in Estonia and are not an important source of out-of-pocket payments, according to recent studies (Josing 2004; CIET 2002). This may be due to the introduction of formal copayments in 2002 or to the generally low level of corruption and informal payment practices.

**Figure 9.5   Estonia: Out-of-Pocket Payments Compared with the EU, 2004**

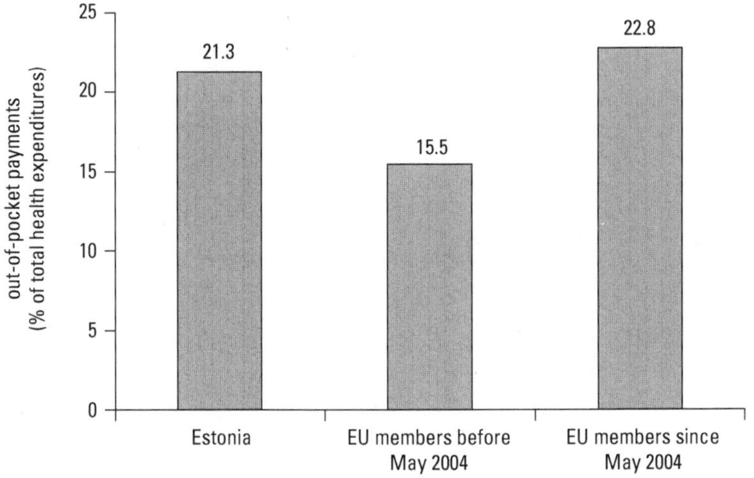

*Source:* Health for All Database 2006.

Private insurance funds plays little role in health care in Estonia. Until recently, the private insurance market consisted mostly of employer-paid health care travel insurance. Since 2002, one private insurer has offered health insurance, but it is not very popular (just a few hundred enrollees) because the benefits package is limited. In addition, the EHIF scheme enables people who otherwise would remain uninsured to enroll in the public health insurance scheme. Eligibility for voluntary coverage by public scheme is restricted to Estonian residents who receive a pension from another country or people not currently eligible for membership, but who were members for at least 12 months in the two years before applying for voluntary membership. Voluntary members pay a contribution based on the previous year's average national salary and benefit from the same coverage as other insured people. These contributions are pooled with the funds covering the other insured people.

## *Allocation of Funds and Purchasing Services*

The schematic overview of the organization of health financing arrangements in Estonia is given in figure 9.6. The core purchaser of health care services is EHIF, which purchases most of the care for insured persons (94 percent of total population), except ambulance service. Ambulance service is financed directly from the state budget and administered by the Health Care Board, an agency of the Ministry of Social Affairs. Emergency care costs for the uninsured are covered from the state budget, but the administrative tasks are delegated to the EHIF, in the interests of efficiency, because the same payment methods and tariffs are used for uninsured and insured persons.

**Figure 9.6  Estonia: Overview of the Health Financing System, 2004**

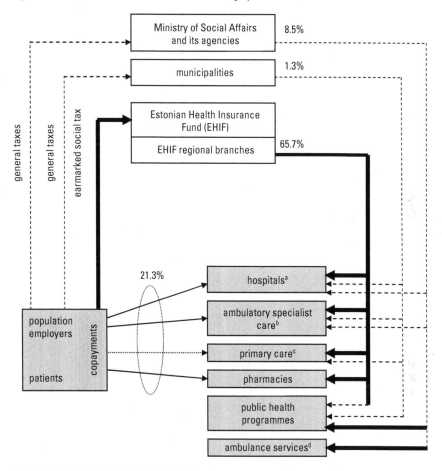

*Source:* Adapted by the authors from Jesse et al. 2004.

*Note:* The bold line represents main sources of revenue.

a. Fee-for-service plus daily rate plus some per case payments. Fifty percent of each case is reimbursed using DRG prices; contracts are close-ended case-volume contracts.
b. Fee-for-service; close-ended case-volume contracts.
c. Weighted capitation plus fee-for-service plus additional fixed payments.
d. General budgets and fixed payment per provider unit.

The EHIF funds are collected centrally to balance regional disparities in income. Pharmaceutical and temporary sick leave benefits (open-ended obligations for the EHIF) are administered centrally, but most health care services funds are allocated to EHIF regional departments (four in 2006) by a crude capitation method, unadjusted for need. For primary health care, however, a more sophisticated formula is used.[9] Overall, 98 percent of the EHIF health care services funds

**Figure 9.7   Estonia: The EHIF Contracting Process**

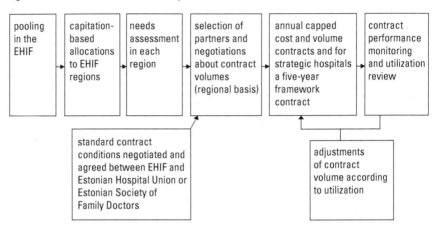

*Source:* Couffinhal and Habicht 2005.

are allocated to the regional branches. The rest remain centrally managed for a few expensive or infrequent procedures for which regional allocation would not be feasible. These include bone marrow transplants, peritoneal dialysis, some areas of oncology, and hematological treatment.

The allocation of funds is further refined during the contracting process. The EHIF contracts with providers (not individual doctors) for all types of care: primary care, specialist outpatient and inpatient care (except ambulance care and emergency care for the uninsured), and all other services in the benefits package. The EHIF contracting process is shown in figure 9.7.

Since 2001, the EHIF has gradually introduced the need assessment as an input for purchasing decisions. Currently, these decisions are based mainly on historical data analysis about health care services utilization and existing queues or waiting times, but there are further plans to use more sophisticated methods. In 2005, the EHIF started to negotiate with medical specialist associations[10] about their assessment of population needs in terms of their specialty to obtain detailed input from specialists and involve them in the planning process. The results of these negotiations are taken into account in EHIF budgeting and contracting processes and benefits package updates. The aim is to broaden the role of the medical profession in long-term direction setting for purchasing decisions.

The next step in the contracting process is selection of prospective providers. Contracts are made only with providers licensed to work in Estonia by the Health Care Board. The EHIF practices selective contracting (choosing not to contract with certain providers). Selective contracting is intended to motivate service quality improvement and to introduce mild market competition into health care provision, but also to buy services for delivery in areas providers perceive as less attractive.[11]

Nevertheless, the EHIF is required to contract with all Hospital Master Plan hospitals (fewer than 20 strategic acute care hospitals), which have a historically determined guaranteed contract volume. The main exception is dental care, which does not systematically contract with the EHIF and provides services privately. Also, 20 percent of outpatient care is purchased using selective contracting, where the EHIF announces public procurements and all providers can submit proposals.

The EHIF negotiates the standard contract conditions yearly with providers representing associations such as the Society of Family Physicians and the Hospital Association. This ensures that once the EHIF and the provider associations agree on the overall contract terms, they are universal, and all provider have to accept them.

After selection of the providers and agreement on the contract, negotiations continue with selected providers of specialist care to determine the service volume (number of cases) and average price per case by specialty. These negotiations do not determine the actual payment method but constitute a planning element aimed at containing costs for each case. In terms of coverage, the agreement on the number of cases is more important. This supports the implementation of the EHIF objective of keeping access to care at least at the same level as in previous year (measured as overall cases per provider). As a result of these negotiations, contract volumes are agreed with each provider. Until 2005, a strict system was applied: if a provider exceeded the agreed volume during the contract period, the EHIF would not pay. This principle was followed to ensure EHIF solvency. Since 2006, additional cases can be covered, but then EHIF pays at reduced rates. In addition if additional revenues materialize or the projected number of cases has to be changed during the year, the contracts can be renegotiated. To keep abreast of real access, the EHIF monitors contract implementation by providers monthly via the Management Information System. That process applies only for specialist care because, for primary care, the contract volume is not negotiable but is determined in accordance with the payment rules.

As mentioned, the actual payment methods, service prices, and benefits package are not determined during the contract negation process (in Estonia they are viewed together in one "health services list," which determines all three). All payment methods used by the EHIF are regulated by government-approved health care services list. Payment method revisions follow the same process as price revisions. Inpatient and outpatient providers of specialized care are paid using a range of payment methods that depend on the type of services provided: fee-for-service, visit fees, per diem, DRG-based, and case-based complex prices. During the late 1990s, a decision was made to move away from detailed fee-for-service payments and their perverse incentives and to increase case-based payments. This was motivated by the fact that the average length of stay was well above the proclaimed objective of 4.5 days for acute care cases. In addition, the bed occupancy rate in acute care hospitals decreased from 80 percent to 65 percent during the 1990s, which indicated that hospital capacity was being used inefficiently. Gradual

**Figure 9.8   Estonia: Payment Methods for Inpatient and Outpatient Specialist Care, 2005, actual share from budget**

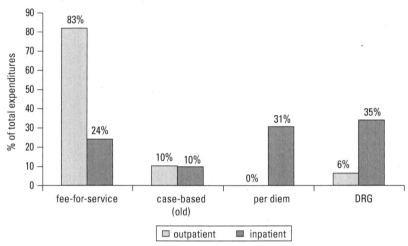

*Source:* EHIF, personal communication, July 2006.

implementation of the diagnosis-related group (DRG) system began in April 2004. The proportion of DRG payment for each case was initially set at a low 10 percent to minimize possible risks under the new system. In 2005, the share was raised to 50 percent. However, several types of payment methods are used at the same time, with the intention of balancing different incentives (figure 9.8).

FPs are paid through a combination of age-adjusted capitation and other types of payment (fee-for-service, lump sum to cover fixed costs) that make up the practice budget (figure 9.9). For capitation payments, FP practices receive monthly prepayments, recalculated twice a year to reflect changes in the patient list. An additional payment instrument was introduced in 2006, a *quality bonus system* in which targets are set at practice level to improve overall health care quality[12] and promote good performers.

Health care service prices are identical for all providers, and there are no adjustments for regional or hospital characteristics such as complexity of services provided or teaching status. In principle, prices cover all costs related to delivering services except scientific and teaching activities, which are funded separately. All prices approved are maximum prices, and providers and the EHIF can agree on lower prices for the contracts with individual providers. Revision of service prices and payment methods can be initiated by provider or specialist associations or by the EHIF. Each service should be evaluated in terms of four criteria: medical efficacy (evaluated by the relevant medical specialist association), cost-effectiveness (evaluated by health economists), appropriateness and compliance with the national health policy (evaluated by the Ministry of Social Affairs), and

**Figure 9.9    Estonia: Payment Methods for Family Physicians, 2005, as share of total budget**

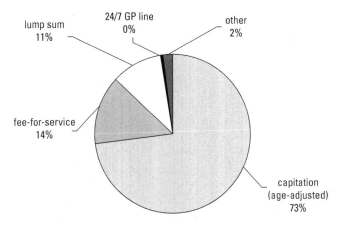

*Source:* EHIF 2006 (http://www.haigekassa.ee).

the availability of financial resources (evaluated by the EHIF). The service list is usually updated annually.

## Benefits Package and Patient Copayments

In Estonia health insurance coverage is mandatory with no opt-out possibility and intended for the whole population. Entitlement to health insurance coverage is based on residence in Estonia and membership in main categories defined by law. In 2004, mandatory health insurance covered 94 percent of the population in four main categories: persons who pay their own contributions as employees or self-employed persons eligible for coverage without contributing, in particular children and pensioners; persons covered by contributions from the state; and persons covered by voluntary agreements. Some minor alterations in entitlement rules have not caused changes in overall coverage.

The EHIF provides two kinds of benefits for the insured: cash benefits (about 20 percent of total EHIF expenditures) and benefits in kind (rest of the budget, health care services paid by the EHIF). The cash benefits (reimbursement for services) include the costs of dental care for adults and some reimbursement for high pharmaceutical expenditures.[13] In addition, the EHIF pays for temporary health-related incapacity for work in different forms as sickness benefits, maternity benefits, adoption allowance, and care allowance.[14]

Since the end of 2002, voluntary EHIF coverage has been extended to persons who might otherwise remain uninsured. Voluntary members pay a contribution of 13 percent of the previous year's national average salary as published by the Statistical Office, and they are entitled to the same benefits as compulsory members. However, the number of voluntary members is still low.

The uninsured (6 percent of the total population) are working-age individuals who are not employed in the formal labor market and are not eligible under other criteria to register as unemployed or disabled. The EHIF does not reimburse the uninsured for any kind of health care cost. The uninsured have the right to emergency care, which is reimbursed through the state budget but administered by the EHIF, which has the lowest transaction costs. Local municipalities used to cover emergency care costs of the uninsured, but this led a situation in which access to treatment was different by municipality. Discussions are ongoing about whether local municipalities should start to cover primary care and essential pharmaceutical costs of the uninsured. Another option on the table is to allow municipalities to buy EHIF coverage for selected vulnerable groups in their constituencies.

The EHIF covers a broad range of health care benefits (in-kind benefits for patients) such as family physician services, in- and outpatient specialist care, long-term care, rehabilitation, dental care for children, and prescription drugs. This feature is in part inherited from the old system in which the state funded and provided universal, comprehensive health care. Some health care services are excluded from the benefits package (for example, cosmetic surgery, alternative therapies, and opticians' services). An attempt has been made to introduce explicit rules for adding new services to the benefits package (see above) and for establishing the appropriate level of user charges.

In addition to health care services, the EHIF finances health prevention and promotion programs. The EHIF administers its special health promotion fund, from which public health institutions, nongovernmental organizations (NGOs), and local activists can apply for funds for one-year projects on preset priority areas. At the same time targeted public procurements are organized in key areas (such as information sharing, guidelines for population). Disease prevention programs funded include school health, reproductive health, screenings (breast cancer, phenylketonuria, and hypothyreosis, cervical cancer, hearing in newborns), specific immunizations, and other activities. This has broadened the scope of services supported by the EHIF from purely curative to preventive services. Since 2007, the health promotion and disease prevention activities are coordinated and advised by merged commission.

Different dental care benefits for children and adults are included in the benefits package. Since 2002, the EHIF has guaranteed free dental care for children and adolescents until the age of 19, including preventive and curative services. Adults must pay for dental care out of pocket but may receive partial reimbursement by the EHIF (US$11.51 per year for most people). The reimbursement rate is higher for some population groups with greater needs, such as pregnant women, mothers in the first year after childbirth, and people suffering from certain diseases that affect their teeth).

The pharmaceuticals covered by the EHIF are defined on a positive list[15] of medicines requiring a prescription from a physician. Guidelines for adding new pharmaceuticals to the positive list have been clarified, and reference prices have been introduced. In addition, efforts have been made to put more generics on the market and promote their utilization. This has been done not only to contain insurance costs, but also to promote cheaper but equally effective medicines for patients, still with a mixed outcome. Medical devices for certain diseases are also included as in-kind benefits and are subject to a coinsurance rate of 90 percent up to a yearly ceiling of US$1,534. Prescription drugs are generally subject to a US$3.82 deductible, and a further coinsurance percentage usually applies (50 percent up to US$15.41). Beyond this ceiling, the user covers all costs. Additional measures attempt to limit the burden for some categories of patients: a positive list of drugs for chronic conditions[16] with 75 percent and 100 percent coinsurance rates and a lower deductible of US$1.59. Additional exemptions apply for children and retired people.

Flat copayments are charged for some types of health care services—primary care physician home visits, outpatient care visits, and hospital bed-days. The general principle has been to move to free primary care without any patient cost sharing. Since 2002, the only copayment that FPs are allowed to charge is a US$3.76 home visit fee. Earlier, a small visit fee (US$0.61) was applied with some exemptions such as children and retired or disabled persons.

For outpatient specialist care, the consultation fee is US$3.82, and this is applied to office visits as well. These fees are defined as maximum, but the provider can decide the actual amount between zero and US$3.82. Providers are not allowed to charge a visit fee for children younger than two years or for pregnant women. Inpatient care providers can charge patients a per diem rate for up to 10 days with a limit of US$2.21 per day. Care for children, pregnancy or delivery-related conditions, and emergency care are exempt. These rules apply to care for which the EHIF reimburses contracted providers. If a patient covers the full cost (as do uninsured patients), providers are allowed to set different user charges to cover treatment costs as long as these charges are "reasonable." Before 2002, there were no such explicit rules, and different providers applied different user charges even when the EHIF was reimbursing the costs.

The health care service list approved in government also sets a maximum ceiling for coinsurance by service type, which the Health Insurance Act says can be up to 50 percent. Most services have no coinsurance except for in-vitro fertilization (30 percent coinsurance), abortion without medical indication (30 percent), and rehabilitation per diem for some illnesses (20 percent).

## Efficiency and Equity Performance of the Health Financing System

In 2004, Estonia spent a relatively moderate 5.1 percent of GDP on health, yet the public share of total health expenditures is high, 76 percent. This allows good financial protection for most of the population. However, out-of pocket payments rose from 13.7 percent in 1998 to 21.3 percent in 2004, and financial protection is increasingly worrisome. In 1995, 0.3 percent of households had health expenditures higher than 40 percent of their budget after buying their food. In 2002,

1.6 percent of households faced health expenditures of that magnitude. (Habicht et al. 2006).

The main objective of health financing system is to improve the people's health. The present health financing organization has been in place for 15 years its long-term objectives are ambitious. Therefore, intermediate objectives such as improving service quality and access to care are more informative indicators of health financing performance. Access to care in terms of waiting times and number of treatment cases has been the most explicit and important objective of the EHIF.

The EHIF is legally obliged to balance yearly revenues and expenditures and so far has done so except in 1999 due to economic crisis.[17] This good performance is partly due to freedom to cut provider contract volumes to operate within diminished revenues. But a more important reason has been the rapidly increasing health insurance tax revenues (allowing increases in contract volumes and service prices). The Health Insurance Fund Act also requires the EHIF to maintain adequate reserves to minimize potential financial risks. The EHIF has to have two types of long-term reserves: legal reserves of 6 percent of its budget and risk reserves of 2 percent. The accumulation of reserves began in 2002, and the reserve requirements were fulfilled in 2003.

In terms of income inequalities, Estonia is a country where income is very unequally distributed. In 2004, the average income in the lowest decile was one-tenth of that in the highest decile. Health expenditures follow same pattern, and the low out-of-pocket spending by the poorest individuals probably reflects financial barriers in access to care. For instance, the usual copayment for a specialist visit (EEK 50, about US$4), represents more than 6 percent of the monthly income in the lowest decile.[18] This assumption is supported by empirical research correlating health care utilization with socioeconomic status (Habicht and Kunst 2005). Controlling for health status, lower-income individuals utilize fewer FP and specialist services, as well as dental care. It is expected that pharmaceutical use follows the same pattern.

Estonian health insurance coverage is mandatory and targeted to the whole population. Still, about 6 percent of population remains uninsured. Because Estonian health insurance is closely related to labor market, the share of insured is dependent on the employment level. The share of uninsured decreased from 6.6 percent in 2000 to 5.5 percent in 2004, a reflection of increased labor market participation. Over the same time period, the unemployment rate decreased from 13.8 percent to 9.9 percent. The uninsured are among the working age population because children and pensioners are all covered. According to the Household Budget Survey 2003 (Statistical Office of Estonia 2004), the uninsured are mainly men (6 percent, 3 percent among women) in the 35 to 54-year-old age group. By socio-economic background, the uninsured are predominantly the less educated. They live in rural areas and poorer municipalities, where the average income is below the country's average.

## Overview of the Health Care Delivery System

The health care delivery system can be divided into primary care and specialist care. The natural parts of the primary care are a well-developed family medicine system, ambulance services, and prescription medicines. Specialist outpatient and inpatient care, mostly at hospitals, is described below. Nursing homes, rehabilitation services, and long-term care are in the early stages of development in Estonia and are not discussed here.

### *Primary Care—Family Medicine*

The introduction of primary care started in 1991 with the redesign of the Soviet-type polyclinic model for delivering primary care. Polyclinics were staffed by working medical school graduates with no specialized training and by pediatricians and other specialists such as cardiologists. The first step in primary care reform was to introduce family medicine as a medical specialty and to start post-graduate training for it in the early 1990s. Now there are enough family physicians to cover the whole population (figure 9.10). Since 1997, all citizens have been required to register with a family physician patient list, and family physicians have been entitled to become independent service providers. For doctors (as practice leaders), a motivation was the capitation fee, defined by the size of the registered list. Any patient who did not register with an FP was assigned to one. In 1996, only 8 percent of the population used a family doctor (EMOR 1996); by 2003, everyone did. The regulatory framework of 2002 stipulates primary care as the point of

**Figure 9.10   Estonia: Number of Family Physicians, 1993–2004**

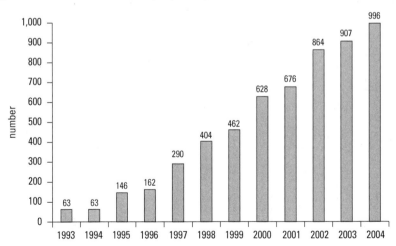

*Source:* Ministry of Social Affairs 2006.

entry to the health system for most conditions.[19] Direct access is maintained for the list of outpatient specialists, for example, gynecologists.

All family physicians are required to work with at least one family nurse in their practice to be contracted by the EHIF. However, there is a shortage of family nurses (fewer than 700 in 2004), who have better employment prospects abroad or in other industries (Atun 2004). This has put some limitations on further development of family medicine in Estonia, although special training programs for family nurses have been launched. Family medicine includes a range of services such as diagnosis, laboratory tests, investigations, treatment, follow-up, and also prevention and promotion activities. A further development in 2004 was the introduction of a family medicine call center funded by the EHIF to provide 24/7 access to advice from a family doctor. This line is free of extra charges for the whole population; and only the regular phone call fee is applied. In the first quarter of 2006, 24/7 took more than 36,000 calls, and use of this family medicine direct line service has been stable.

Family physicians can operate as sole proprietors or as companies (general partnerships or limited partnerships) with a list of registered patients. Despite the private practice option, the majority of family physicians have a contract with the EHIF.[20] As mentioned, each family physician has a list of registered patients, which cannot contain fewer than 1,200 or more than 2,000 patients.[21] The average practice size was around 1,600 persons in 2005. The practices are organized around one family doctor with a nurse, but group practices have been springing up for efficiency gains in resource use (both equipment and human).

The patient is free to choose and change a family physician. In 2005, only 13 percent of the population changed doctors and the main reason was a change in their place of residence. The family physician can refuse to register a person only if the practice list has reached the maximum size or if the applicant does not permanently reside in the practitioner's service area. Family physicians are required to have at least 20 visiting hours a week, and practices are to be open at least 8 hours a day.[22] Patients should be able to see their family physician within one day for acute problems and within three days for care of chronic conditions. In actuality, around half the patients requesting an appointment can see the family doctor the same day (regardless of the condition), and the majority make the visit within three days. Good access and the services available at the family medicine level has increased patient satisfaction with the family medicine system. In 2005, about 90 percent of the population was satisfied with the family medicine system, as compared with 80 percent in 1999.[23]

The system for reimbursing family physicians is designed to provide incentives for giving preventive care, as well as for taking more responsibility for diagnostic services and treatment. Therefore, a mix of payment methods is used (capitation, fee for service, lump sum) to balance the financial risk associated with different incentives. Management of key chronic conditions at primary care level has improved in recent years (Atun et al. 2006).

## Primary Care—Ambulance Services

The ambulance services organization in Estonia was inherited from the previous system with strong emphasis on prehospital care, as in many East European countries. This is the mixed model, where the ambulance has dual roles: to diagnose and provide onsite treatment and to transport the patient to the hospital. Forty percent of the ambulance teams are led by a doctor and other 60 percent, by a specialized nurse. Thus, the service can often be provided on site, and transportation to the hospital is not needed. As provider organizations, 80 percent of ambulance service providers belong to other institutions (e.g., hospitals), and 20 percent specialize in emergency care.

The ambulance services have gone through several stages in terms of financing schemes and services. From the early 1990s through 1996, ambulance services were financed by regional sickness funds with some additional transfers from the state budget. Insurance coverage defined entitlement to the services, and the provider billed for them. In 1997, financing was centralized in the Central Sickness Fund, but coverage was still governed by insurance status. However, centralization removed regional differences in service financing practices. In addition, the incentive to provide services changed because the payment for each visit was linked to the preparedness to act of the emergency care teams, headed by either a doctor or a specialized nurse. The general budget is used, and its size depends on the number of teams and their composition.

Since 1998, ambulance services have been financed from the state budget (managed by the Ministry of Social Affairs). This ensured that everyone in Estonia (citizens as well as temporary residents) are entitled to the services. Previously, access to ambulances was related to insurance status. Although the number of teams (90 in 2005) and cars (126 in 2005) has decreased slightly, service availability has not. In the late 1990s, 230,000 calls for ambulances were answered, 240,000 in 2005. In 2002, responsibility for purchasing and monitoring ambulance services was shifted from the ministry to the newly created Health Care Board under ministry supervision. Ambulance services and family medicine thus, to some extent, balance and fill in for each other to provide comprehensive access to services.

## Outpatient and Hospital Specialist Care

Since the beginning of the 1990s, Estonian specialist health care has undergone broad reforms including centralization of highly specialized services and decentralization of outpatient specialist services. Currently, outpatient specialist care is provided by health centers, hospital outpatient departments, and specialists practicing independently. Both public and private specialists can be contracted by the EHIF.

Estonia inherited an excess of hospital beds from the 50-year Soviet era. In the early 1990s when health insurance system was established, a clear purchaser-provider split was introduced. The hospital sector was restructured, and lower-level

**Figure 9.11   Estonia: Number of Hospitals and Acute Care Admissions, 1985–2003**

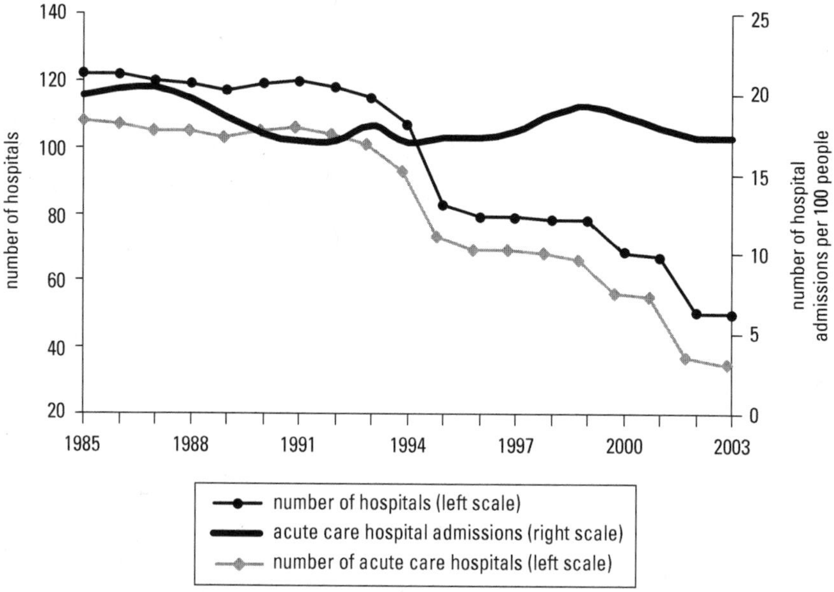

*Source:* Ministry of Social Affairs 2006 (www.sm.ee).

or lower-quality facilities were closed (figure 9.11). Quality standards were set and a licensing system introduced. Still, because many aspects remained unsolved in the changing regulatory framework, hospital sector reform was reinitiated in late 1990s, when the Ministry of Social Affairs commissioned the Hospital Master Plan 2015[24] to make projections about future hospital capacity. The plan projected a three-fourths decrease (from 68 to 15) in the number of hospitals through mergers and other types of restructuring, a two-thirds reduction in the number of acute care inpatient beds, and concentration of acute inpatient care in 15 large hospitals by 2015. Complementing the reduction in the number of acute care beds, a system for rehabilitation and long-term care was to be developed. Criteria used for planning hospital capacity included sufficiently large population pools to support minimum service volume for quality and efficiency, development of medical technology, demographic and epidemiological projections, and accessibility (not more than 70 kilometers away, an hour's drive by car).

According to a recent study using data from the late 1990s, access barriers were lower for 3.4 percent of the population living farther than 30 minutes from acute care hospitals (Roovali and Kiivet 2006). Despite some variations, hospital care is accessible for different population groups in rural and urban areas (figure 9.12). Further reforms centralizing high-technology services would affect a quarter of the population. Access to general services will decrease for 10 percent of the pop-

**Figure 9.12    Estonia: Access to Medical Care, by Residence**

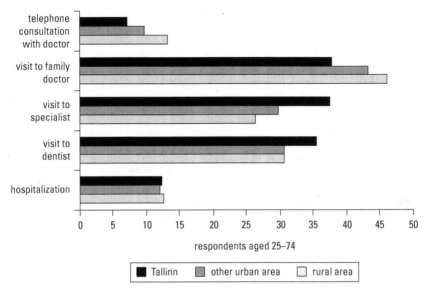

*Source:* Kunst et al. 2002.
*Note:* The proportions of respondents (age 25 to 74) in 1999 who had a telephone consultation with a doctor; visited a doctor, specialist, or a dentist in the previous six months; or was hospitalized in the previous 12 months.

ulation, but the development of outpatient care and strengthening of the primary care already available can compensate for this decrease.

This Hospital Master Plan was also an important input to the development of the Health Service Organization Act of 2001,[25] which clarified the legal environment for service provision (hospitals but also all service providers in the health care sphere). All hospitals (public and private) have to operate under private law as foundations or joint-stock companies. This means that even hospitals owned by the central or local government must be run as private companies, with full managerial rights over assets, residual claimant status, and access to financial markets. Hospitals are governed by supervisory boards, composed of members named by the owners or founders who are mainly from the public sector. All hospitals must be licensed by the Health Care Board. Licenses for meeting minimum standards are issued for five years.

Estonia has succeeded in reorganizing the hospital sector to improve efficiency and systemic responsiveness. In 1990, Estonia had about 120 hospitals and 14,000 acute care beds. The number of acute care beds had fallen to 8,600 by 1998 and to about 6,000 by 2003. The contraction is related to the establishment of the hospital licensing system under which small hospitals providing predominantly long-term care lost their acute care status and were turned into nursing homes. Other

**Figure 9.13   Estonia: Number of Doctors and Nurses per 100,000 Inhabitants, 1998–2004**

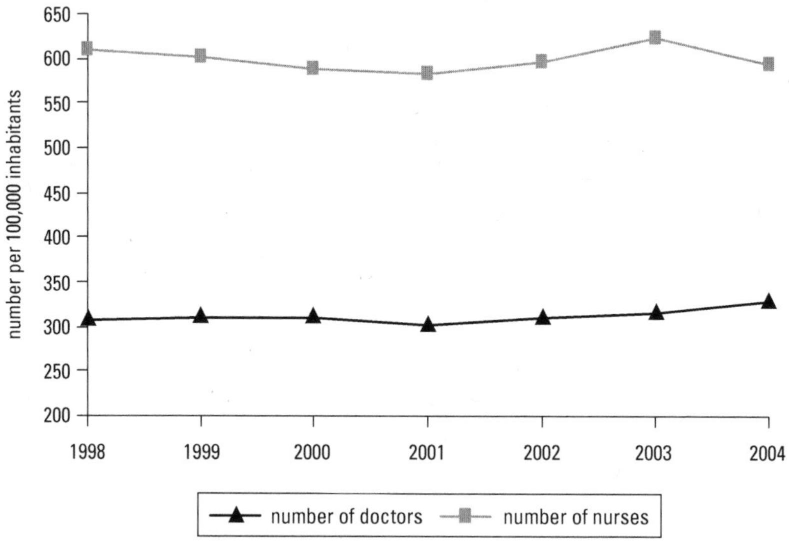

*Source:* Ministry of Social Affairs 2006 (http://www.sm.ee).

hospitals have been turned into primary care centers for outpatient care. In terms of hospital closures, access to care as measured by acute care hospital admissions has remained same (figure 9.12). The reduction in the number of acute beds has been due to hospital mergers. The average length of stay was been reduced from 14 days in 1990 to 6.4 days in 2003, but the bed occupancy rate is still low—68 percent in 2003 compared with 77 percent in 1994.

One of the most critical aspects of the Estonian health system is human resource planning, and the number and quality of health care professionals. Since the early 1990s, the entire health workforce has been independent and outside the public service. This means that doctors and nurses are free to contract with providers such as hospitals for their services. This freedom has provided motivation for professionals but has also made long-term planning difficult.

At the beginning of health care reforms in the early 1990s, it was assumed that there was an oversupply of doctors, particularly in certain specialties. At the same time, there was and still is a shortage of nurses (figure 9.13), and specialist services are unevenly distributed around the country. After independence, underinvestment in health facilities and human resources was a major source of cost savings, resulting in relatively low salaries and poor morale among doctors and nurses. More recently, salary increases have improved staff motivation. The prospect of free movement of medical professionals within the EU has put further pressure on human resources in the Estonian health system. This has been reflected in the high number of documents processed by the Health Care Board for health care professionals wanting to work outside Estonia (more than 300 doctors and around 150 nurses in 2004). In 2004–05, 4 percent of Estonia's doctors and 1 percent of its nurses left. However, in 2006, the outflow slowed, and professionals now leaving are seeking short-term work aboard rather than stays of several years. The current challenge, in addition to the migration of professionals, is the aging of professionals, where the medium-term impact would be higher.

### Pharmaceuticals

The pharmaceutical sector was reformed during the 1990s with the aims of establishing a drug regulatory authority, creating a modern legislative framework, introducing a system for reimbursing drugs and privatizing pharmaceutical services (e.g., pharmacies). During the 1980s, the range of pharmaceuticals available was 20 years behind the times, and only a few, privileged patients had access to contemporary medication. The new reimbursement scheme for medicines was introduced in 1993. Since then the reimbursement category is determined by disease severity, medication efficacy, and the patient's ability to pay. Whereas the lack of effective medication was the main issue until 1992, the increased of cost of medicines has become a major driving force for reforms (figure 9.14). The cost of medicines in Estonia has gone up for three main reasons. First, medication use has

**Figure 9.14   Estonia: Cumulative Increase in EHIF Pharmaceutical and Health Care Services Expenditures, 1993–2006**

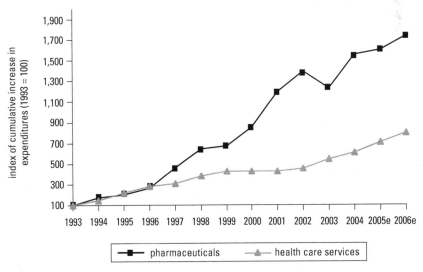

*Source:* EHIF 2006 (http://www.haigekassa.ee).

a. Forecast for 2005 and 2006.

**Figure 9.15  Estonia: Use of Cardiovascular Medicines, by Groups, 1994–2005**

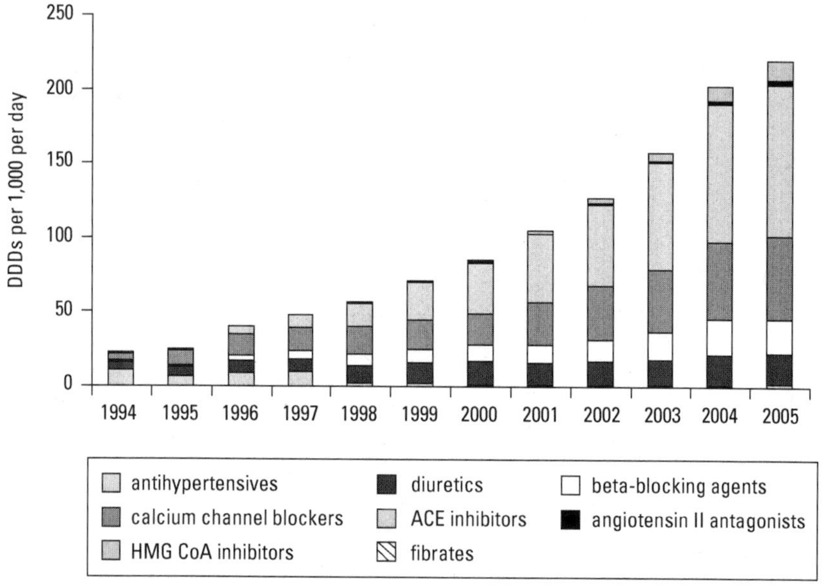

*Source:* State Agency of Medicines, Annual Statistics on Medicines 2006.

increased—triple the 1990s' budgets. Second, older drugs are being replaced by more effective, but more expensive, medications. And third, new pharmaceuticals, previously unused or unavailable in Estonia, have been introduced (Kiivet and Harro 2002).

The last two qualitative changes have expanded drug coverage and allow the prescribing doctor to use more effective and safe medicines. In volume terms, the amount of prescription pharmaceuticals used per capita doubled during the 1990s: from 314 defined daily doses (DDDs) per 1,000 per day in 1994, to 574 in 1999 and 754 in 2004. In monetary terms, the pharmaceutical market increased 2.5 times between 1999 and 2005. Examples of important changes in medicine use patterns in Estonia include treatments for ulcers, hypertension, depression, and inflammatory joint diseases, all targeting more chronic conditions needing continuous medication.

Looking only at the treatment of hypertension (figure 9.15), a move toward evidence-based prescription can be observed. ACE inhibitors are used more widely, almost as much as the European average, and use of other evidence-based pharmaceuticals has at least doubled. The changes in general were driven by opening the market to new medicines, by the targeted insurance reimbursement system embodied in the positive list, and by information sharing on evidence-based practice with service providers and public.

Thus, pharmaceuticals of known quality and proven efficacy have been made available, and the well-functioning reimbursement system supports public access to them. The State Agency of Medicines under the Ministry of Social Affairs is fully responsible for the control of all pharmaceutical activities—registration, quality control, and other activities involving drugs for veterinary as well as human consumption.

Until 2003, EHIF led the pharmaceuticals initiative. Since then, the Ministry of Social Affairs, with its special policy unit for medicines, has been responsible for all pharmaceuticals reimbursement policies. For prescription pharmaceuticals, reimbursement is either 90 percent or, for drugs used to treat more serious diseases, 100 percent. Over-the-counter pharmaceuticals, vitamins, mineral supplements, herbal remedies, and the like are not reimbursed. All pharmaceuticals used in hospitals are free for inpatients, similar to other inpatient services for insured persons.

Since the development of the first essential drug list for Estonia in 1992, the list has been used as a guide for medicine usage and reimbursement. Later, hospitals used it to develop their own formularies. In hospital, all medicines are free for patients covered by the EHIF.

## Health Coverage Reforms

Since regaining independence in 1991, Estonia has been going through extensive health care reforms to expand services and insurance coverage. These reforms can be evaluated against two main goals: to ensure access to high-quality services and to provide financial protection (through insurance coverage with a broad benefits package and limitations on out-of-pocket payments).

Chronologically, Estonian health care reforms can be divided into four phases: the early 1990s, the mid-1990s, the late 1990s and early 21st century, and the current system. In this section, the last 15 years of health care reforms and their impact on health coverage are described chronologically in terms of the two main goals. The reform milestones are depicted in figure 9.16.

**Figure 9.16  Estonia: Milestones in Health Sector Reform, 1992–2003**

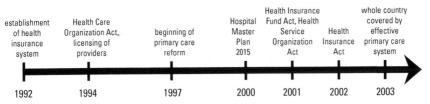

*Source:* Authors.

## The Early 1990s: Establishing the Social Health Insurance System to Ensure Sustainable Financing

During the 1980s, when Estonia was part of the Soviet Union, health care coverage was virtually universal in terms of breadth. In reality, the depth of coverage varied among population groups. Services were well developed in some specialties such as maternal and child health, but in other areas, the use of modern technology or clinical methods for treatment lagged practice in West European countries.

The first health care reform, before Estonia became officially independent, began with financing. The objective was to build a health insurance system to secure sustainable financing for the health care sector. From the centralized integrated state model of Semashko, the system would be shifted to a decentralized social health insurance model, protecting health funds through earmarked taxes and enhancing systemic efficiency and responsiveness. Preparations began in the late 1980s when changes were foreseen and need to establish a functioning health system emerged. The first Health Insurance Act was approved by Parliament, also before Estonia's official independence.

The Estonian Medical Association (representing the majority of doctors) played a significant role in successful implementation of health insurance reform. It saw in the insurance system a possibility to ensure sustainable funding for medical care in a new economic environment. This support was important in streamlining the reform. Another important success factor was the consensus and commitment of political parties to the system between 1993 and 1995 after independence and during a period of political stability.

The health insurance system was designed around regions, where 22 noncompeting sickness funds were established. This was one part of the health care decentralization plan. The sickness funds were organized by county or city governments authorized to approve the sickness fund statutes and rules for calculating health care benefits. The Ministry of Social Affairs exercised a supervisory role over the health insurance system. To enhance national coordination, the government set up an Association of Sickness Fund.

One reason for establishing a Bismarckian type of health insurance system was to ensure a sound revenue base for the health care system. Another important rationale was to relate health insurance closely to the labor market to give people incentives to participate in the formal labor market. Thus, the health insurance tax was introduced with a contribution, set at 13 percent of employees' salaries, paid entirely by employers. Other contribution rates were set for different kind of entrepreneurs. The 13 percent rate on salaries still applies, but due to changes in the legal environment, other types of entities (e.g., self-employed farmers) have been reorganized but pay the same 13 percent rate. At first, the health insurance tax was a separate tax. In 1994, it was incorporated in the social tax as a share earmarked for the health care system.

In the early stages, the regional sickness funds collected the health insurance tax, and there was no central pooling or any risk adjustment of funds. Therefore, more deprived areas had lower revenues, which curtailed their access to care. Recognition of this shortcoming of regional organization impelled administrative changes.

The established health insurance system was mandatory with no opt-out exceptions, but people were allowed to buy supplementary private insurance for uncovered expenditures. From the beginning, insurance coverage was almost universal because as most population groups were eligible.

Out-of-pocket payments for health care services were almost nonexistent during the Soviet era. Formal out-of-pocket payments were not introduced at first. In 1993, Estonia introduced the prescription pharmaceuticals reimbursement system, based on the positive list principle[26] and limited cost-sharing.

The introduction of a purchaser-provider split was seen as one tool for facilitating downsizing of the provider network. Sickness funds were contracting with service providers to ensure necessary care for insured persons in their region. Providers were paid according to the price list approved by Ministry of Health (later the Ministry of Social Affairs). The price list was based on the German price list, where fees for different services were adjusted for local prices.

Before 1995 copayments were US$0.38 per prescription for medicines on the positive list with a coinsurance rate of 100 percent (defined by disease groups and pharmaceutical names) and for population groups such as disabled persons, children under three years old, and people over 70 years of age. Similar copayments were applied for medicines with a coinsurance rate of 90 percent, and slightly higher copayments for prescription medicines with a coinsurance rate of 50 percent. The policy resulted in a small share for kept the share of private expenditures low in the early 1990s and access to medicines good.

This first wave of reform laid the base for a functional health system by establishing a sustainable and fully operational health financing system, an inevitable prerequisite for the later reforms. The health insurance system was crucial to ensure breadth and depth of coverage after the collapse of the Soviet system while Estonia started to build up a social security system. An important change while expanding depth of coverage was the introduction of new reimbursement system for prescription medicines, which made medicines available with limited out-of-pocket payments. Another important change was the introduction of a purchaser-provider split to obtain transparent contractual arrangements for achieving efficient use of resources.

## Mid-1990s: Decentralizing the Provider Network to Ensure Access to Modern, High-Quality Health Care

Reorganization of the provider network marked the second phase of reforms. After the introduction of the purchaser-provider split, health care organizations were gaining more autonomy than they had had under the Semashko type of system. The new freedom opened space for incentives for restructuring the provider network to improve systemic responsiveness and efficiency. When the Health Service Organization Act came into force in 1994, the health service planning function was delegated largely to the municipalities to dilute the central government's role. In 1991, the provider licensing system had been enhanced, an important precondition for decreasing hospital network capacity and ensuring quality. In 1994, after a detailed review of all providers, substandard providers were closed. However, legislation enacted up to that point did not provide for supervision and accountability.

In line with hospital sector reorganization, primary health care reform was initiated. The first step in primary health care reform was to introduce the family medicine as a separate medical specialty (in 1993) and to start postgraduate training at the University of Tartu, the only university providing training for future doctors. Respecialization training had been introduced in 1991. The basic framework for family medicine, set up in the Health Service Organization Act, was amplified in the Family Practice Act during 1994, but the act remained a draft and reform slowed down, because there were no appropriate incentives. In 1997, the primary care reform plan was reinitiated by ministerial decree.

Administrative changes were also going on in the health insurance system. The first years of experience showed that a fully decentralized, uncoordinated system of sickness funds was too fragmented. Revenue collection was also fragmented, lacked the vital central pooling and risk-adjustment arrangements, and contributed to widening inequalities between regions. To strengthen central functions such as planning, redistribution of revenues between regions, and control of financial resources, the Central Sickness Fund was established in 1994 and the regional sickness funds were subordinated to it. The revenue collected was pooled centrally and reallocated to the regions on capitation basis. The regional sickness funds were cut to 17 in an attempt to improve resource use efficiency.

Jointly with introduction of Central Sickness Fund, the State Health Insurance Council (SHIC) was established. The SHIC consisted of 15 members,[27] nominated by the organizations represented on the council and mandated to serve for three years. The main SHIC responsibilities were to approve the state health insurance budget and to develop the price list for health care services. The role of the SHIC was mainly advisory. Concurrently with establishment of the SHIC, Regional Health Insurance Councils were also established to advise each of the regional sickness funds. Although their role was advisory, they had a remarkable influence on contracting processes.

Changes were also made in health insurance eligibility criteria by defining more precisely the groups eligible for health insurance without contributions. As a result, some segments of the working-age population remained uninsured.[28] The motivation behind this change was to give clear incentives to participate in the legal labor market and to decrease the share of informal payments, a serious concern due to the ongoing privatization and other radical changes in the economic environment.

Another important amendment of the Health Insurance Act was to allow regional sickness funds financial discretion only to the extent resources were available. In the early years when resources were plentiful, this provision was not so important. The providers' capacity to deliver enough services was the challenge at that time, but it was feared that, as provider capacity expanded, the health insurance system might be unable to cover all expenses. Regional fund managers have strictly followed this principle of balanced revenues and expenditures, Only once, in 1999, did operating expenditures exceed revenues, and the deficit was covered from central sickness fund reserves. The balanced budget principle was followed mainly because of the funds' desire to demonstrate independence from the state budget and ability to function autonomously in the health sector. Since the early 1990s, Estonia's general fiscal policy has always supported balanced budgets in every sector. This commitment is bound by strict regulation and generally conservative fiscal policy, which disapproves of public sector deficits.

In 1995, patient copayments for primary care and specialist visits were introduced. The copayments were low (EEK 5, less than US$0.50) and many population groups were exempt. The copayments were introduced mainly to decrease informal payments, which were common during the Soviet era, and to rationalize health care service utilization by eliminating unnecessary visits. However, this decision was politically sensitive because people were used to free medical care and their willingness, but also their ability, to pay for medical care was limited. After 1995 cost sharing for pharmaceuticals was also increased by raising copayments and putting ceilings on EHIF-covered benefits. Copayments for pharmaceuticals continued to increase modestly in the mid-1990s but more rapidly in the late 1990s and in the current century.

The second wave of reforms ensured further development of service provision. The primary health care system was strengthened through family medicine reform, and ambulance services were separated from the health insurance system, ensuring access to ambulance care for the whole population. To ensure the quality of the provider network, a clear licensing system was created that resulted in closure of substandard providers. As a result, the number of hospitals decreased, enabling more efficient use of resources and securing service quality.

## Late 1990s and Early 21st Century: Recentralizing to Enhance Depth of Coverage

After Estonia regained independence, the health care system was widely decentralized to municipalities and counties. The weakness of implemented reforms lay in the lack of preparation in terms of staff training, accountability procedures, and guidelines for policy sustainability. In the health insurance system, some recentralization was already going on in 1994, with the establishment of the Central Sickness Fund. But it was evident that the provider network restructuring needed reinforcement. Municipality-level planning of provider-related functions did not work. Protecting the interests of local providers often took precedence over system-level efficiency and accountability, and the municipalities, as administrative units, lacked the necessary revenue base and competences. Some functions clearly had to be recentralized and the legal status of providers established. The Ministry of Social Affairs had to take the stewardship role in planning the provider network.

The important milestone in the third reform phase was the Hospital Master Plan 2015. This was a necessary accelerator for continuing hospital sector reform with clear targets.

Until 1998, primary care was provided mostly in polyclinics and ambulatories, owned by the municipalities, and by a few private providers. In 1998, some primary care planning functions were recentralized from municipality to county. To foster the primary care reforms, the Ministry of Social Affairs introduced the primary care reform plan in 1997 with goal of providing the whole population with family physician services by 2003. Ensuring access to primary care has been seen as important precondition for centralizing specialist care and downsizing hospital network capacity. All Estonian inhabitants, insured and uninsured, must be registered with a family physician. A new mix of payment methods for family physicians was introduced. To encourage physicians to retrain and become certified as family medicine specialists, they were offered an incentive of about US$80 per month.

Overall coverage, including the ambulance services, has been expanding. Entitlement was broadened to the whole population, and service quality was improved, even with the smaller number of teams available. These accomplishments contributed to the overall development of the health care sector with centralized hospital services, new opportunities for high-quality services, and access to doctors and nurses at the primary care level.

In the meantime some administrative changes were made in health insurance system. In 1999, the social tax collection function was assigned to the Tax Agency, which transfers the revenue earmarked for health care to the health insurance fund. This allows the health insurance fund to concentrate on the purchasing function. Tax revenue collections have also increased.

Over the decade, as Estonia's own legal system evolved, the legal status of sickness funds grew fuzzy, with some features of public independent legal person and some of a state agency related to the Ministry of Social Affairs. In 2001, the establishment of the EHIF as a public, independent legal body with seven regional departments enabled clarification of the roles of central and regional departments. The legal status of service providers was also defined more precisely, clarifying relations between purchaser and providers. In 2003, seven regional departments were merged into four departments as a natural step in centralization, each covering 200,000 to 500,000 insured persons. In 2002, the Health Insurance Act clarified the regulation of all aspects of the health insurance system, including benefits, reimbursement lists and levels for health services and drugs, maximum levels of cost sharing for insured people, and contractual relations between the EHIF and providers.

The most important feature of the third wave of health coverage reforms has been the tidying up the overall regulatory framework for the health financing system and provider network. In terms of breadth of coverage, changes were made in insurance eligibility criteria, and some population groups were excluded. However, the share of uninsured population has not increased, because employment has strengthened. The third phase has also been marked by growing out-of-pocket expenditures for pharmaceuticals and for dental care, which was excluded from the benefits package for adults and replaced with a low yearly monetary compensation. In addition, maximum ceilings for patient copayments were set for specialist visits and hospital stays, keeping FP visits free of charge for the insured population, but leaving the uninsured to cover all costs but emergencies out of pocket.

## *Further Directions and Challenges*

The fundamental changes to build a wide-coverage health care system in Estonia were made in the early stages of reform, the early 1990s. The further incremental arrangements were made to support the primary health care and hospital sector reforms and to strengthen the EHIF purchasing function. Now some fine tuning of the system is needed to improve performance.

One continuing subject of debate concerns the low level of health expenditures in relation to GDP. Additional funding could be one answer. In the long term, however, financial sustainability is a big concern because the care of an aging population will absorb more and more health resources. In terms of public financing, the broadening of the health insurance revenue base (taxing other incomes in addition to salaries) is one option. A second option is to persuade local municipalities to increase their financing by expanding their responsibilities, for example, by providing health care services for the uninsured. Because both alternatives demand strong political commitment, it is doubtful that radical changes will be made any time soon. The only decision made in 2006 was to increase the state's contribution rate, which will increase the budget by less than 2 percent and affects only 4 percent of the insured.

Another topic under discussion is an expansion of private financing by fostering more favorable conditions for private insurance or by increasing out-of-pocket payments. Out-of-pocket payments have been creeping up in an attempt to activate macro-level cost-containment in public funding by rationalizing use of health care services and pharmaceuticals. Therefore, the impact of rising out-of-pocket payments on different social groups should be evaluated, considering that current evidence shows that access to medicines may already be difficult. Introducing targeted exemptions could be considered, especially for people with chronic conditions. In addition, supply-side measures such as prescription budgets, active feedback to doctors, and rational prescribing training programs have also been discussed. Nonetheless, in the absence of a strong commitment to contain costs, funding has mounted every year.

The uninsured are the most vulnerable population group in terms of high out-of-pocket health expenditures. Currently the insurance eligibility policy for the working-age population is deliberately tied to labor policy, and health insurance is seen as one incentive for landing a job in the formal market, subject to payroll taxes. This link is unlikely to be cut in the near future, thus barring the way to fully universal coverage.

In terms of service delivery, fine tuning presents the biggest challenges. The strengths of the current delivery system are strong family medicine centered on primary health care. This system covers for a wide range of first-tier services without copayments and with minimal waits. It is complemented with the ambulance services for care outside normal working hours and on weekends, which now counts as a fourth of all health care visits. This slight overuse of this service can be considered a weakness in the delivery system, because many of those "visits" turn out to be cases treatable by family physicians or just calls for transportation (National Audit Office 2004). That was one of the reasons for opening the increasingly popular 24/7 primary care call line, in late 2005.

The challenge lies in making the delivery system more patient centered and in coordinating care at the primary level with development of additional nursing and rehabilitation services. This would enable more efficient use of resources and ensure better access and quality of care. Continuity of care presents another challenge: having outpatient care and high-quality hospital services close to patients without long waits. All this hinges on the availability of human resources, particularly nurses, who for several years have been migrating to neighboring countries or leaving nursing for other jobs.

## Health Coverage Reforms: Lessons for Other Countries

Health care coverage has improved in Estonia over the last 15 years, and health financing reforms have played a key role. The main enabling economic, political, and institutional factors are summarized in this section, together with some lessons learned in the reform process that may be useful to other countries.

### Successes and the Reasons

Estonian health financing reform has succeeded in establishing a health insurance system that ensures nearly universal coverage, The society's commitment to radical changes, the medical profession's support, and political consensus have been the most important enabling factors of health financing reform. In the late 1980s and early 1990s, the entire population was open to change and willing to move away from the Soviet system to a market economy. Politicians as well the general public were open to radical changes, and there was political consensus for establishing a social health insurance system. Another vital factor for the development of the health insurance system has been robust economic growth,[29] allowing continuous expansion of health insurance revenues and restructuring and scaling up of the health system. These factors have guaranteed stability and continuity long enough to build an institutionally sound social health insurance system.

Support from the medical profession early in the reform was crucial. Doctors, nurses, and other health workers saw in the new health insurance system, with yearly revenues from the earmarked tax, a sustainable way of financing health care, contrary to budget allocations in Soviet times. The health insurance contribution rate (13 percent of salary) was decided upon after looking at examples from other social health insurance systems, but calculated in a way that would bring in more revenues than projected to be needed in the early 1990s. This cushion ensured enough resources in the early years of change—to the medical profession's satisfaction.

## Some Unresolved Issues

Because Estonia was emerging from a Semashko-type centralized health care system, the incentive to decentralize was strong. Thus, in the early years of reform, both the financing system and the provider network were decentralized. However, the regions' varying capacity to conduct all necessary functions soon led to recentralization. In 1994, the Central Sickness Fund was established to supervise the regional sickness funds. The service delivery planning function was also decentralized, and the role of Ministry of Social Affairs decreased. However, the regions needed central oversight to organize and plan service delivery, and the ministry had to enhance its stewardship role. The correct balance has not yet been struck between the stewardship role and direct control of functions in an environment in which neither service providers nor the medical profession are under the direct control of government.

## Some Lessons for Other Reformers

For low- and middle-income countries, nine lessons can be derived from Estonia's experience with health coverage reforms.

**1. *Health system revenue collection should be in line with a country's general fiscal policy and take into account labor market policies and trends.*** In Estonia, the mainly salary-based health insurance system is closely related to the labor market. At the same time, solidarity makes the system cohesive and comprehensive; some noncontributing groups are covered: children, pensioners, and some special groups (e.g., disabled persons, mothers on job leave). For the working-age population, the eligibility criteria for health insurance are set in such a way as to give strong incentives to participate in the formal labor market. Therefore, a part of the working-age population (the informally employed) remains uninsured. The underlying rationale has been to support overall labor market policies, focused in the 1990s, on decreasing the size of the informal labor market, but now emphasizing increased labor market participation, particularly among the long-term unemployed.

The revenue collection arrangement, payroll taxes, has supported privatization, labor market development, and decreased unemployment. It has also ensured a stable resource base for the health insurance system and has allowed the Estonian Health Insurance Fund to provide a broad benefits package. In the long run, however, relying solely on salary-related contributions could jeopardize financial sustainability as the economy develops and the population ages. Therefore, to broaden the revenue base, diversification options should be considered when the system is designed. Although the system has ensured sustainable funding in Estonia so far, its relation to fiscal policies and labor market patterns should be continuously evaluated.

*2. Formalization of the labor market and the economy as part of efforts to decrease corruption also has positive impacts on the health sector.* Informal payments (money for services) were common in Estonia until the early 1990s. When health care reforms began, these informal payments were a serious concern. To formalize payments so both patients and doctors know where they stand, copayments for primary and specialist care were introduced by regulation in the mid-1990s. Lately, however, informal payments have resurfaced as an issue, especially in some specialties, but patients are not complaining publicly. These considerations prompt the conclusion that economic formalization and clear regulation are not enough to clear away invisible barriers to care posed by informal payments. Patients have to be informed about their rights, and processes have to be set up for them to make complaints about violations.

*3. Out-of-pocket payments play a large and growing role in health financing but should not be allowed to become a barrier to care for the less well-off.* The Estonian health financing system relies mainly on public resources, which enables it to protect most of the public from illness-related financial hardships, but the growth of out-of-pocket expenditures poses a risk. To some extent, this growth is related to increased incomes and changing consumption patterns. Out-of-pocket payments are used to ration health care and are an important source of revenue for many countries' health systems. For some people, however, out-of-pocket expenditures are a serious access barrier to necessary care, especially for prescription medicines. Their impact on access for different population groups should therefore be evaluated and monitored. If necessary, income- or health-related targeted exemptions should be introduced.

*4. All levels of government need to be involved in designing the health financing system so that rational, transparent allocations can be made among competing uses.* When the health insurance system was introduced in Estonia, the central government and local municipalities were expected to continue financing health care at their historic levels. In practice, they gave other development sectors greater priority and less funding to health care. Now most of the public funds for health care come through the health insurance system. Therefore, countries planning to introduce a mandatory health insurance system should be aware that this may send a signal to the central and local governments that they can reduce their financial support to the health sector, with adverse effects on long-term sustainability of the health finance. Once again, building the finance system on diverse revenue sources can ensure better sustainability in transition economies and in countries where demographic changes are taking place.

5. *In a changing environment, roles and functions throughout the health care system have to be constantly watched and adjusted to improve performance.* To keep up with changing times, Estonia has already had to make some adjustments in its new health care system. The mandatory social health insurance system, as conceived, was decentralized. Noncompeting, regional sickness funds collected the insurance tax and bought services, each for its own enrollees. After only a year, it was obvious that an organization with a pool of less than 1.5 million is administratively ineffectual and that the lack of risk-adjustment mechanisms would widen disparities between regions because of differences in regional wealth. Therefore, the Central Sickness Fund was established. Now, funds collected regionally are pooled centrally and allocated to each region based on capitation. Centralization enabled improvements in administrative efficiency and central pooling of funds.

Centralization of other functions has continued. Client services and relations with insured persons have been developed further at the regional level and moved into Internet-based services. Now, for example, an insured person can check on the validity of its insurance, using Internet-based banking services. Planning and overall monitoring are done centrally. Purchasing and service-quality monitoring by trustee doctors is performed by regional branches of the insurance fund. Functions of this kind need to be analyzed in each country and tailored to its particular health system. The ability to make necessary structural changes to improve systemic performance should be built into the design.

6. *Centralization has enabled strengthening of the purchasing function and efficiency improvements in resource use.* One strong purchaser wields much more market power over providers than many disconnected local sickness funds. Consolidation of purchasing power was also an important enabling factor for restructuring the provider network, because the hospital network also had to be merged and restructured. The EHIF purchasing process facilitated that restructuring. Without it, the process would have been complicated by dealings with the all the independent regional sickness funds and their individual local interests.

7. *Delineation of clear, transparent, contract obligations was the basis for achieving cost containment, service quality, and access to care.* The health insurance fund has devoted considerable effort to enhancing the purchasing function. Besides planning, needs assessment, and monitoring, contracts have been an

important component of that effort and the foundation for the purchasing function. In Estonia, unlike some societies, contracts have always been considered serious agreements between parties. This tradition of respect for contracts was the basis for accountability in honing the purchasing function. Standard contract conditions are now negotiated with provider associations (not single providers), which streamlines the contracting process and makes it transparent. Estonia's experience shows the importance of insurer-provider contracts that specify the responsibilities on both sides for improving performance in terms of access and quality of care. The contracts have also been a vital cost-containment mechanism, because they specify the minimum number of treatment cases and the upper limit of volume.

**8. For equitable service coverage, a comprehensive provider network should be put in place for every level of care.** Estonia did this by developing family medicine centered on primary care, restructuring ambulance services, and reorganizing the hospital sector by introducing high-technology services and providing access to modern medicine. These changes were sequenced. Health financing reforms supported the development of the provider network by developing appropriate financial mechanisms (as incentives for primary care). With the development of the provider network, a new balanced system was achieved, providing coverage for a wide range of services.

New issues have arisen related to continuity of care and integrating disease prevention and health promotion services into the current system. The ongoing challenge has been to improve coverage, step by step (e.g., by providing new curriculums, staff training, equipment and facilities, and financial incentives) at different levels of care.

**9. Information technology has played an important role in helping providers and health financing institutions extend and improve their service.** Estonians are receptive to IT technologies, not least in the health sector. In the mid-1990s, the providers used to send the health insurance fund bills on paper. Now all health care providers have personal computers, and electronic communications are used between the EHIF and its partners (patients, employees, providers) to increase data processing efficiency and speed up outcomes. Today all transactions between health care providers and pharmacies are also done electronically. Electronic data transmission, besides making transactions more efficient, enables collection of high-quality data for assessing provider performance and service use by the insured.

## Endnotes

1. World Bank. World Development Indicators. 2006.

2. The tax wedge for low-income workers was 37.2 percent in Estonia in 2004, compared with the European Union average of 36.4 percent (Eurostat 2006, http://europa.eu.int/comm/eurostat/).

3. Ministry of Social Affairs 2006, http://www.sm.ee.

4. Ministry of Social Affairs 2006, http://www.sm.ee.

5. According to latest data available (October 2007), there were almost 6,200 HIV-positive individuals (Health Protection Inspectorate 2007, http://www.tervisekaitse.ee).

6. The inflation rate was 3.0 percent in 2004 and 4.1 percent in 2005 (Ministry of Finance 2006, http://www.fin.ee).

7. According to Health Care Services Organization Act (2001), in Estonia *emergency care* means health services provided by health care professionals in situations where postponement of care or failure to provide care may cause death or permanent damage to the health of the person requiring care.

8. In 2005, the share of health expenditures from total budget varied from 8 percent to 0 percent by municipalities.

9. Age-adjusted capitation plus additional allocations through fee-for-service and lump-sum payments.

10. In 2005, pulmonology and oncology were priority areas.

11. The criteria for provider selection are: the proximity of service provision to patients; the share of provision of services in day care; the experience in the last contracting period (rejected claims for reimbursement, complaints by patients); and the price of services (lower price offer winning EHIF preference).

12. The expected outcome is improvements in the quality and effectiveness of preventive services and monitoring of chronic diseases. Specific outcome indicators have been agreed and are being monitored. The first "round" of quality bonuses was paid in 2007 on the basis of results for 2006.

13. Insured people who spend more than a given amount out of pocket on listed drugs in a year can claim partial reimbursement. Since 2003, additional financial protection has been provided to those who face high pharmaceutical expenditures: the EHIF reimburses 50 percent of a yearly cost between US$460 and US$767, and 75 percent beyond, up to a limit of US$1,534. Any additional cost is not covered.

14. For details, see the Health Insurance Act, http://www.legaltext.ee.

15. Developed by Ministry of Social Affairs and updated as needed.

16. The government-approved list of eligible conditions is available in Estonian at https://www.riigiteataja.ee/ert/act.jsp?id=1008084.

17. The deficit was then covered by fund's own reserves, and no extra allocations from state budget were made.

18. According to Income and Living Conditions Survey 2003, 7 percent of the adult population did not get needed FP care for economic reasons (mostly uninsured, who face out of pocket payments), long waiting times, and long travel distances. For specialist and dental care, these shares were, respectively, 8 percent and 15 percent. Access barriers are bigger for lower socioeconomic groups and rural dwellers.

19. If a specialist is contacted directly, the patient has to bear the full cost of services (except in some narrow specialties such as selected infectious diseases, fertility and gynecology related cases, and traumas).

20. If the FP has no contract with the EHIF, the patient bears the full cost of service.

21. Exemptions are allowed in some regions if a county governor and the EHIF agree.

22. This is monitored by trustee doctors under a system developed by the EHIF for quality control through, for example, visiting practices, reviewing clinical work, auditing, and checking on access.

23. TNS EMOR (1999–2003), Faktum (2004–05).

24. The HMP 2015, done by Swedish consultants in 1999, was published in April 2000 (SC Scandinavian Care Consultants AB. 2000). The plan, used as a basic planning exercise, was developed further in 2002 and 2006.

25. The regulation covers all health care service provision in Estonia (previous legislation from mid-1990s with updates) from primary care to hospital services. In addition, patient-provider relations are regulated by the Obligations Act, and provider-purchaser relations by insurance regulations and contracts.

26. The positive list included a list of pharmaceuticals reimbursed at different levels of copayment (with a small deducible).

27. One representative each from the Ministry of Social Affairs and the State Social Insurance Board, one county doctor, one municipal doctor, one provider representative, five representatives of employer unions, and five representatives of insureds' unions.

28. Data on coverage from this period are not available.

29. GDP growth in real terms was 7.1 percent in 2003, 8.1 percent in 2004, and 10.5 percent in 2005.

## References

Atun, R. A. 2004. "Advisory Support to Primary Health Care Evaluation Model: Estonia PHC Evaluation Project." Final Report, WHO Regional Office for Europe, Copenhagen.

Atun, R. A., N. Menabde, K. Saluvere, M. Jesse, and J. Habicht. 2006. "Introducing a Complex Health Innovation—Primary Health Care Reforms in Estonia (Multimethods Evaluation)." *Health Policy* 79: 79–91

CIET International (Community Information, Empowerment and Transparency International). 2002. "Curbing System Leakages: The Health Sector and Licensing in Estonia." CIET International, Tallinn.

Couffinhal, A., and T. Habicht. 2005. "Health System Financing in Estonia: Situation and Challenges in 2005." HSF Working Document, Health Systems Financing Programme, WHO Regional Office for Europe, Copenhagen.

Faktum. 2004. *Elanike rahulolu arstiabiga 2004* [Population satisfaction with health care]. Survey. Tallinn: Faktum.

Faktum. 2005. *Elanike rahulolu arstiabiga 2005* [Population satisfaction with health care]. Survey. Tallinn: Faktum.

Habicht, J., K. Xu, A. Couffinhal, and J. Kutzin J. 2006. "Detecting Changes in Financial Protection: Creating Evidence for Policy in Estonia." *Health Policy and Planning* 21: 421–31.

Habicht, J., and A. Kunst. 2005. "Social Inequalities in Health Care Services Utilization after Eight Years of Health Care Reforms: A Cross-Sectional Study of Estonia, 1999." *Social Science and Medicine* 60: 777–87.

Jesse, M., J. Habicht, A. Aaviksoo, A. Koppel, A. Irs, and S. Thomson. 2004. "Health Care Systems in Transition: Estonia." WHO Regional Office for Europe for the European Observatory on Health Systems and Policies, Copenhagen.

Josin, M. 2004. *Korruptsiooni ja varimajanduse levik Eestis* [Corruption and the black market in Estonia]. Tallinn: Estonian Institute of Market Research.

Kiivet, R., and J. Harro, eds. 2002. *Health in Estonia 1991–2000.* Tartu, Estonia: University of Tartu.

Kunst, A. E., M. Leinsalu, A. Kasmel, and J. Habicht. 2002. *Social Inequalities in Health in Estonia.* Main Report. Tallinn: Estonian Ministry of Social Affairs.

Rooväli, L., and R. A. Kiivet. 2006. "Geographical Variations in Hospital Use in Estonia." *Health and Place* 12(2): 195–202.

Ministry of Social Affairs, Estonia. 2006. "Years Lost Due to Burden of Disease: Links with Risk Factors and Cost Effectiveness to Reduce Risks." Report [in Estonian], Tallinn.

SC Scandinavian Care Consultants AB. 2000. "Estonian Hospital Master Plan 2015." Summary Report. Tallinn.

Statistical Office of Estonia. 2004. "Household Living Niveau 2004." Special data query provided by Statistical Office, Talinn.

TNS EMOR. 2003. *Elanike rahulolu arstiabiga 2003* [Population satisfaction with health care]. Survey. Tallinn: EMOR.

———. 2002. *Arstiabi kasutamine elanike poolt 2002* [Utilization of health care services by the population]. Survey. Tallinn: EMOR.

———. 2001. *Arstiabi kasutamine elanike poolt 2001* [Utilization of health care services by the population]. Survey. Tallinn: EMOR.

vices by the population]. Survey. Tallinn: EMOR.

———. 1999. *Arstiabi kasutamine elanike poolt 1999* [Utilization of health care services by the population]. Survey. Tallinn: EMOR.

———. 1996. *Arstiabi kasutamine elanike poolt 1996* [Utilization of health care services by the population]. Survey. Tallinn: EMOR.

National Audit Office of Estonia. 2004. "First-Level Emergency Care Organization" [in Estonian]. Tallinn.

# 10

# The Kyrgyz Republic: Good Practices in Expanding Health Care Coverage, 1991–2006

*Melitta Jakab and Elina Manjieva*

## Background

*The Kyrgyz Republic is a small (191,300 sq. km), landlocked, mountainous, low-income Central Asian country. Its population (5.2 million) is predominantly rural (CIA 2006). In 2004, per capita GDP was US$431 (Recent Economic Development, Jan–Dec 2004, WB). The Kyrgyz Republic devotes 5.6 percent of GDP to health care, about average for its income level. Some 41 percent of health spending is public, but out-of-pocket payments (formal and informal) account for 50 percent of health expenditures, a higher proportion than in comparable countries. In terms of health outcomes, it does slightly better, with a life expectancy of 68.*

*In 1991, at the time of the breakup of the former Soviet Union (FSU), the Kyrgyz Republic had a norm-driven, centrally planned, general revenue–financed health system in which free health care was every citizen's right. Between 1991 and 1996, the Kyrgyz economy collapsed, and GDP contracted by more than half with equivalently large reductions in government funding for the health system. As a result, the Kyrgyz Republic found itself saddled with an inefficient and unaffordable health system and gradual erosion of health benefits coverage. Coverage erosion manifested itself in increased out-of-pocket payments both formal and informal.*

*Reforms starting in the mid-1990s diversified health sector financing, centralized the flow of public funds into a national pool, clarified entitlements to health benefits, introduced provider payment reforms, strengthened primary care, rationalized the delivery of hospital services, updated treatment protocols, and broadened consumer choice.*

*The Kyrgyz reforms were successful at halting the process of coverage erosion and at reversing the earlier trends in some areas by 2004. At the heart of the reforms was the recognition that efficiency gains had to be made before coverage and equity issues*

**269**

*could be directly addressed due to tight resources and excess physical capacity. Although changing the provider payment mechanisms and restructuring service delivery are usually recognized as instruments for improving efficiency, they became critical preconditions for improving equity in the Kyrgyz context. Recognition of the interlinked nature of efficiency and equity meant that the reform instruments were realistic, appropriately sequenced and relied on internal resources in the system rather than on injection of additional government or donor funds.*

*Several factors explain why coverage reform featured strongly in the Kyrgyz health system agenda: availability of data and information on the erosion of coverage and use of this information through advocacy; linking health reforms to the wider poverty reduction agenda, stressing to the connections between erosion of coverage and poverty; support of the president in the early phases of the reforms; support of the international community; and the equity orientation of the health reform architects and their recognition of the reality of the limited fiscal space.*

## Introduction

This section provides the economic, demographic, social, and political context for the health sector reforms discussed in this chapter. The extent of economic downturn and its impact on government spending for social services, including health care, are highlighted This trend provides a vital contextual factor for understanding why efficiency and equity were seen as inseparable goals of the reforms in the Kyrgyz context where equity could be achieved only through increased efficiency and not through injection of external resources.

### Economic Environment

The Kyrgyz Republic, one of the poorest republics in the Soviet Union, depended heavily on subsidies from Moscow.[1] The loss of subsidies and the economic consequences of disintegration led to a painful transition process. Between 1991 and 1995, GDP declined by more than 50 percent. Strong economic growth in 1996 and 1997 was not enough to noticeably improve most peoples' standard of living. GDP per capita has still not recovered to the preindependence level (figure 10.1). The growth spurt of 1996 and 1997 was followed by another downturn in 1998, attributed largely to the spillover effects of the Russian financial crisis. Since then, the GDP growth rate has stabilized at around 5 percent a year.

Extreme poverty[2] continued to increase during the early years of transition, reaching a rate of 23.3 percent in 1999. The absolute poverty rate[3] was also high and rising, from 52 percent in 1996 to 64 percent in 1999 (World Bank 2001). However, in 2000 both extreme and absolute poverty started to decline: extreme poverty fell by half, and absolute poverty fell from 63 to 49 percent in 2000 and 2003 (World Bank 2005a). Measured against the international poverty line of US$2.15 per day, however, poverty in the Kyrgyz Republic is significantly higher: in 2003, it was estimated at 70 percent. Unfortunately, the lack of consistent interna-

**Figure 10.1** **The Kyrgyz Republic: Key Economic Indicators, 1990–2004**

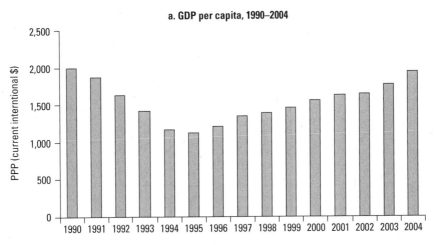

a. GDP per capita, 1990–2004

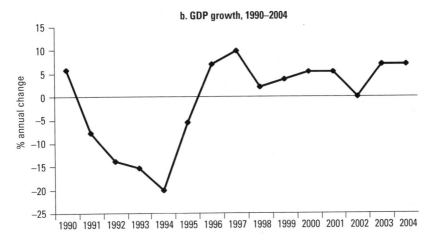

b. GDP growth, 1990–2004

*Source:* WDI Dataset, 2006.

tional poverty line estimates before 2000 makes longitudinal comparisons difficult, but recent health and education indicators seem to reflect overall improvement in the well-being of the population.

The Kyrgyz Republic became the first state in Central Asia to be welcomed into the World Trade Organization (WTO), in December 1998. The growth recovery was led by agriculture, gold mining, and trade. In 2004, gold exports represented 40 percent of total exports. Apart from gold, the Kyrgyz Republic relies on a few other exports such as cotton, electricity (bartered for natural gas and coal), and tobacco, making it vulnerable to changes in commodity prices (World Bank

2005b). More than half of the population is employed in the agricultural sector, which has a low productivity[4] and, consequently, low wages.

## Political Economy

The Kyrgyz Republic is a *unitary state* with a strong central government. It is divided into eight regions *(oblasts)*, including the capital city, which are sub-divided into 43 districts *(rayons)* (Oxford Policy Management 2006). The president appoints the regional governors subject to the approval of local councils. The Law on the Basic Principles of the Budget (No. 78, June 11, 1998) establishes revenue assignments (including a tax-sharing system and local revenue options) and defines expenditure responsibilities between the national and subnational governments.[5] However, there is a mismatch between subnational public service responsibilities and available revenue-raising instruments. The system of intergovernmental fiscal transfers is such that subnational and subregional governments have limited control over revenue sources and few incentives to raise their own revenues. This, coupled with large differences in regional fiscal bases, results in chronic underfunding of services for which local governments are responsible, except in the capital city Bishkek and a few other relatively rich districts. Until 2006, health and education were considered local government responsibilities, which contributed to geographical disparities in the quality of those services. In 2006, financing of health services was transferred to the central budget, with the exception of the capital city.

## Demographic, Epidemiological, and Social Environment

Although two-thirds of Krygyzstan's population is still rural, there is a high rate of rural to urban migration and emigration that is not officially registered. Life expectancy at birth fell in the early transition years from 68.3 years in 1990 to 65.7 years by the mid-1990s but began to recover and by 2004, at 68.2 years, was close to its pretransition level (WDI Dataset, 2006). The adult literacy rate is over 90 percent. Gross enrollment ratio in secondary schools is also improving after the record low of 85 percent in the mid-1990s (NSC Dataset 2005).

The Kyrgyz Republic has a fairly young population: 31 percent of the total population is under 15 years of age. However, as shown in figure 10.2, the population is gradually getting older: the total fertility rate and the child dependency ratio have both declined in the last 15 years (from 3.69 to 2 births per woman, and from 65 to 50 children per 100 working age adults).

Similarly to other countries in Central Asia and the Caucasus, the Kyrgyz Republic is confronted with a dual challenge of controlling high rates of both communicable and noncommunicable diseases at the same time. In addition to high childhood mortality due to infectious diseases, countries in this region are struggling with staggering adult mortality due largely to cardiovascular diseases, cancer, and injuries (World Bank 2004a). Control of TB and HIV present a further challenge to governments in this region.

**Figure 10.2    The Kyrgyz Republic: Population Pyramids, 1990 and 2005**

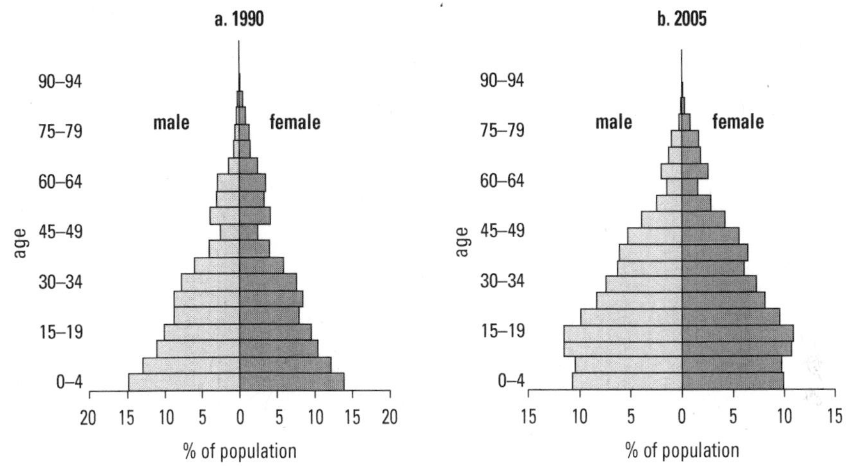

Source: United Nations Population Division 2004.

The leading cause of mortality and morbidity among both men and women in the Kyrgyz Republic is cardiovascular disease (table 10.1), and the largest gain in life expectancy in the Kyrgyz Republic, 4.52 years, will come from reducing that toll (World Bank 2004a). In terms of years of life lost due to premature mortality and disability, as measured by disability-adjusted life years (DALYs), neuropsychiatric

**Table 10.1    The Kyrgyz Republic: Leading Causes of Mortality and Disability, 2002**

| Disease | Total deaths (thousands) | Share (%) | Disease | Total DALYs (thousands) | Share (%) |
|---|---|---|---|---|---|
| Cardiovascular diseases | 21 | 47 | Cardiovascular diseases | 199 | 17 |
| Malignant neoplasms | 4 | 9 | Neuropsychiatric conditions | 164 | 14 |
| Respiratory diseases | 3 | 7 | Unintentional injuries | 121 | 11 |
| Infectious and parasitic diseases | 3 | 7 | Infectious and parasitic diseases | 98 | 9 |
| Unintentional injuries | 3 | 6 | Perinatal conditions | 93 | 8 |
| Other | 11 | 24 | Other | 465 | 41 |
| Total (all causes) | 45 | 100 | Total (all causes) | 1,140 | 100 |

Source: WHO Global Burden of Disease Dataset 2004 (http://www.who.int/healthinfo/bodestimates/en/index.html).

**Figure 10.3    The Kyrgyz Republic: Leading Causes of Infant Mortality, 2004**

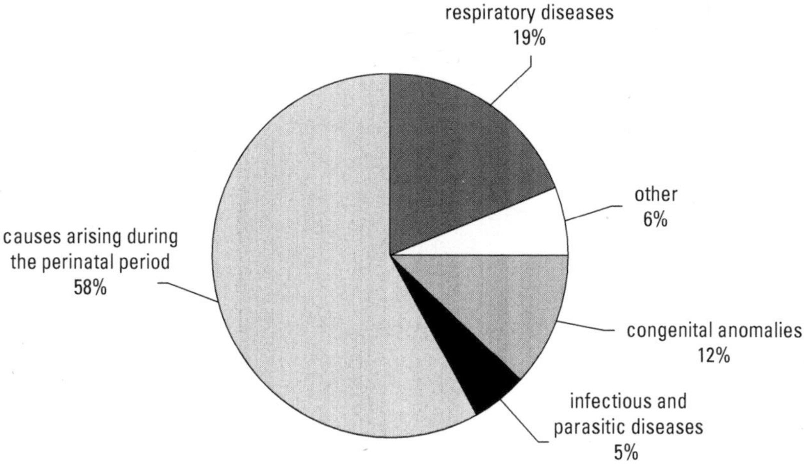

*Source:* RMIC 2004.

conditions are the second most important cause of disability after cardiovascular diseases; however, cancer is the second most important cause of death.

Child mortality indices in the Kyrgyz Republic have been steadily improving. The infant mortality rate (IMR) declined from 28.2 per 1,000 live births in 1997 to 20.9 in 2003.[6] Under-five (U-5) mortality during the same time period improved from 42.1 to 27.6 per 1,000 live births. However, these improvements hide large intra-country disparities with some regions showing almost no improvement. According to Ministry of Health (MOH) data for 2004, the high/low IMR ratio is 2.1 (RMIC 2004). One of the largest contributors to infant mortality in the Kyrgyz Republic is respiratory disease. Regardless of recent declines, deaths from respiratory diseases still account for almost one-fifth of all infant deaths (figure 10.3). Infectious and parasitic diseases accounted for 16 percent of infant mortality in 1999. However, their share has been steadily declining, reaching 5.3 percent in 2004. As infectious and parasitic causes of infant deaths have declined in importance, the share of causes arising during the perinatal period (including asphyxia, infection, and premature deliveries) has increased, from 33 percent in 2000 to 58 percent in 2004 (RMIC 2004). This trend highlights the need for continued attention to prenatal care programs in primary health care (PHC) and the quality of care for management of deliveries and newborns.[7]

Although the infant mortality rate due to respiratory infections decreased significantly in all regions between 1997 and 2004 (table 10.2), the pace of improvement has been varied. The Issyk-Kul and Osh regions had similar indicators in 1997, but by 2004, they showed stark differences: 25.3 deaths per 10,000 births in Issyk-Kul as compared with 81.3 deaths per 10,000 births in Osh.

**Table 10.2 The Kyrgyz Republic: IMR from Respiratory Infections, 1997–2004 (per 10,000 births)**

| Country/locality | 1997 | 2001 | 2003 | 2004 | Percent change, 1997–2004 |
|---|---|---|---|---|---|
| Kyrgyz Republic | 122.6 | 67.9 | 61.6 | 48.0 | –60.9 |
| Bishkek | 31.3 | 25.2 | 26.0 | 14.4 | –54.1 |
| Batken oblast | 150.4 | 105.7 | 106.3 | 77.8 | –48.3 |
| Jalal-Abad oblast | 145.7 | 78.7 | 65.1 | 4202 | –71.1 |
| Issyk-Kul oblast | 131.6 | 34.2 | 30.1 | 25.3 | –80.8 |
| Naryn oblast | 118.3 | 68.1 | 51.7 | 61.1 | –48.4 |
| Osh oblast | 136.1 | 84.6 | 90.4 | 81.3 | –40.3 |
| Talas oblast | 150.5 | 71.6 | 57.0 | 51.4 | –65.9 |
| Chui oblast | 60.5 | 38.0 | 39.9 | 25.2 | –58.4 |
| Osh City | — | — | 38.2 | 40.0 | — |

*Source:* RMIC, Health of the Population and Performance of Health Facilities in the KR. 1997–2004.

*Note:* — = not available.

## Political Context

The Kyrgyz Republic, in the early years of independence, was viewed by the international community as one of the few success stories of economic and political reform in Central Asia and the country became known as an "island of democracy."[8] In contrast to the other Central Asian states, independent media, nongovernmental organizations (NGOs), political parties, and civil society organizations were allowed to develop. However, starting in the mid-1990s, President Akaev began to tighten his grip on power, reducing the powers of parliament and curbing the activities of some political parties, mass media, and NGOs. Growing opposition to the president's powers brought the country close to a crisis on several occasions (Institute for War and Peace 2003).

By 2005, the Akaev had lost support among citizens and alienated some of his former allies and key national and regional elites. Parliamentary elections in February to March 2005 were widely perceived as unfair and caused the initial wave of protests conducted mostly by supporters of individual candidates. Over the following two weeks, the wider opposition joined in, and the agenda broadened to national issues. As the protests reached the capital, the president fled the country with his family and eventually resigned from the post he had held for 15 years.

The new government, formed in 2005, has not yet met expectations of further democratization, increased transparency, and accelerated economic and social development, leading to widespread popular disillusionment. Economic and political reforms are slowly progressing, but the overall political uncertainty creates an unpredictable policy environment not conducive to long-term structural reforms.

## Overview of Health Financing and Coverage

This section describes the development of the health financing system under the Manas Health Sector Reform Program. Health financing trends, the evolution of coverage, and how financing and payment reforms aimed to increase coverage of health benefits are discussed. The discussion of the financing and payment reforms in two parts corresponds to two phases of the reforms. The first phase (1997–2000) was a preparatory phase with piloting of elements of the future health financing system and intensive capacity building. The second phase (from 2001 and continuing to this date) focused on the nationwide implementation of major structural reforms. At the end of the section, several indicators of equity and efficiency the reforms aimed to improve are reviewed.

### Trends in Health Care Financing

Public spending on health declined from 4.0 percent of GDP in 1995 to a low of −1.9 percent of GDP in 2001, improving to 2.2 percent in 2003 (World Bank 2004b). At the same time, out-of-pocket expenditures rose steadily (table 10.3). There are no reliable estimates of out-of-pocket expenditures prior to 2000, because most of these were informal and thus not officially acknowledged.

According to most assessments, health expenditures declined both as a share of GDP and as a share of total government expenditures, showing that the decline in public spending resulted not only from the decline in public expenditures in general, but also from changes in government spending priorities. The share of health expenditures in both republican (central) and local budgets has declining since 1996 (figure 10.4).

Declining public expenditures translated into budget shortfalls for covering the costs of existing structures and previous activity levels. As a result, patients were asked to contribute toward the cost of their care for basic items such as medicine, syringes, IV tubes, bandages, notebooks, light bulbs, linen, and food. These expenses were in addition to informal payments to health care personnel. In contrast to the "free" health care services provided during Soviet times, health care services had become expensive by 2000 for the average Kyrgyz household. By 2000, the mean out-of-pocket spending was KGS 337 (US$8). Conditional on reporting any contact with the health system (visit, hospitalization), the mean out-of-pocket payment was KGS 1,846 (US$46), the equivalent of five times monthly per capita consumption. Total out-of-pocket expenditures were composed of expenditures for outpatient visits (14 percent), outpatient drug purchases (58 percent), and payments associated with hospitalization (28 percent).

### Depth of Benefits Packages

In Soviet times, the coverage of health services was both wide and deep. Publicly funded and provided services were available to all citizens. There was no explicitly defined benefits package, and there was no private sector (Sargaldakova et al.

**Table 10.3   The Kyrgyz Republic: Key Health Financing Indicators, 2000–2007**

| | 2000 | 2001 | 2002 | 2003 | 2004 | 2005 | 2006 | 2007 |
|---|---|---|---|---|---|---|---|---|
| **In nominal terms** | | | | | | | | |
| **Total health expenditures (million som)** | | | | | | | | |
| Budget | 1,248 | 1,335 | 1,478 | 1,528 | 1,809 | 2,148 | 2,421 | 3,706 |
| MHIF | 105 | 120 | 142 | 197 | 338 | 255 | 467 | 581 |
| OOP | 1,521 | 1,885 | 2,254 | 2,628 | 3,091 | 3,491 | 3,922 | 4,406 |
| SWAp | | | | | | | 253 | 457 |
| Total | 2,875 | 3,340 | 3,874 | 4,354 | 5,238 | 5,893 | 7,062 | 9,150 |
| **Per capita health expenditures (in som)** | | | | | | | | |
| Budget | 255 | 270 | 297 | 305 | 353 | 419 | 473 | 707 |
| MHIF | 21.5 | 24 | 29 | 39 | 66 | 50 | 91 | 111 |
| OOP | 310.8 | 382 | 453 | 524 | 604 | 682 | 766 | 841 |
| SWAp | | | | | | | 49 | 87 |
| Total | 587 | 677 | 779 | 869 | 1,023 | 1,151 | 1,379 | 1,745 |
| **As share of total health expenditures** | | | | | | | | |
| Budget | 43.4% | 40.0% | 38.2% | 35.1% | 34.5% | 36.4% | 34.3% | 40.5% |
| MHIF | 3.7% | 3.6% | 3.7% | 4.5% | 6.5% | 4.3% | 6.6% | 6.3% |
| OOP | 52.9% | 56.5% | 58.2% | 60.4% | 59.0% | 59.2% | 55.5% | 48.2% |
| SWAp | | | | | | | 3.6% | 5.0% |
| Total | 100.0% | 100.0% | 100.0% | 100.0% | 100.0% | 100.0% | 100.0% | 100.0% |
| **As share of GDP** | | | | | | | | |
| Budget | 1.9% | 1.8% | 2.0% | 1.8% | 1.9% | 2.1% | 2.2% | 2.7% |
| MHIF | 0.2% | 0.2% | 0.2% | 0.2% | 0.4% | 0.3% | 0.4% | 0.4% |
| OOP | 2.3% | 2.6% | 3.0% | 3.1% | 3.3% | 3.5% | 3.5% | 3.2% |
| SWAp | | | | | | | 0.2% | 0.3% |
| Total | 4.4% | 4.6% | 5.2% | 5.3% | 5.8% | 6.1% | 6.3% | 6.6% |
| **In real terms** | | | | | | | | |
| **Total health expenditures** | | | | | | | | |
| Budget | 1,248 | 1,244 | 1,449 | 1,469 | 1,721 | 2,005 | 2,217 | 2,990 |
| MHIF | 105 | 112 | 139 | 190 | 322 | 238 | 428 | 468 |
| OOP | 1,521 | 1,757 | 2,210 | 2,527 | 2,941 | 3,259 | 3,592 | 3,555 |
| SWAp | | | | | | | 231 | 369 |
| Total | 2,875 | 3,113 | 3,798 | 4,186 | 4,984 | 5,502 | 6,236 | 7,382 |
| **Per capita health expenditures** | | | | | | | | |
| Budget | 255 | 252 | 291 | 293 | 336 | 392 | 427 | 570 |
| MHIF | 22 | 23 | 28 | 38 | 63 | 47 | 82 | 89 |
| OOP | 311 | 356 | 444 | 504 | 574 | 637 | 692 | 678 |
| SWAp | | | | | | | 45 | 70 |
| Total | 587 | 631 | 764 | 835 | 973 | 1,076 | 1,246 | 1,408 |

*Source:* Adyljan Temirov et al., Policy Research Paper #48, CHSD, Bishkek, April 2008; FMR for 2007, MOH, March 2008.

*Note:* GDP deflator 2000=100 (in som). Private expenditures for 2007 are projected based on the growth rate between 2005 and 2006. OOP = out-of-pocket.

**Figure 10.4 The Kyrgyz Republic: Health Expenditures as Share of the State Budget, 1995–2003**

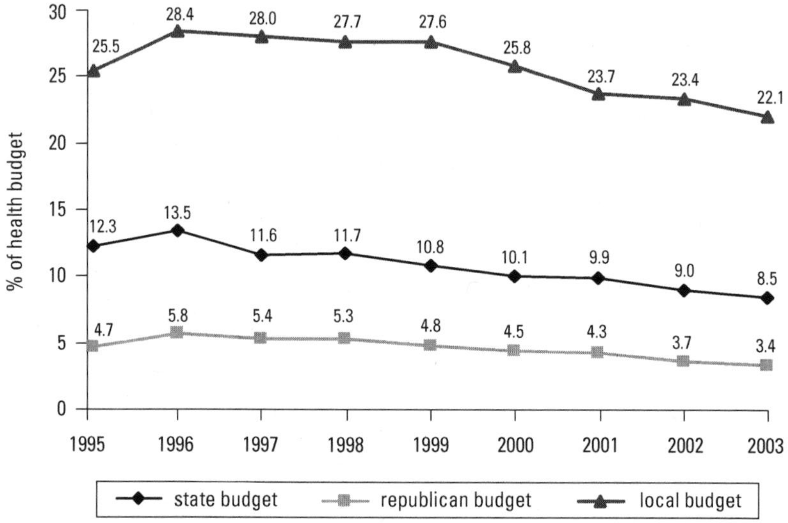

Sources: Treasury data; WHO staff calculations.

2000). Health services, including inpatient drugs, were largely free of charge at point of service. The only exception was outpatient medicines and occasional gifts to providers. The Soviet health system provided high levels of financial protection. The provider network was extensive at both primary and secondary care levels, and geographic access for the population was good. The only official rationing of services was through waiting lists where several privileged groups of patients (e.g., war veterans, families of military servicemen or employees of the Ministry of Interior, pregnant women, disabled individuals, residents of high-altitude areas) received preferential treatment.

As a legacy of the Soviet health system, all Kyrgyz citizens were entitled to the same benefits when the transition began. However, these benefits increasingly went unfunded after the drastic loss of budgetary revenues during the 1990s. According to laws existing at the time, health facilities could not, by charging official fees, cover the growing funding gap between their budgets and the cost of inherited benefits. They could charge only for services that were not part of the "guaranteed volume of services" and provided only by highly qualified specialists (Meimanaliev 2003). At the same time, the definition of what constituted "guaranteed volume of health services" was vague and undefined. Thus, declining budgets and vague laws spawned informal charging practices. To continue delivering services, physicians began to ask patients to contribute to the cost of their care by buying medicines and supplies and paying medical personnel. These informally charged payments, unrecorded in accounting books, grew throughout the 1990s at the discretion of medical personnel, unregulated by the state or even by hospital management. Although entitlements did not change during the transition period, drastic budget cuts and the emergence of informal payments led to a de facto reduction in the depth of coverage.

From 1996 on, the Kyrgyz government became seriously engaged in health sector reform. From a health financing perspective, the reform consisted of two phases. The first phase lasted from 1997 to 2001 with the introduction of the Mandatory Health Insurance Fund (MHIF) and a small complimentary payroll tax. The second phase was launched in 2001 with a complete reform of the fund-flow and purchasing mechanisms, benefits packages, and service delivery structure. Both phases are described in greater detail below.

Phase 1 began in 1997 with the introduction of the MHIF. A small payroll tax contribution was collected from the economically active (employed, self-employed, and agricultural workers). Pensioners and the registered unemployed were funded out of the pension and unemployment funds, respectively. Collection of these contributions was entrusted to the Social Fund, which was to make appropriate transfers to the MHIF (Law on Insurance Contributions for the State Social Insurance 1998; Law on Medical Insurance 1999). In the first three years after the introduction of the mandatory health insurance scheme, coverage reached 30 percent (Meimanaliev 2003). The main impediments to increasing enrollment were lack of trust in the insurance system, limited employment in the formal sector, and low tax compliance. The rate of coverage by the medical insurance scheme increased as new financing sources were added. Thus, in 2000, coverage had reached almost 70 percent when the republican budget started funding insurance contributions for children under 16 years of age (including full-time students under 21) and social welfare recipients (Kutzin et al. 2001).

By 2001, 83 percent of the population was covered by the mandatory health insurance. The remaining 17 percent were primarily unemployed individuals who failed to register as such. A large part of this group consisted of housewives, because insurance provided to formal sector employees did not cover their families unless they were covered as a member of some other group; for example, as recipients of welfare benefits paid to women with more than five children. The insurance status of students (18 to 21 years old) has been left unclear. According to legislation on the books, they are insured by the state, but the annual budget law has yet to provide funding for this group.

In terms of depth of coverage, the introduction of the MHIF did not significantly change entitlements. The benefit offered by the MHIF to the insured relative to the uninsured was access to free drugs during inpatient care when the drugs were subject to user fees (table 10.4). As described above, however, because most out-of-pocket payments in hospitals were informal, this benefit was notional. At the same time, the additional public financing channeled to hospitals was meant to reduce formal or informal payments by patients. There is no direct evaluation of whether this occurred, but the effect was likely small because the share of the

**Table 10.4** **The Kyrgyz Republic: Coverage in Phase-1 (1997–2001): Population Groups, Sources of Financing, and Benefits**

| Population group | Year | Source of financing | Services provided/Depth of coverage |
|---|---|---|---|
| Formal sector employees, except civil servants | 1997 1998 2000 | 2% from the wage bill administered by the Social Fund (SF) | Drugs at hospital level, salary bonuses Emergency care at the primary level[a] Additional/outpatient drug package |
| Civil servants | 1998 2000 | 2% from the wage bill administered by the SF | Drugs at hospital level, salary bonuses Emergency care at primary level Additional/outpatient drug package |
| Pensioners | 1997 1998 2000 2003 | Value of 1.5 x minimum salary administered by the SF (Pension Fund) Republican budget | Drugs at hospital level, salary bonuses Emergency care at primary level Additional/outpatient drug package Coverage unchanged |
| Registered unemployed | 1997 1998 2000 2002 | Value of 1.5 x minimum salary administered by the SF (Unemployment Fund) Republican budget | Drugs at hospital level, salary bonuses Emergency care at primary level Additional/outpatient drug package Effectively not covered: no funding provided this group by Republican budget |
| Children and students under 21 | 2000 | Value of 1.5 × minimum salary Republican budget | Drugs at hospital level, salary bonuses Emergency care at the primary level Additional/outpatient drug package |
| Welfare benefits recipients | 2000 | Value of 1.5 x minimum salary Republican budget | Drugs at hospital level, salary bonuses Emergency care at the primary level Additional/outpatient drug package |
| Farmers | 1997 2002 | 2% of the land tax administered by SF (5% in 2000, 6% in 2003) Health insurance policies (400 KGS = US$10/year) administered by MHIF | Drugs at hospital level, salary bonuses Emergency care at primary level Additional/outpatient drug package Coverage unchanged |
| Self-employed | 1998 2000 2002 | 2% of the value of 3 x minimum salary Health insurance policies (400 KGS = US$10 / year) administered by the MHIF | Drugs at hospital level, salary bonuses Emergency care at primary level Additional/outpatient drug package Coverage unchanged |

*Sources:* Law on Insurance Contributions for the State Social Insurance for 1998, 1999, 2000, 2003; Law on Medical Insurance of the Citizens of the Kyrgyz Republic, October 18, 1999, with amendments from April 21, 2003, and July 15, 2003.

*Note:* The reimbursement principles: primary level, per capita for emergency care (1998); hospital care, per treated case for drugs and salary bonuses (1997).

a. By law emergency care at the primary level is to be provided to the entire population but per capita reimbursement is provided only for the insured.

health sector budget allocated through the MHIF was less than 5 percent of total public expenditures on health in 1998 (Kutzin et al. 2001). The real benefit from the introduction of the MHIF in this first phase was institutional, allowing step-by-step introduction of population and output-based purchasing mechanisms in a previously input-based environment.

Phase 2, launched in 2001, marked the introduction of significant health financing and service delivery reforms after a long preparatory and piloting period (5 to 6 years). A key instrument of these reforms was explicit definition of entitlements to coverage through the State Guaranteed Benefits Package (SGBP). The primary role of the SGBP was to enumerate the rights and obligations of patients and the state with regard to provision of health services and clarify the entitlements of different population groups (Government Decree No. 98, February 25, 2002). The SGBP specifies the following:

- Primary care is provided free of charge for the entire population with certain lab and diagnostic tests against copayment.
- Hospital care is provided against formal copayment. Copayment is a flat fee payable upon admission.
- Copayments vary with insurance status, exemption status, case type (delivery, surgery, medicine), and referral status (required written referral from primary health care physician.
- Exemption categories were designed based on categorical targeting and disease types to protect populations with high expected health care use. Providers receive a higher payment for treating exempt patients to prevent selection.
- An additional outpatient drug benefit was also introduced to subsidize the price of medicines for primary care sensitive conditions in order to reduce unnecessary hospitalizations (e.g., anemia, ulcers, pneumonia, hypertension).

The use of copayment is regulated. Twenty percent can be used to complement the salary of personnel, and 80 percent must be used for key inputs such as medicines, medical supplies, laboratory supplies, and food. Copayment collections are reported monthly to the MHIF (Oblast Departments); use of copayment revenues, quarterly.

The SGBP and the associated copayment system were not aimed specifically at any income group or geographic area. Copayment rates vary with insurance status, exemption status, case type (delivery, surgery, medicine), and referral status (see, for example, tables 10.5 and 10.6). Two exemption categories were designed, based on categorical targeting and disease types to protect populations with high expected health care use:

- *Targeting based on social categories.* Assistance was intended to reach economically vulnerable groups, but they were defined largely in terms of social and demographic characteristics, whereas, for example, war veterans, people over

**Table 10.5    The Kyrgyz Republic: Copayment Rates for Surgery, 2004 (KGS)**

| Locality | Exempt | Insured | Uninsured | Without referral |
|---|---|---|---|---|
| Bishkek, without Republican HF | 260 | 900 | 1,602 | 2,330 |
| Bishkek, Republican HF | 260 | 1,080 | 1,440 | 2,730 |
| Chui | 260 | 780 | 1,130 | 2,120 |
| Issyk-Kul | 260 | 780 | 1,130 | 2,070 |
| Naryn | 260 | 690 | 1,040 | 2,060 |
| Talas | 260 | 690 | 1,040 | 1,900 |
| Osh | 260 | 560 | 920 | 1,550 |
| Osh City | 260 | 650 | 1,020 | 1,740 |
| Jalal-Abad | 260 | 650 | 1,020 | 1,720 |
| Batken | 260 | 560 | 920 | 1,640 |

*Source:* Law on State Guaranteed Benefits Package for 2004.

**Table 10.6    The Kyrgyz Republic: Copayments for Treatment without Surgery, Diagnosis, Minor Surgery, 2004 (KGS)**

| Locality | Exempt | Insured | Uninsured | Without referral |
|---|---|---|---|---|
| Bishkek, not Republican HF | 200 | 690 | 970 | 1,790 |
| Bishkek, Republican HF | 200 | 830 | 1,110 | 2,100 |
| Chui | 200 | 600 | 870 | 1,630 |
| Issyk-Kul | 200 | 600 | 870 | 1,590 |
| Naryn | 200 | 530 | 800 | 1,580 |
| Talas | 200 | 530 | 800 | 1,460 |
| Osh | 200 | 430 | 710 | 1,190 |
| Osh City | 200 | 500 | 780 | 1,340 |
| Jalal-Abad | 200 | 500 | 780 | 1,320 |
| Batken | 200 | 430 | 710 | 1,260 |

*Source:* Law on State Guaranteed Benefits Package for 2004.

75 years of age, and the disabled regardless of their income were fully exempt from any fees.

- *Targeting based on medical condition/disease type.* Interventions to prevent and cure diseases with important public health consequences and externalities were also exempt from charges (TB, AIDS, syphilis, polio, diphtheria).

Hospitals set up reserve funds to subsidize copayments for the uninsured very poor that did not fall under any of the exemption categories. These funds were to be financed by setting aside 10 percent of copayments. About 9.5 percent of patients in Chui and Issyk-Kul received free treatment, 43 percent of them funded from hospital reserve funds from March to December 2001 (Ibraimova 2002). However, there is no systematic monitoring of the functioning and impact of these reserve funds.

The Outpatient Drug Benefit Program, also called the Additional Drug Package (ADP), was introduced in 2000 as a small pilot test in seven pharmacies and gradually rolled out to the entire country by 2003. The ADP allows insured patients to buy prescribed drugs at discount prices at pharmacies under contract to the MHIF. The subsidy amount, based on a reference price, is about 50 percent of the reference price. The fund reimburses the difference between retail price and the patient pays the pharmacy. By 2004, the number of participating pharmacies and drug sales outlets more than doubled, to 800, up from 357 in 2002 (MHIF Dataset, 2006). However, the geographical disparity in distribution noted earlier is also present here: the high/low ratio between oblasts is 8.8 (excluding the capital). For example, in 2004, in Jalal-Abad oblast there were 35 pharmacies as compared with only 4 in Talass oblast (MHIF Dataset, 2006).

The list of ADP-reimbursed drugs was carefully selected from the essential drug list to include those necessary for managing primary care–responsive conditions (Meimanaliev 2003). A constant effort is being made to improve cost-effectiveness and to include as many generic drugs as possible. The share of generic drugs prescribed by doctors has increased to more than 90 percent, and the package includes 74 generics (MHIF Dataset, 2006). According to a recent evaluation of the outpatient drug benefits program in the Kyrgyz Republic (Ibraimova, Kadyrova, Jakab, draft), the introduction of the ADP has led to reductions in overall prices and in price variations across the geographical areas for covered medicines (e.g., atenolol for management of hypertension).

In itself, the SGBP did not change the de facto coverage gap that emerged because of lack of public funding, but it did clarify entitlements. It made it clear that public funds would cover about 50 percent of hospitalization costs and patients were responsible for paying for the rest. Out of necessity, this was the prevailing practice, but physicians were free to charge whatever they liked. The introduction of the SGBP aimed to end this practice and match entitlements to available public funding and eliminate unfunded mandates. The success of these reforms is examined later.

## Financing and Payment

Revenue collection, pooling, and purchasing fall into three distinct periods: pre-1997, 1997 to 2000, and 2001 to 2006.

***Revenue collection, pooling, and purchasing prior to 1997.*** Prior to 1997, health services were funded from general tax revenues and out-of-pocket payments. Public funding was fragmented along administrative structures: republican-level (central-level) providers were funded from national taxes; oblast (region) facilities, from oblast taxes; city facilities, from city taxes; and rayon (municipal) facilities, from rayon taxes. There was no funding and decision making across these administrative boundaries. This fragmented system of resource allocation led to overlapping population coverage in most urban centers and undercoverage in rural areas. For example, residents of Bishkek had access to both the republican and city health systems, while rural dwellers had direct access only to rayon health facilities unless they traveled to Bishkek or an oblast center. In addition, the capital and oblast centers had more resources than the other areas to fund their health systems. The need to eliminate this duplication of services became acute urgency with the sharp decline in the state health budget when 75 percent of government spending went for staff and infrastructure, leaving little for direct medical expenditures. The resulting savings could be allocated to underserved areas and variable costs, but first resource allocation had to be changed.

According to the input-based budgeting then current, annual budget allocations for health facilities depended on the number of beds and staff positions no matter what the output. Eighteen input categories were used for budgeting (e.g., personnel, drugs, utilities), and managers could not reallocate across line-item categories if need or opportunity arose without a long procedure of obtaining permission from the Ministries of Health and Finance. Moreover, there was no mechanism for reinvesting savings. For instance, if a health facility managed to decrease its utilities costs, it could not reallocate those savings to increase staff salaries or buy medicine. The input-based budgets, allowing no managerial authority to move funds across different line items, had to be replaced to give managers incentives to increase throughput with the minimal amount of resources. Most important, however, this could increase the depth of coverage because resources freed up through increased efficiency would allow health managers to acquire more drugs and medical supplies that patients would otherwise have to cover.

*Revenue collection, pooling and purchasing 1997–2000.* The revenue collection and pooling arrangements changed slightly with the introduction of the MHIF in 1997. Most revenues remained as described above, and the resources managed by the MHIF were added to the revenue mix as a small complementary public resource allocation mechanism. In 1998, the general tax–funded share of the health sector amounted to 95 percent of public expenditures on health, while revenues pooled through the MHIF made up the remaining 5 percent (Kutzin et al. 2001). During this phase, there was no change through the budget in the purchasing mechanisms, which remained based on historical line-item budgets.

The real significance of this reform period was to create the foundation for the second phase in the new MHIF institutional structure and allow it to learn purchasing and use of prospective provider payment mechanisms using small amounts of funds. The MHIF began to contract with a small number of providers and in two years had contracts with all central district (rayon) hospitals. For these contracted facilities, the MHIF introduced new reimbursement procedures: case-based payment to hospitals and capitation-based payment to primary-level health facilities. These will be described further in the next section, because they gained in importance as the MHIF-managed resources grew.

*Revenue collection, pooling, and purchasing 2001–06.* The introduction of significant health financing reforms began in 2001 in two oblasts. The reforms were systematically rolled out to the rest of the country by including two more oblasts every year, gradually changing the health financing system by 2004. In the Kyrgyz Republic, these reforms are referred to as the "Single-Payer Reforms," capturing well their main intent: to end fragmentation of the pooling mechanism by creating regional purchasing pools.

Oblast purchasing pools were established as departments of the MHIF, pooling all oblast, rayon, and city tax revenues. Oblast finance departments transferred all tax revenue allocated for health into the oblast departments of the MHIF. These tax revenues were complemented by the payroll tax revenues collected by the MHIF and transferred to providers using the same payment mechanism. This change created an opportunity to reallocate resources across city-rayon boundaries within oblasts.[9]

The role of the MHIF changed dramatically with the introduction of single-payer reforms because it was made responsible for pooling state budget funds as well as health insurance premiums at the regional (oblast) level. Thus, it became the sole purchasing agency for health care services in every region. It also gained additional roles in quality assurance and the development of health information systems because these were considered part of the contract-monitoring functions.

Once oblast purchasing pools had been created, the old line-item provider payment mechanisms had to be replaced. Once pooled at the oblast level, public funds were transferred to capitation-based outpatient care and to hospitals on a per-case basis. Payment rates per case were defined prospectively, and payment to hospitals was made retrospectively (monthly). The system for grouping cases is modeled on the U.S. diagnosis-related-groups (DRGs) but was created from Kyrgyz utilization and cost data. The case-based payment system introduced the concept of output-oriented payment to the Kyrgyz health system. According to Kutzin and others (2002: 12), "in doing so, the MHIF challenged one of the fundamental weaknesses of the former system: low productivity." This change gave providers incentives to downsize within their facility.

The capitation rate for PHC facilities is based on the available budget and the estimated number of insured persons that will be enrolled in family group practices (FGPs) for the coming year. Previously, citizens were assigned to a district physician according to their place of residence. The new regulation allows them to choose the FGP in which they want to enroll and to switch at each annual registration period. So, in theory, practices that attract more patients receive more capitation funds, an incentive to provide high-quality and user-friendly services to attract users (Atun 2005). In practice, this works only in large urban settings because rural areas and small towns have relatively few providers. Allocation of primary care resources based on a capitation formula adjusted by coefficients for rural, small towns, and mountainous areas allows equalization of resources across the country.

Beyond the financing mechanism, these reforms have important institutional dimensions. The MHIF was established as a parastatal social insurance fund under the Ministry of Health. It was important to create the oblast purchasing pools outside the core public bureaucracy and establish them as part of this parastatal entity. Had centralization of pooling taken place within the confines of regular oblast budgets, prospective payment could not have been implemented. Because public administration and budgeting was (and still is) governed by the same rigid input-based, line-item budgeting mechanisms as during Soviet times, the incentives for downsizing and savings would not have materialized. Pooling alone without changing provider payment mechanisms would not have changed resource flows and allocation patterns.

From 2006, the oblast purchasing pools were further centralized into one national purchasing pool. This shift offers further scope for cross-subsidization across regions and should lead to further improvement in geographical equity. It also expands the risk pool to the national level, a positive development for a country with a small population. The changes made as a result of this new pooling arrangement do not have direct implications on any other elements of the system, such as source of funds, collection, or purchasing methods (Kutzin, O'Dougherty, Jakab 2005). This is important because it means no significant additional training is required for administration of the system—which could expose the key stakeholders to "reform" exhaustion.

## Equity

The drop in public funding and the growth of out-of-pocket payments affected demand for health services. By 2000, significant inequalities in utilization emerged, leading to a disproportionate capture of public expenditures by the rich and consequently poor targeting. The utilization ratio of the PHC and outpatient specialist services among the poorest quintile as compared with the richest quintile was about 2:5 (figure 10.5). The difference in utilization by income was slightly smaller in case of hospitalization: the ratio of the poorest quintile to the richest quintile was about 3:5.

Limited data are available on how these trends affected the distribution of health outcomes. The 1997 DHS Survey is the only data point on the distribution of health outcomes in the period prior to reforms, and it does show the expected poor-rich gradient. According to the survey, infant mortality was 1.8 times higher in the poorest quintile than in the wealthiest, child mortality was almost twice as high, and the stunting rate was 2.4 times higher among children from the poorest quintile than among the richest. Considering the pronounced growth in poverty during the 1990s, it is difficult to disentangle causality and attribute the emerging health inequalities to deterioration of general household welfare or to health system factors such as erosion of coverage.

**Figure 10.5    The Kyrgyz Republic: Access to Health Services, by Income Level, 2000**

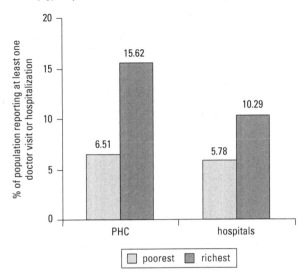

*Sources:* NSC HBS 2001, and HSC HIS 2004; WHO staff calculations.

## *Efficiency*

Limited resources and excess capacity were general features of the health sector in all FSU countries, and the Kyrgyz Republic was no exception. As shown in figure 10.6, the Kyrgyz Republic had a large hospital infrastructure even compared with wealthier countries. The number of hospital beds per 100,000 in the Kyrgyz Republic exceeded the number of hospital beds in the European Union (EU) by more than 25 percent (863.6 against 687.9). Figures for the average length of stay and hospital admission rate were also higher for the Kyrgyz Republic than in the EU member countries, both old and new, but lower than the CIS average.

The increase in inequality demonstrated earlier and the erosion of coverage were inexorably linked to health system inefficiencies. First, two-thirds of the health sector budget was spent on expenditures related to utilities and personnel. This was due to the combination of the ponderous infrastructure inherited from Soviet times, which was sucking away a bigger and bigger piece of a shrinking health care budget. As a result, fewer resources were left for other inputs, such as medicines and supplies, also needed for good quality medical care. So until downsizing could be finished, the inefficiencies manifested in the large hospital infrastructure meant that coverage would remain shallow and patient contributions high.

Second, in addition to poor technical efficiency outlined above, there were problems with allocative efficiency in distributing health expenditures between primary and hospital care. Resources were allocated disproportionately to hospital-

**Figure 10.6    The Kyrgyz Republic: Comparative Indicators of Hospital Efficiency, 1995**

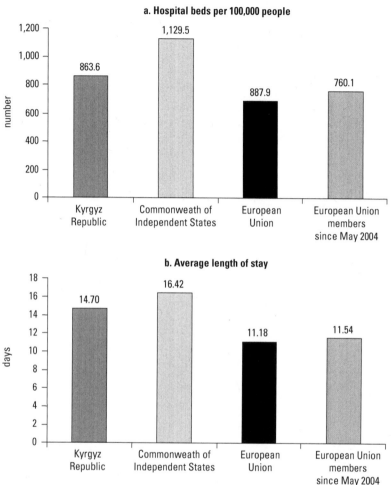

**a. Hospital beds per 100,000 people**

**b. Average length of stay**

based curative care while primary health care was neglected. Primary care did not fulfill the gatekeeper function, and there was a strong tradition of self-referral by patients to specialists and hospitals. In 2001, when the major reforms in health care financing were launched, only 15 percent of total health expenditures went to primary care facilities. Hospitalizations were frequent for conditions that could be treated in primary care (e.g., hypertension, ulcers, anemia, and pneumonia). This inefficiency also added to the financial burden on patients and contributed to increasing inequality in use patterns presented above.

**Figure 10.6    The Kyrgyz Republic: Comparative Indicators of Hospital Efficiency, 1995 *(Continued)***

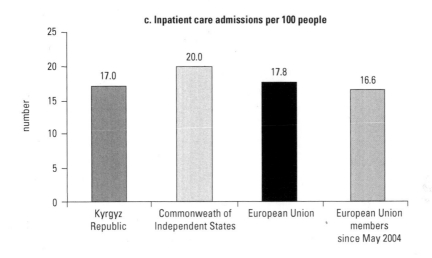

c. Inpatient care admissions per 100 people

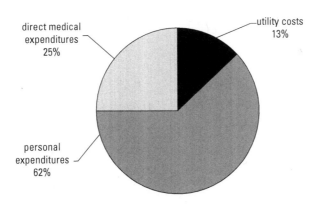

d. Health expenditures, by category

*Sources:* WHO Health for All Database; Central Treasury data quoted in G. Purvis et al. 2005.

It was widely recognized that tackling inefficiencies by reducing hospital capacity and shifting treatment for primary care–responsive conditions out of hospitals was a precondition to improving coverage and equity in the health system. In light of postindependence economic developments, the inherited infrastructure and care patterns were not sustainable. Efficiency gains in the health system were the only possible way to increase coverage in this fiscal context.

## Overview of Health Delivery System

To achieve efficiency gains, service delivery had to be restructured and reoriented. This section focuses on the changes in the inherited Soviet service delivery system (Atun 2005; Kutzin 2002; and Meimanaliev 2003).

### Supply and Organization of Hospitals, Physicians, and Public Health Programs

This section describes primary, secondary, and tertiary care service delivery systems and reforms, including organization, physical infrastructure, and human resources. The section concludes by showing the impact of the changes on the efficiency of service delivery as seen in the allocation of public expenditures between the fixed and the variable costs.

*Primary health care.* There are three types of primary health care providers in the Kyrgyz Republic: Feldsher-Obstetrical Ambulatory Points (FAPs), family group practices (FGPs), and family medicine centers (FMCs). FGPs are the main providers of PHC. An FGP usually consists of three to five doctors. There are three organizational forms of family group practices: freestanding and autonomous, a unit within a free-standing polyclinic (in urban areas), and a unit within a hospital-based polyclinic. FGPs have to meet licensing and accreditation criteria before they can be contracted by the MHIF (Atun 2005). Of the 701 FGPs in the country, 670 are part of FMCs (RMIC Dataset, 2006).

FAPs, which are health care facilities in remote rural areas, offer the most basic services such as antenatal and postnatal care, immunizations, and health education. The 875 FAPs across the country each serve between 500 and 2,000 people (RMIC Dataset, 2006). FMCs are the largest outpatient health facilities, staffed by 10 to 20 medical professionals. They offer services ranging in scope from general care to specialized care and instrumental diagnostics, thus combining primary care services and secondary outpatient care. FMCs, renamed oblast- and rayon-level polyclinics, are now staffed by general practitioners and specialists, who also work in outpatient departments. There are now 85 FMCs in the country, which include 670 FGPs and 816 FAPs (RMIC Dataset, 2006).

PHCs are generally accessible, even in rural areas. Primary health care facilities are located close to patients' homes, with a median distance of 1 to 2 kilometers (Atun 2005). For most patients (73 percent) the travel time to the nearest health facility is less than a half hour. Most patients walk, and only one in three incurs travel expenses when attending health facilities (26 percent in Bishkek to 43 percent in Batken) (Atun 2005). However, the physical presence of a FAP or an FMC does not always translate into access to health services because of shortages of basic medical supplies and, increasingly, health professionals willing to work in rural areas. Poor living conditions, low salaries, and a rising demand for health workers in more prosperous neighboring countries such as Kazakhstan and Russia are the main factors behind the growing problem of unfilled vacancies in many rural health facilities (MOH 2006).

Soviet medicine put heavy emphasis on hospital care, and primary care was neglected. Primary care facilities did not have independent legal and administrative status and functioned mostly as hospital subdivisions. The result was low-quality and underfinanced primary care providing a narrow range of services and limited gatekeeper function. To address this, early health system reforms in the mid-1990s focused on replacing the system of district doctors with family practitioners along the following main lines:

- Primary care was organizationally and financially separated from hospital care. Independent FGPs were set up. The population was required to enroll with an FGP of their choice.

- Human resources training was overhauled in an attempt to institutionalize family medicine training at three levels: undergraduate training; postgraduate training (two-year clinical internship for graduates of higher medical education institutions); continuous training (training trainers, such as doctors and nurses, in family medicine; retraining doctors and nurses in family medicine; and qualifications upgrading of practicing specialists and trainers in family medicine). Most family doctors and nurses (between 60 and 70 percent) participated in retraining in the field of family- and evidence-based medicine under different programs supported by ZdravPlus, Scientific Technology and Language Institute (STLI), the Swiss Cooperation Office, and the World Bank.

- On the basis of evidence-based medicine, 162 clinical protocols on the most prevalent diseases were developed and introduced.

- The State Guaranteed Benefits Package (SGBP) was introduced, specifying people's health care benefits and payment obligations. Within the framework of the SGBP, all citizens, irrespective of their insurance and enrollment status, are entitled to free primary health care services.

- An ADP was introduced, entitling insured individuals to drugs for primary care–responsive conditions at reduced prices.

- Primary health care began to receive additional funding from payroll taxes through the MHIF.

- New provider payment methods were successfully introduced for FGPs based on per capita financing, including partial fund-holding for medicines in the ADP. Capitation payments are a more equitable way of distributing resources at PHC level than line-item financing based on historical performance.

- Outreach activities have been initiated to improve relations with the public and involve local communities in the decision-making process relating to PHC services.

*Secondary and tertiary care.* Secondary care is provided by oblast merged hospitals at oblast level and territorial hospitals at the level of rayons and cities. The structure of all in-patient care facilities at oblast and rayon levels is similar and consists of an administrative-logistical unit (management, human resources, planning, economic, and accounting departments), outpatient diagnostic department (ODD) and treatment units. The main difference between the territorial and oblast hospitals is in the number of treatment units—that is, in the variety and complexity of conditions that can be treated on site. There are 51 territorial hospitals (former city- and rayon-level hospitals), including 1 children's hospital in Bishkek, and 7 oblast hospitals (one per region).

Tertiary care is provided in eight central-level hospitals, including the National Center for Oncology, the National Cardiology and Therapy Center, and the National Center for Surgeries. These facilities provide highly specialized services and are meant to serve the entire country, although studies of referral patterns show that 90 percent of patients reside in the capital and neighboring Chui oblast. The medical personnel at these hospitals also are better educated and more experienced than staff members working in secondary-level hospitals (Meimanaliev 2003).

According to Article 4 of the Law on Health Care Organizations (August 13, 2004), there are two types of ownership of health care organizations: private and public. The private sector has a marginal role in service delivery, specializing mostly in optic and dental care services, gynecology, and urology. Privately owned health facilities are concentrated in the capital. The limited evidence available suggests a growing, though small, number of private sector providers.

As explained above, hospital network downsizing was essential to improve technical and allocative efficiency. This was achieved through centralizing the pooling mechanism and changing provider incentives and administrative mechanisms. Introducing case-based payment created incentives for downsizing, and pooling created the opportunity to rationalize across administrative boundaries.

As most hospitals were built on a pavilion design, operating in 15 to 20 small buildings, within-facility downsizing had great potential for savings on fixed costs. The unnecessary buildings were demolished, rented out (e.g., to pharmacies), or transferred to other public uses (e.g., health promotion cabinets). In 2001–04, physical capacity in the hospital sector was reduced from 1,464 buildings to 784, and the square footage was reduced by 39.6 percent with corresponding changes in the total operational area, utility costs, and maintenance costs (Purvis et al. 2005). Simultaneously, personnel were cut by about 30 percent. At the same time, across-facility downsizing involved merging facilities serving overlapping populations through administrative mechanisms. This allowed reallocation of expenditures from fixed costs (personnel, infrastructure, and maintenance) to direct medical expenditures (drugs and supplies) (figure 10.7).

**Figure 10.7    The Kyrgyz Republic: Reallocation of Public Expenditures in the Single-Payer System from Fixed Costs to Variable Costs**

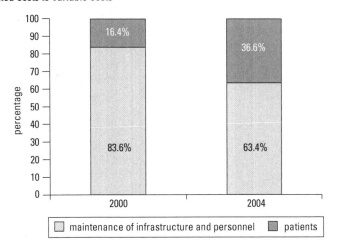

*Source:* MHIF Dataset in Purvis et al. 2005.

## Regulatory Framework

The Law on Health Protection (January 9, 2005) established the general legal framework and articulated roles and responsibilities of state bodies involved in health care service provision. It is a key legal document that regulates the quality of health services, including licensing and accreditation processes for health professionals and organizations (Article 81). The Medical Accreditation Commission (MAC) was established in 1997 as an independent agency responsible for accreditation of health organizations. At its current capacity, the MAC can carry out 50 accreditation surveys a year. Accreditation for health facilities is voluntary. The validity periods vary according to the score received. The Medical Insurance Law (October 18, 1999) provided a basis for financing the health care system through compulsory and voluntary medical health insurance.

According to the Law on Health Care Organizations (August 13, 2004), "state and municipal health organizations have financial autonomy within the boundaries set out in their organizational charter," which is approved by the owner (Article 35). Organizational charters are developed on the basis of standard charters that are approved by a Ministry of Health order. These charters allow health facility management to make decisions on allocation of resources across different inputs. Moreover, management is allowed to maintain commercial bank accounts for copayments retained by the facility. Retention by the facility is particularly important: previously all officially collected user fees were turned over to the central budget where they could be reallocated to other needs. The lack of "own resources" contributed to the rise in informal payments and lack of transparency in financial management of health facilities.

## Other Components of the Delivery System

Medical education, pharmaceuticals, medical technology, and health information systems are other vital parts of the delivery system.

*Medical education.* Until the recent closures, eight higher educational facilities provided medical education in the Kyrgyz Republic. Recognizing the growing problem of poor quality of medical education, a joint commission led by the Ministry of Education closed five institutions and one pharmaceutical education department—none of them accredited. This action was welcomed as an attempt to reduce surplus capacity in medical education and improve the quality of remaining training programs. Graduate and postgraduate training is provided by the Kyrgyz State Medical Academy (KSMA), and the Kyrgyz State Medical Institute for Retraining and Continuing Medical Education (KSMIRCME).

Family medicine principles have been introduced into undergraduate curriculums, but undergraduate programs have not been reoriented toward general practice, and students still choose their specialized educational track the first day of medical school. Teaching remains largely theoretical and didactic, with limited clinical opportunities for medical students to supervise patient care, and no unified educational standards across educational institutions. KSMA and KSMIRCME are participating in regional efforts that have been initiated with donor assistance to begin to move toward the World Federation of Medical Education accreditation standards. As part of the National Health Reform Strategy for 2006–10, a working group has been set up to review the undergraduate medical curriculum and develop a strategy to improve both its content and the teaching/educational processes used to teach it.

Strengthening family medicine programs and making them more attractive for students has a direct impact on ensuring access to health care services, particularly for the rural population. As noted in the discussion of health service delivery, the lack of family doctors, particularly in rural areas, is increasingly problematic. There is also a constant shortage of applicants to family medicine programs. In 2005, KSMA offered 70 clinical residencies but filled only 7 places; in 2006, it offered 50 residencies and filled only 14.

There are 14 medical (nursing) colleges located throughout the Kyrgyz Republic where nurses and feldshers[10] are trained. In 2005, 2,365 people were graduated from medical colleges. The nursing curriculum has been revised, the training period extended to three years, and new disciplines introduced (e.g., introduction to law, reproductive health and family planning). New government educational standards have been developed for eight specialties for mid-level medical personnel, including pharmacists.

*Pharmaceutical sector.* The pharmaceutical sector changed dramatically in 1997 with the adoption of a new drug policy that allowed privatization of pharmacies (Meimanaliev 2003). Simultaneously, the MOH established a Department of Pharmaceutical Provision and Supplies as the main regulatory body responsible for accreditation of pharmacies, regardless of the ownership, and licensing of pharmacists and pharmaceutical organizations (Government Decree No 556, September 26, 1997). By 2000, there were 1,285 pharmacies and drug outlets in the Kyrgyz Republic (MOH Report 2004). However, they are unevenly distributed across the country, because running a drug outlet in remote rural areas is unprofitable. To address this issue, the MOH allows personnel with clinical backgrounds, after a month of training, to sell drugs in villages that do not have a private pharmacy. Two laboratories control the drug quality. Currently, 70 percent of imported drugs must be tested, and all of them are tested. The remaining 30 percent come from reliable manufacturers and are exempt from testing (GMP certified).

*Medical technology.* The use of advanced medical technology is limited first and foremost, by the highly constrained resource environment. In 2002, recognizing that sustainable, transparent, and equitable mechanisms had to be instituted for providing expensive, high-technology medical care, the government created the High-Technology Fund (Government Decree No 287, May 7, 2002). The fund is financed from four sources: the republican (central) budget, external donors, private charitable organizations, and humanitarian assistance. Since its creation, however, it has been chronically underfinanced and has had little impact on patients' access to high-technology services. The shortage of financing, at least from external donors, is partly due to lack of clear operational guidelines for the fund. The decree is vague on basic rules of access to services. The government has yet to decide on the maximum amount allowed per service or procedure, rules for allocating the available budget across types of procedure, rules for determining eligibility (clinical and financial needs), and the extent of and any exemption from copayments.

*Health information system.* The Kyrgyz Republic has a well-developed health information system for a country of its income level. The system has three main levels: national, the MHIF; oblast, the oblast departments of the MHIF; and provider level. This system feeds information into five databases: the MHIF database on the insured population; the enrollment database with primary care facilities to enable capitation-based payment; the hospital admission database with case coding to enable case-based payment managed by the Republican Medical Information Center; the outpatient care utilization registry also managed by the RMIC; and the Additional Drug Package.

However, because the health management information system development was driven largely by the needs of health care financing reforms, it has largely ignored other important areas. Thus, information on health status and quality of care indicators is not always consistent and reliable. Also, financial resources needed for system maintenance are lacking. High telecommunication costs also pose a significant barrier to further HMIS development.

## The Health Coverage Reforms

Depth of coverage was the problem that emerged in the Kyrgyz Republic during the transition period. At the start of transition, the entire population was entitled to free health services of every kind, with the exception of a few specialized services and outpatient drugs for which small fees were charged. During Soviet times, these entitlements were funded, and an extensive service delivery infrastructure reached most rural areas, at least with paramedical if not primary health care posts. Until 1991, coverage was high—both in terms of breadth and depth.

The dramatic loss of budget revenues after independence from the Soviet Union made these entitlements unaffordable and increasingly unfunded. In the early transition years (1991–95), providers were left to their own devices to find a way to adjust to this dramatically reduced financing. At the time, the input-based budget formation process, which rewarded capacity, gave no incentives for efficiency. Thus, the adjustment took place by introducing informal charging practices. Patients were required to pay for medical personnel, medicines, medical supplies, and even nonmedical supplies. Although entitlements did not change on paper during this time, the depth of coverage eroded, marked by increasing out-of-pocket payments. There was a mismatch between de jure and de facto entitlements, and a deep sense of disillusionment with the health system.

In the 1990s, the Kyrgyz Republic emerged as the second poorest country in the FSU. Poverty rates hovered around 50 percent, and the potential for fast economic growth was crippled. It became clear that the fiscal context would remain limited, at least in the short run, and that the depth of coverage could not be restored to pretransition levels from the depleted public coffers. Reforms to create a transparent and sustainable system of coverage required two difficult steps: (1) eliminating the mismatch between the de jure and de facto entitlements by clarifying the respective roles of the government and individuals in funding health services within the prevailing fiscal space, and (2) downsizing the inherited service delivery infrastructure to achieve and rechannel efficiency gains from fixed costs to variable costs and lighten patients' financial burden.

Because the coverage problems and their causes were entangled in a broad web of performance problems and inadequacies of the inherited Soviet health system, a systemic approach was necessary. The ensuing reforms had to encompass the entire spectrum of the health system; they could not address isolated reform objectives or use single instruments. The reforms thus reposed on four main pillars:

- *Clarification of entitlements through the introduction of the State Guaranteed Benefits (SGBP) package.* The primary role of the SGBP was to define the rights and obligations of patients and the state with regard to provision of health services and clarify the entitlements of different population groups. In itself, the SGBP did not change the de facto coverage gap that emerged due to lack of public funding, but it did clarify entitlements. It was based on the acknowledgment that public funds were sufficient to cover only about 50 percent of hospitalization costs and that patients were responsible for paying for the other 50 percent. Out of necessity, this was the prevailing practice but charging practices were left entirely to the discretion of physicians. The introduction of the SGBP aimed to end this practice, match entitlements to available public funding, and eliminate unfunded mandates.

- *Centralization of previously fragmented pooling arrangements.* Oblast purchasing pools were created in 2001 in two oblasts and gradually introduced nationwide by 2004. The new system replaced the previously compartmentalized financing arrangements with city revenues funding city hospitals, rayon revenues funding rayon hospitals, and oblast revenues funding oblast hospitals. In this fragmented context, the service delivery system could not be restructured across these rigid administrative boundaries. Thus, pooling reform was a precondition for reconfiguring the service delivery structure and thus to achieve efficiency gains. In 2006, the pooling arrangements were further centralized at the national level, moving to one pool for purchasing most health services and promising great potential for equalizing funding across the country.

- *Replacement of historical line-item, capacity-linked budgeting with population- and output-based provider payment mechanisms.* Pooling was a necessary but insufficient condition to initiate restructuring of the hospital sector. As long as the budgeting process was based on capacity and the payment mechanism was based on rigid line items, there were no incentives to downsize. The introduction of case-based payments was a milestone in this regard. The health sector became unique in the public administration by severing the link between inputs and budgets.

- *Restructuring of service delivery with strengthened primary health care and more efficient and streamlined hospital care.* Pooling and payment reforms created an enabling environment for downsizing hospital capacity. Downsizing was not left entirely to the discretion of hospital management. The MHIF, the newly formed Hospital Association, and a qualified consulting company worked closely with each hospital to demonstrate the benefits of downsizing and develop a restructuring plan. Outside the capital city, significant downsizing took place, as described above, with documented reductions in fixed costs. Simultaneously, arduous efforts were made to strengthen primary care and broaden the scope of services. To reduce unnecessary hospitalizations, particular attention was devoted to primary care–responsive conditions such as ulcers, pneumonia, hypertension.

In sum, the Kyrgyz coverage reforms were closely linked to an overall reform agenda trained on the creation of an efficient and sustainable health system.

## Chronology

The Kyrgyz health system reforms described above became known as the Manas National Health Care Reform Program (1996–2005). The reforms were implemented in two main phases. Phase 1 (1996–2000) focused on refining the reform design; building capacity in the health sector for policy development, implementation, and evaluation; launching primary care reform; establishing the MHIF; and piloting new financial mechanisms. Phase 2 (2001–05) involved major structural changes in health care financing and service delivery (box 10.1).

In 2006, a follow-on phase was introduced with the Manas Taalimi National Health Care Reform Program (2006–10). In this phase, the achievements of the Manas reforms will be taken forward, the remaining weaknesses addressed, and a new generation of reforms introduced.

---

**B O X  10.1**  *The Kyrgyz Republic: The Manas National Health Care Reform Program*

| 1997–2000 **Establishment of the Mandatory Health Insurance Fund and piloting of reforms** | 2001–05 **Development and Implementation of Single-Payer System** |
|---|---|
| 1. Approval of the Manas National Health Care Reform Program (1996)<br>2. Family group practices enrollment campaign in Issyk-Kul oblast (1996)<br>3. Law on Drugs (1997)<br>4. Licensing and accreditation process started (1997)<br>5. Case-based payment to hospitals from insurance funds introduced, rolling-out of primary health care reforms to three additional oblasts and the capital city Bishkek (1997–98)<br>6. Case-based payment from budgetary funds to selected hospitals introduced in Bishkek (1999)<br>7. Laws on Interpretation of the Law on Principles of the Budget and the Law on Local Self-Governments, laying the foundations for the single-payer system:<br>  (a) Pooling of rayon/city funds to finance health care allowed at higher levels;<br>  (b) "Copayment" introduced in the health system that is outside of the Treasury system and is tax exempt (2000). | 1. Government Decree on Introduction of a New Health Care Financing Mechanism in Health Facilities (2001)<br>2. Government Decree on Program of State Guarantees fo Issyk-Kul and Chui Oblasts (2001)<br>3. Piloting of the Outpatient Drug Benefits Package in Bishkek (2001)<br>4. Transfer to output-based financing in Issyk-Kul and Chui oblasts (2001)<br>5. Single payer system joined by Naryn and Talas, followed by Batken, Jalal-Abad, and Osh oblasts (2002–03)<br>6. Countrywide introduction of Outpatient Drug Benefits (2003)<br>7. Countrywide coverage with State Guaranteed Benefits Package (2004)<br>8. Law on Single-Payer System in Health Care Financing (2004)<br>9. Law on Health Care Organizations (2004)<br>10. Law on Health Protection (2005)<br><br>*Source:* Authors' compilation. |

## Evaluations

The financial protection impact of the Kyrgyz reforms is still being evaluated, but already it is clear that they are associated with a declining financial burden of hospital care, especially for the poor, and increasing transparency. In addition, utilization of both outpatient and inpatient health services has become more equal. Nonetheless, large out-of-pocket payments for health care still put a sizeable financial burden on households nationwide.

Interpretation of national trends has been hampered by the phased introduction of the reforms. What drives nationwide results is unclear: is it the lack of reforms in late-reform areas or the reforms themselves in the early areas? The preliminary results of an ongoing evaluation to separate these effects shows evidence that the financial burden associated with hospital care has been lightened and informal payments are less prevalent in the early-reform oblasts than in the late reformers. Concomitantly, growing expenditure on outpatient medicines has emerged as a next generation coverage/financial protection problem. These findings are expanded below, but a definite assessment of reform benefits has to await analysis of the household survey of 2007.

*Depth of coverage.* Analysis of the 2001 and 2004 household surveys show that nationwide, out-of-pocket expenditures continued to grow (figure 10.8). Out-of-pocket payments include payments in outpatient settings for outpatient drugs and

**Figure 10.8   The Kyrgyz Republic: Trends in Out-of-Pocket Payments, 2000–03 (KGS)**

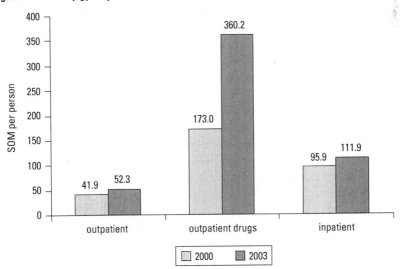

*Sources:* NSC 2001; Household Budget Survey, Health Module, NSC, 2004; Kyrgyz Integrated Household Survey, Health Module; WHO staff calculations.

both formal and informal payments at the time of hospitalization. This increase is fueled by spending on outpatient medicines. People consume more drugs, and drugs cost more. The large increase is due to both a price and a quantity effect.

Analysis of out-of-pocket patterns by consumption quintiles shows that the share of out-of-pocket payments in household resources grew significantly among the poorest quintile to 7 percent by 2003. The second, third, and fourth quintiles also spent more of their resources on health in 2003 than in 2000. In all four quintiles, spending on outpatient medicines drove the results. The richest quintile experienced a slight reduction, mainly because the better-off are using less health care.

Because the reforms were introduced in phases, they had been implemented in only four of the eight oblasts when the follow-up survey was done. Thus, these nationwide trends do not allow identification of cause and effect. An ongoing evaluation of the Kyrgyz reforms on financial protection uses a difference-in-difference approach to isolate the prereform effect. According to preliminary results, out-of-pocket payments for hospitalization were similar in reform and control oblasts prior to the introduction of the reforms, controlling for many other observable household characteristics. During the reform period, out-of-pocket payments increased significantly in control oblasts by nearly SOM 600 (US$15). In contrast, out-of-pocket payments increased by only SOM 200 (US$5) per individual in reform oblasts during the same period. This leads to a difference-in-difference estimate of the reform effect of minus KGS 393 (US$10), equivalent to 29 percent of the prereform out-of-pocket payments in reform oblasts. The results show that the reform effect has benefited mostly the lower-income groups. This suggests that the reforms have been successful at limiting the increase in out-of-pocket payments for hospitalization, and the effect size is quite large (Jakab 2007).

In sum, whether the reforms have improved depth of coverage is not yet a clear. Nationwide data show that out-of-pocket payments still put a sizeable burden on households seeking treatment, but a more refined evaluation of the reform effect shows that the reforms have considerably improved financial protection, at least for hospital care.

*Equity in access to care.* Despite an increase in the burden of out-of-pocket payments, utilization of health care services across socioeconomic groups has become more equal over the 2000–03 time-period for both outpatient and inpatient care (figure 10.9). In 2000, the richest 20 percent of the population used outpatient services twice as frequently as the poorest 20 percent. By 2003, the visit rate dropped, but only among the richer half of the population. The poorest quintile experienced no change in their rate of visits, and the visit rate for the second income quintile increased significantly. Similar trends were observed for hospitalizations. The hospital utilization rate declined for all socioeconomic groups. For the poorest, it declined only marginally while for the richest it declined by 40 percent. As a result, the rich are using hospital care only slightly more frequently than

**Figure 10.9   The Kyrgyz Republic: Access to Outpatient Care and Hospital Care, 2000 and 2003**

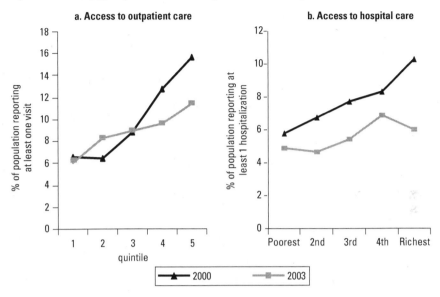

*Sources:* NSC 2001; Household Budget Survey, NSC 2004; Kyrgyz Integrated Household Budget Survey; WHO staff calculations.

*Note:* Outpatient care includes primary and specialist care. The population was grouped into five quintiles using consumption data and quintile data calculated by the National Statistical Committee. Each quintile group contains 20 percent of the population ranked from poorest to richest.

the poor. On the whole, the reforms appear to play an equalizing role on utilization across the country and across socioeconomic lines.

*Transparency.* The single-payer system has improved health system transparency for the population by creating a clear system of benefits and entitlements through the SGBP and the copayment policy. Previously, confusion about entitlements, coupled with great pressure on providers to make up for a drastic decline in public funding, gave rise to a widespread system of informal payments, in particular for hospital care. At the time of hospitalization, most patients had to make informal to payments to physicians for medicines and other supplies. However, there was no formula for regulating the contribution (in-kind and in-cash) that patients were required to contribute, and physicians could decide for themselves how much and whom to charge according to their own understanding of social justice. Various surveys indicate that patients found this system opaque, subjecting them to unpredictable financial demands at the time of illness. The cost of hospitalization was not known in advance, not even at the time of admission, and expenditures mounted steadily during the course of a hospital stay.

**Figure 10.10   The Kyrgyz Republic: Mean Payment by a Public Hospital Patient, 2000 and 2003**

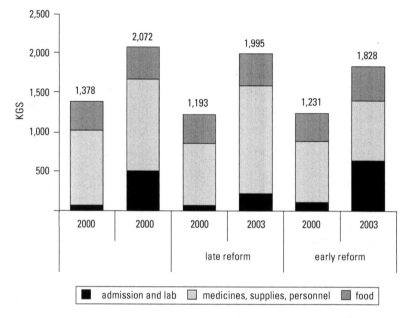

*Source:* NSC 2001; Household Budget Survey, NSC 2004; Kyrgyz Integrated Household Budget Survey; WHO staff calculations.

*Note:* "Early reform" includes Issyk-kul, Chui, Naryn and Talas; "late reform" includes Osh, Jalal-Abad, Batken. Medicines, supplies, and personnel covers unequivocally informal payments, because patients should receive these services free of charge against their copayment. In 2000, also largely informal admission and lab payments, because there was no charge at that time for admission. In 2003, admission and lab payments are in early reform oblasts is a formal copayment, but in Bishkek and late-reform oblasts it reflects a mix of copayment and informal payment due to the varied timing of these policies.

The reforms clarified entitlements, but problems remain. Figure 10.10 shows a breakdown of out-of-pocket payments for hospitalization, by category. The payment amount reflects the mean payment per episode of hospitalization among patients admitted to a public hospital at least once in the year preceding the survey. The dark solid area is formal and informal payments made upon admission and for lab tests; formal and informal payment that cannot be separated based on this survey. The checkered area represents payments for medicines, supplies, and personnel, all of them informal payments. The white area is the amount paid for food.

The figure shows that the overall out-of-pocket payments at the time of hospitalization grew the most slowly in early-reform oblasts. This indicates that the reforms did slow the growth of out-of-pocket and the resultant burden on households. In areas where single-payer reforms and copayment were introduced latest, informal payments increased, by 73 percent in the late-reform oblasts of Osh, Jalal-Abad, and Batken, and by 24 percent in Bishkek. In contrast, informal payments decreased by 2 percent in the early-reform oblasts of Issyk-kul, Chui, Naryn, and Talas where the reforms had more time to take hold.

As the evaluation above shows, depth of coverage, equity of access, and transparency have tangibly improved. However, some issues still need to be addressed before the benefits of the reforms reach the entire population. A key impediment to reaching this goal is lack of awareness of entitlements among vulnerable groups. Although the SGBP clearly regulates entitlements, many people do not know that primary care is free or that insured individuals have a right to the Outpatient Drug Benefits Package. At the hospital level, many patients continue to pay informally, despite publicly displayed copayment schedules. Lack of awareness of rights is a particular problem among internal migrants who do not know that their health insurance benefits are portable and that their enrollment with a family group practice is not linked to a permanent place of residence (World Bank 2005c).

## Scaling-Up

The Kyrgyz reforms were piloted and the introduced in phases. Although in many contexts, pilots do not get scaled up for nationwide implementation, the Kyrgyz experience is positive from this perspective. The reforms were introduced in two additional oblasts each year between 2001 and 2005, when the entire country was finally covered. In the interim, resistance grew and side effects began to show. To carry out these politically sensitive, unpopular reforms, strong political ownership was essential. Gradual implementation allowed learning-by-doing, which is critical when introducing completely new financing and institutional mechanisms. In addition, phased implementation also allowed policy makers to devote sufficient attention to the oblasts and providers that were next in line.

## Lessons for Other Countries

The successes of the Kyrgyz health reform are due in part to the focus on a comprehensive approach rather than on isolated instruments or "magic bullets." The Kyrgyz reforms did not attempt to find a magic bullet to achieve every health system objectives such as the "right" benefits package or the "right" provider payment reform. The reforms involved a coordinated package of changes in pooling, purchasing, design of the benefits package, and patient copayments. A key element of this package was a carefully structured and well-aligned financial incentive system on both the provider and the patient sides. In addition, reforms of health care financing were complemented with harmonization of the organization and structure of service delivery at both the macro- and microlevels. This included restructuring of facilities and extension of provider autonomy.

## Enabling Factors

***Complex reforms require careful sequencing of various reform steps.*** The Kyrgyz reforms stand out in this regard. First, it was implicitly acknowledged that, without efficiency improvements through downsizing, other health system objectives such as equity and quality cannot be improved, given the fiscal constraints. By combining financing and service delivery reforms, the Manas reforms were extremely successful in achieving efficiency gains, which paved the way for focusing on other health system objectives in the next phase. Second, the health financing reform measures were also carefully sequenced. Changes in revenue collection and pooling were the initial steps to ensure optimal flow of public funds first. Then, new purchasing arrangements to provider incentives were introduced. These steps brought transparency to the public sector. The last step, introduction of a benefits package, created a transparent social contract between the people covered and the government providing coverage through taxation.

*Close attention to the institutional aspects of the reforms was important to ensure sustainable results.* Progress on efficiency and quality would have been much more difficult had the MHIF not been formed as a parastatal agency in charge of purchasing. The single-payer system has successfully incorporated "strategic purchasing" in its day-to-day operations. This included output-based payment mechanisms, cleverly structured incentives for referrals and exemptions, the ADP and regular monitoring of quality. All these tools provided explicit incentives for efficient and high-quality delivery of health care. Had the MHIF not been set up outside the core public sector, it would not be able to purchase services "strategically" and would have had to rely on hierarchical line-item input control as other organizations in the core public bureaucracy. This type of input-based budgeting was a major source of inefficiency in the system inherited from the USSR, and it could it not have been overcome without changing purchasing methods.

*Phased implementation and successful piloting were an effective implementation approach that helped build capacity and stakeholder support and allowed learning by doing.* The Issyk-kul Intensive Demonstration Site provided an opportunity for the basic health reform model to be developed. Many of the early adjustments and fine-tuning of the reforms had already taken place in Issy-Kul. Also, Issy-Kul became a visible symbol of reform, greatly assisting the expansion of these reforms to other parts of the country and the further expansion of the family group practice model. Issyk-Kul continues to serve as a demonstration site for the country as the reforms here have been deepened over time. For example, the inpatient copayment policy was first implemented in Issy-Kul and Chui (another oblast where the reforms have been ongoing for at least five years). The finding that the greatest and most sustained reduction in informal payments occurred in Issyk-kul is likely to be due to this longer experience with the reforms, which allowed capacity building and commitment to reform principles.

*Strong MOH coordination and collaboration with the development partners facilitated harmonized activities for reform design and support.* Donor presence in the health sector is strong in the Kyrgyz Republic. However, experience from other highly donor-dependent countries indicates that donor support is often fragmented and overlapping. That means that the health sector often benefits less from donor support than it should and has fewer results to show at the end of a long period of donor support. This was not the case in the Kyrgyz Republic where donor collaboration has been strong. The activities of most major donors in the health sectors were well aligned with the government's reform plan and the donors made an effort to harmonize their procedures and positions. Having a well-articulated sector strategy facilitated this unified approach. The donors supporting the same health sector strategy became important political advocates for its continued implementation and success. By gradually moving to a "single voice" on many policy issues, they provided powerful political support and contributed to the continuity of the Kyrgyz reforms over a decade. Due to the successful alignment and harmonization of donor support over a decade, the Kyrgyz health sector has moved to a Sector-Wide Approach (SWAp) in 2006 for the first time in the region.

## Key Financing Factors

***The decline in public expenditures during reform implementation limited the impact on financial protection and transparency.*** Oblast funding began to decline after successful restructuring. Oblast-level pooling and output-based payment have achieved their intent: the Kyrgyz health system underwent significant downsizing and became slimmer between 1996 and 2003 with resultant reductions in utility and maintenance costs. The rest of the public sector has not taken the same giant steps as the health sector to move to output-based payment of public providers. Declining staff and beds triggered the well-instilled response of the Soviet budgeting system: if inputs decline, so too should public funds. This mechanistic response has removed savings from the health sector, reducing provider incentives to embark on painful downsizing processes elsewhere. The introduction of copayment also had a crowding-out effect on public spending. The period of accelerated decline in public funding, especially at oblast level, coincided with the introduction of copayment. This seemed to create a crowd-out effect in budget negotiations, and marginal resources were allocated to sectors that did not have a chance to collect additional revenues through copayments.

***The slow pace of reforms in the overall public finance system created a challenging operating environment for the health sector and limits its ability to achieve efficiency, quality, and equity gains.*** The health sector gradually but firmly moved away from input-based, line-item budgets and administrative control mechanisms and began to switch to performance management and output-based payment of public providers. These changes have vastly improved transparency and efficiency in public health sector management. At the same time, these ideas remained revolutionary within the overall public system, which still operates largely on the inherited principles of input-based budgeting and strict line items. This mismatch between the pace of public finance reform and health finance reform has created significant problems for the health sector in the annual budget negotiation process.

## Key Political Economy Factors

*Due to political pressures to eliminate copayment without a commensurate increase in public funding, unfunded mandates have returned to the health sector in recent times.* In the 2006 revision of the SGBP, copayment was eliminated for children under five, deliveries, and pensioners over 75 years of age. This move, a result of political pressure from the new government, was not accompanied by any clear and transparent calculations of the cost and affordability of the policy. As a result, commensurate funding is not likely to be available to compensate providers for the loss of official copayments, and this will usher in the return of informal payments and deterioration of hard-won improvements in transparency. The impact of this policy is currently under evaluation.

## Replicability in Low- and Middle-Income Countries

The Kyrgyz reform in its entirety is particularly applicable in transition economies confronted with excess capacity and drastically reduced fiscal space. The main logic of the Kyrgyz reforms was to squeeze efficiency gains out of the system and use the savings to improve the depth of coverage. This set and sequencing of reform instruments have less relevance in countries without significant excess capacity in infrastructure and staff.

## Endnotes

1. Unless otherwise noted, economic and poverty data in this section are taken from the World Development Indicators (WDI) Dataset, 2006.
2. The *extreme poverty rate* is defined as the proportion of the population with insufficient expenditures (or consumption) to purchase a food basket of 2,100 calories.
3. The *absolute poverty rate* is defined as the proportion of the population too poor to obtain the proper amount of food and necessary nonfood consumables.
4. The share of agriculture in GDP is 34 percent, according to WDI.
5. Government functions are funded from the central budget and mixed functions, from the central and local budgets. *Local functions* are defined as expenditure obligations of local self-governments.
6. IMR increased to 25.7 in 2004, but it is not strictly comparable to earlier years because the government introduced new live birth criteria to conform with the international standards.
7. For more details, see Asymbekova, unpublished report.
8. This description of the political situation is based on two reports by the International Crisis Group (2001; 2005).

9. The centralization of financing reforms was completed in 2006 with oblast purchasing merged into one purchasing pool for the entire country, further increasing the scope from cross-subsidization and transfers.

10. A *feldscher* is equivalent to a physician's assistant or nurse practitioner in the United States. The following definition of feldscher is the correct one: Feldsher or Obstetrician Posts are primary rural health facilities that provide basic predoctor services such as first aid, preventive care and antiepidemic work, sanitary and hygiene promotion, early detection of and initial measures against infectious outbreaks. FAPs have only mid-level health personnel (up to three people), such as obstetricians, doctor's attendants and nurses.

## References

Asymbekova, Gulnara. "Analysis of Maternal Mortality for 1999 in the Kyrgyz Republic." Unpublished report for the Ministry of Health. Bishkek: MOH.

Atun, Rifat. 2005. *Evaluating Manas Health Sector Reform (1996–2005): Focus on Primary Health Care*. Policy Research Papers. Bishkek: WHO-DfID Manas Health Policy Analysis Project.

CIA (Central Intelligence Agency). 2006. *World Fact Book*. Washington DC: CIA. https://www.cia.gov/cia/publications/factbook/geos/kg.html.

Ibraimova, Ainura. 2002. *Report to the Government of the Kyrgyz Republic on the Activities of the MHIF for 2001*. Bishkek: Mandatory Health Insurance Fund.

Ibraimova, Ainura, Ninel Kadyrova, Melitta Jakab. Washington, DC: CIA. Draft. *Contracting Mechanism to Improve Access to Essential Drugs—the Kyrgyz Outpatient Drug Benefit*. Bishkek: WHO-DfID Manas Health Policy Analysis Project.

International Crisis Group. 2005. *Kyrgyzstan: A Faltering State*. Asia Report. Bishkek/Brussels: International Crisis Group.

———. 2001. *Kyrgyzstan at Ten: Trouble in the "Island of Democracy."* Asia Report. Bishkek/Brussels: International Crisis Group.

Institute for War and Peace Reporting. 2003. "Bishkek Braced for Aksy Anniversary." News Report RCA No. 188, March 4. http://www.iwpr.net/?p=rca&s=f&o=177056&apc_state=hruirca2003

Jakab, Melitta. 2007. "An Empirical Evaluation of the Kyrgyz Health Reform: Does It Work for the Poor?" PhD dissertation, Harvard University, Cambridge, MA.

Kutzin, Joseph. 2000. "Toward Universal Health Care Coverage: A Goal-Oriented Framework for Policy Analysis." Working Paper, World Bank, Washington, DC.

Kutzin, Joseph, Ainura Ibraimova, Ninel Kadyrova, Gulaim Isabekova, Yevgeniy Samyshkin, and Zainagul Kataganova. 2002. *Innovations in Resource Allocation, Pooling and Purchasing in the Kyrgyz Health System*. Policy Research Papers. Bishkek: WHO-DfID Health Policy Analysis Project.

Kutzin, Joseph, Ainura Ibraimova, Ninel Kadyrova, Tilek Meimanaliev, and Tobias Schüth. 2001. *Addressing the Informal Payments in Kyrgyz Hospitals*. Policy Research Papers. Bishkek: WHO-DfID Health Policy Analysis Project.

Kutzin, Joseph, Sheila O'Dougherty, and M. Jakab 2005. *Fiscal Decentralization and Options for the Kyrgyz Health Financing System: Reflections on Three Options*. Policy Research Papers. Bishkek: WHO–DfID Manas Health Policy Analysis Project.

Meimanaliev, Tilek. 2003. *Kyrgyz Model of Health Care System*. Bishkek: Uchkun.

Meimanaliev, Adilet-Sultan et al. 2005. *Health Care Systems in Transition: Kyrgyzstan.* Copenhagen: European Observatory on Health Care Systems.

MHIF (Mandatory Health Insurance Fund). 2006. Dataset provided upon request.

MOH (Ministry of Health), Kyrgyz Republic. 2006. *Manas Taalimi Health Reform Strategy.* Bishkek.

NSC (National Statistical Committee). 2004. *Kyrgyz Integrated Household Budget Survey.* Bishkek.

———. 2001. *Household Budget Survey*. Bishkek.

———. 2005. Dataset provided upon request.

Oxford Policy Management. 2006. "Kyrgyz Republic: Public Financial Management Assessment." Final Report, January 18, 2006. Oxford Policy Management, Oxford, U.K. http://siteresources.worldbank.org/INTECAPUBEXPMAN/Resources/PFMkyrgyz ReportFinal090806.pdf.

Purvis, George, et al. 2005. *Evaluating Manas Health Sector Reforms (1996-2005): Focus on Restructuring*. Policy Research Papers. Bishkek: WHO-DfID Manas Health Policy Analysis Project.

RMIC (Republican Medical Information Center). 1997–2005. *Health of the Population and Performance of Health Facilities in the Kyrgyz Republic.* Bishkek: Ministry of Health of the Kyrgyz Republic.

———. 2006. Dataset provided upon request.

Sargaldakova, Acelle, et al. 2000. *Health Care Systems in Transition: Kyrgyzstan.* Copenhagen: European Observatory on Health Care Systems.

United Nations Population Division. 2006. *World Population Prospects: The 2004 Revision Population Database*. http://esa.un.org/unpp/index.asp.

World Bank. 2006. *World Development Indicators*. Washington, DC: World Bank.

———. 2005a. *Kyrgyz Republic Poverty Update: Profile of Living Standards in 2003*. Washington, DC: World Bank.

———. 2005b. *Kyrgyz Republic: Country Economic Memorandum.* 2 vols. Washington, DC: World Bank.

———. 2005c. *Operationalizing the Health and Education MDGs in Central Asia: Kyrgyz Republic Health Education Case Studies.* 2 vols. Washington, DC: World Bank.

———. 2004a. *Millennium Development Goals for Health in Europe and Central Asia: Relevance and Policy Implications*. Washington, DC: World Bank.

———. World Bank. 2004b. *Public Expenditure Review*. 2 vols. Washington, DC: World Bank.

———. 2001. *Poverty in the 1990s in the Kyrgyz Republic*. Washington, DC: World Bank.

———. 2006. World Development Indicators (WDI) Database. World Bank, Washington, DC.

WHO (World Health Organization). Various years. Health for All Database. http://data.euro.who.int/hfadb.

———. 2004. Global Burden of Disease Estimates, 2002. http://www.who.int/healthinfo/bodestimates/en/index.html.

## Legal Norms

Government Decree No. 98 on Copayment for Drugs, Food and Certain Medical Services Provided by State Health Facilities, February 25, 2002.

Government Decree No.556 on Establishment of the Department of Drug Provision and Medical Equipment under the Ministry of Health, September 26, 1997.

Government Decree No. 287 on High-Technology and Expensive Medical Services, May 7, 2002.

Law on the Basic Principles of the Budget, June 11, 1998.

Law on Health Care Organizations, August 13, 2004.

Law on Health Protection, January 9, 2005.

Law on Insurance Contributions for the State Social Insurance for 1998, January 17, 1998.

Law on Insurance Contributions for the State Social Insurance for 1999, December 26, 1998.

Law on Insurance Contributions for the State Social Insurance for 2000, January 18, 2000.

Law on Insurance Contributions for the State Social Insurance for 2003, February 15, 2003.

Law on Medical Insurance of the Citizens of the Kyrgyz Republic, October 18, 1999, with amendments on April 21, 2003, and July 15, 2003.

Law on State Guaranteed Benefits Package for 2004.

# 11

# Sri Lanka: "Good Practice" in Expanding Health Care Coverage

*Ravi P. Rannan-Eliya and Lankani Sikurajapathy*

## Background

*Sri Lanka, a rainy, 66,000-square-kilometer island in the Indian Ocean near the equator, is in the South Asia Region of the World Bank. Only 15 percent of Sri Lanka's 20 million people live in cities. It is a lower-middle-income country, with GDP per capita of US$965 in 2004.*

*The expansion of health care coverage in Sri Lanka, with its focus on the poor, dates from the 1930s, and many of the initial motivations continue to be important influences. By far the most important one for health services has been democracy. In the 1920s, conditions in the island were much like those in most other British colonies. Government intervention in health was limited to providing health care to a small urban population that operated the colonial infrastructure and administration and an equally small workforce involved in export agriculture, and to a sanitary regime designed to control major epidemic threats such as cholera. Democracy based on universal suffrage was introduced in 1931 expressly to empower the poorer groups in society and women and to put pressure on the elites to pay closer attention to social and health conditions.*

*After 1931, the political economy of the island changed irrevocably as the political power base shifted from urban residents to the majority rural population. The impact of democracy on health was accentuated by the emergence of competitive politics along a left-right dimension with two-party competition well embedded by the late 1950s, a rural bias in the delimitation of electorates where each national legislator typically represented fewer than 10,000 voters in the 1930s, and a single-member constituency system that encouraged politicians to engage in parish-pump politics to maximize the government infrastructure built in their districts. The introduction of democratic politics forced successive governments to continuously expand free public health services into rural areas where voters wanted the same standards established earlier for the urban population.*

*Once democracy had served to establish a widely dispersed government health infrastructure, accessible by all, it then acted to ensure its survival under often difficult, fiscal conditions. Subsequently, successful market-oriented and reform-minded governments in Sri Lanka have generally understood that the cost of adequate public sector health services accessible to the poor was a small fiscal price to pay for the political support that they engender to enable other more important economic reforms.*

## Introduction

Sri Lanka's distinctive history, economy, people, politics, and health conditions have contributed to impressive achievements in health care over the past 50 years.

### Economic Environment

Sri Lanka's economy was historically based around agriculture, primarily rice cultivation, but several centuries of active trade resulted in a society that was more open to outside influences and interactions than most Asian countries. Prior to British occupation of the island in the late-18th century, large-scale irrigation agriculture and later spice exports provided a base for government taxation and dictated key aspects of government organization, and a tight, state-led social organization.

The British introduced coffee, tea, and rubber cultivation, and by the end of the 19th century a classic dualistic export economy emerged (Snodgrass 1966). Cash crop exports brought prosperity and a trade surplus, and their taxation gave the government a ready revenue source. After independence in 1948, Sri Lanka's economy was highly trade dependent, although most of its people were involved in subsistence rice cultivation. Tea, rubber, and coconut made up more than 95 percent of exports, and living standards were the highest in South Asia. Relative prosperity continued until the Korean War commodity boom in the 1950s. Then, declining commodity prices and a failure to diversify exports led to economic stagnation, ever-tighter import controls, and inward-oriented import-substitution policies (Bruton 1992). Income stagnated and unemployment was high (more than 20 percent). Mounting social tensions contributed to two Maoist insurgencies and an ethnic-based separatist conflict after 1970, which have presented major challenges for Sri Lanka's economy.

Under a new government in 1977, Sri Lanka became one of the first developing countries to embark on economic liberalization, pursued ever since. Trade was liberalized, export taxes on cash crops removed, and the economy opened up. In return, Sri Lanka benefited from substantial Western aid inflows for more than a decade. These policies led to substantial improvement in economic growth (table 11.1), averaging 3 to 4 percent real per capita income growth ever since, despite the series of debilitating internal conflicts that started in the early 1970s. Growth has been led by export-oriented manufacturing, initially concentrated in gar-

Table 11.1   Sri Lanka: Economic Indicators 1930–2005

| Year | GDP per capita (1990 US$) | GDP per capita (1990 PPP$) | Revenue (% GDP) | Expenditure (% GDP) | External Debt (% GDP) | ODA (% GDP) |
|------|------|------|------|------|------|------|
| 1930 | 180 | 945 | ~10 | ~10 | ~0 | ~0 |
| 1950 | 273 | 935 | 16 | 20 | 3 | 0 |
| 1970 | 316 | 1,130 | 20 | 27 | 18 | 1.7 |
| 1990 | 577 | 1,935 | 22 | 31 | 72 | 5.7 |
| 1995 | 704 | 2,636 | 20 | 31 | 67 | 4.5 |
| 2000 | 844 | 3,626 | 17 | 27 | 55 | 0.4 |
| 2005 | 962 | 4,390 | 16 | 24 | 48 | 3.4 |

*Source:* Central Bank of Sri Lanka (2006); Institute for Health Policy databases; estimates of pre-1950 GDP originally prepared by author for Rannan-Eliya and de Mel (1997).

*Note:* ~ = approximate.

ments but now diversifying. By the 1990s, more than 75 percent of Sri Lanka's exports were industrial products. Continuing economic growth in recent years has pushed unemployment to less than 7 percent of the workforce, raised income in 2005 to more than US$1,000 per capita, and modestly reduced the number of Sri Lankans living in poverty (table 11.2). More substantial reductions in poverty have not occurred, because recent economic growth has been associated with increasing income inequality, and living standards for the lowest income quintile have hardly changed. Although official development assistance (ODA) remains significant, private foreign direct investment (FDI) is now more important for growth, but not to the same extent as in other Southeast Asian economies.

Table 11.2   Sri Lanka: Social Indicators 1930–2005

| Year | Population (millions) | Poverty head count (<PPP$1 per day) | Poverty head count (<PPP$2 per day) | Literacy (%) | Infant mortality rate | Life expectancy |
|------|------|------|------|------|------|------|
| 1930 | 5.3 | — | — | — | 175 | 40 |
| 1950 | 7.7 | — | — | 69 | 82 | 55 |
| 1970 | 12.5 | — | — | 82 | 47 | 65 |
| 1990 | 16.3 | — | — | 88 | 19 | 71 |
| 1995 | 17.3 | 2.5 | 31.3 | 90 | 16 | 72 |
| 2000 | 18.5 | 2.3 | 31.5 | 91 | 13 | 73 |
| 2005 | 19.6 | 2.3 | 22.7 | 92 | 11 | 73 |

*Sources:* Central Bank of Sri Lanka (2006); IHP databases; Medical Statistician of MOH; de Silva (2007).

*Note:* — = not available.

A key element in the post-1977 economic liberalization was the removal of export taxes, followed by further tax reductions. This led to a collapse in government revenues, and caused a structural fiscal deficit that has averaged between 7 percent and 9 percent of GDP in the past decade (table 11.1). Cuts in government spending have not led to fiscal improvements, because tax revenues have fallen apace. Much of the pressure to cut taxes in recent years appears to have been ideologically driven by key donors, despite fiscal realities that point to the need to increase taxation to achieve fiscal balance. Currently, taxation is predominantly from a mix of indirect taxes, including value-added taxes and excise taxes, with smaller contributions from import taxes. Direct income taxes on individuals contribute to a small fraction of revenues. The fiscal deficit has resulted in mounting public debt, constant pressure on the exchange rate, and the inability of the government to increase social expenditures or to invest in needed physical infrastructure. As a consequence, government policy is now focused on raising taxes, recognizing that there is no room for more substantial spending reductions.

## Demography and Health

Until recently, Sri Lanka had no significant rural-urban migration, largely because social services in rural areas were good. However, with increasing industrialization in the past decade, more people are migrating into urban areas.

Sri Lanka is a multiethnic, multilinguistic, and multireligious society. Three-quarters of the population are Sinhala-speaking; most are Buddhist, and the rest are Catholic and Protestant Christians. The rest comprise three distinct ethnic groups: the Tamil-speaking Sri Lankan Tamils (13 percent), Muslims (7 percent), and Tamil-speaking Indian (or Estate) Tamils (5 percent). The first is mostly Hindu, with a significant Christian minority, and the latter is predominantly Hindu also. There are also small Eurasian Burgher, Malay, and Indian communities (less than 1 percent).

Sri Lanka's health indicators were worse than much of South Asia's in the 1920s (Langford and Storey 1993), but its health reforms in the 1930s quickly reduced mortality rates (Langford 1996). After World War II, mortality rates rapidly fell for a decade, before entering a slower but still rapid and continuing phase of decline. Prior to the 1990s, substantial reductions in infant, child, and maternal mortality were responsible for most of the decline. Life expectancy has continuously risen, but gains, since the 1970s, have been confined largely to women and male life expectancy has stagnated (table 11.3). Life expectancy is 71 years, and the infant mortality rate is less than 13 per thousand live births. The main drivers of these remarkable health gains have been policies that have ensured widespread easy access to medical services for the whole population, the emphasis on universalism, mass female education that has enabled women and mothers to make use of these services, and a continuous policy-driven process of behavioral change that has made Sri Lankans highly sensitive to illness and predisposed to make

**Table 11.3   Sri Lanka: Demographic and Health Indicators, 1930–2003**

| Year | Infant mortality rate | Life expectancy at birth (female) | Life expectancy at birth (male) | Maternal mortality rate | Total fertility rate | Population growth rate (%) |
|------|------|------|------|------|------|------|
| 1930 | 175 | 39 | 41 | 21 | — | 1.4 |
| 1950 | 82 | 55 | 56 | 6 | 5.3 | 2.8 |
| 1970 | 47 | 67 | 64 | 2 | 4.2 | 2.2 |
| 1990 | 19.5 | 73 | 67 | 1 | 2.2 | 1.0 |
| 1995 | 16.5 | 75 | 68 | <1 | 1.9 | 1.1 |
| 2000 | 13.3 | 76 | 70 | <1 | 1.9 | 1.4 |
| 2003 | 11.2 | 77 | 71 | <1 | 1.8 | 1.3 |

*Source:* Data kindly provided by Medical Statistician of MOH, Department of Census and Statistics; De Silva 2007.

*Note:* — = not available.

ready use of modern medical treatment when ill (Caldwell 1986; Caldwell et al. 1989; De Silva et al. 2001; Rannan-Eliya 2001; Rannan-Eliya 2004).

From 1950 through the 1970s, mortality fell and the population grew rapidly. Eventually, fertility rates began to drop, and the total fertility rate (TFR) fell below replacement level by 1993. The TFR is now less than 1.9, and may drop as low as 1.5, according to some projections (De Silva 2007). The population size may stabilize at 22 million by 2030 and decline thereafter, without substantial immigration. With low fertility rates and high life expectancy, population growth, a major concern in the 1960s and 1970s, is giving way to concern about population aging. The number of elderly is rapidly increasing; the number of children, falling. Sri Lanka will be one of the most rapidly aging societies in Asia in coming decades. This demographic shift is already reflected in the age structure of the population, which is no longer pyramidal as in most developing countries (figure 11.1).

Sri Lanka's mortality transition is largely complete, and its mortality patterns resemble those of a developed country. Few die of infectious diseases such as cholera, measles, malaria, and TB, and mortality from communicable disease is declining. Noncommunicable diseases (NCDs) and accidents dominate mortality, and ischemic heart disease is the largest single cause of death (table 11.4). Sri Lanka faces growing epidemics of diabetes, ischemic heart disease and cerebrovascular disease, which affect particularly adult males.

The mortality trends are indicative of the underlying morbidity in the country, with a high prevalence of noncommunicable disease in the adult population. However, reliable morbidity data are not available or routinely collected. Table 11.5 presents the morbidity profile of inpatients at government hospitals and of outpatients in a recent study of private clinic doctors. This profile can be considered representative of the morbidity pattern seen by health care providers, but not necessarily of the overall disease burden.

**Figure 11.1   Sri Lanka: Population Pyramids 1991, 2006, 2026, and 2051**

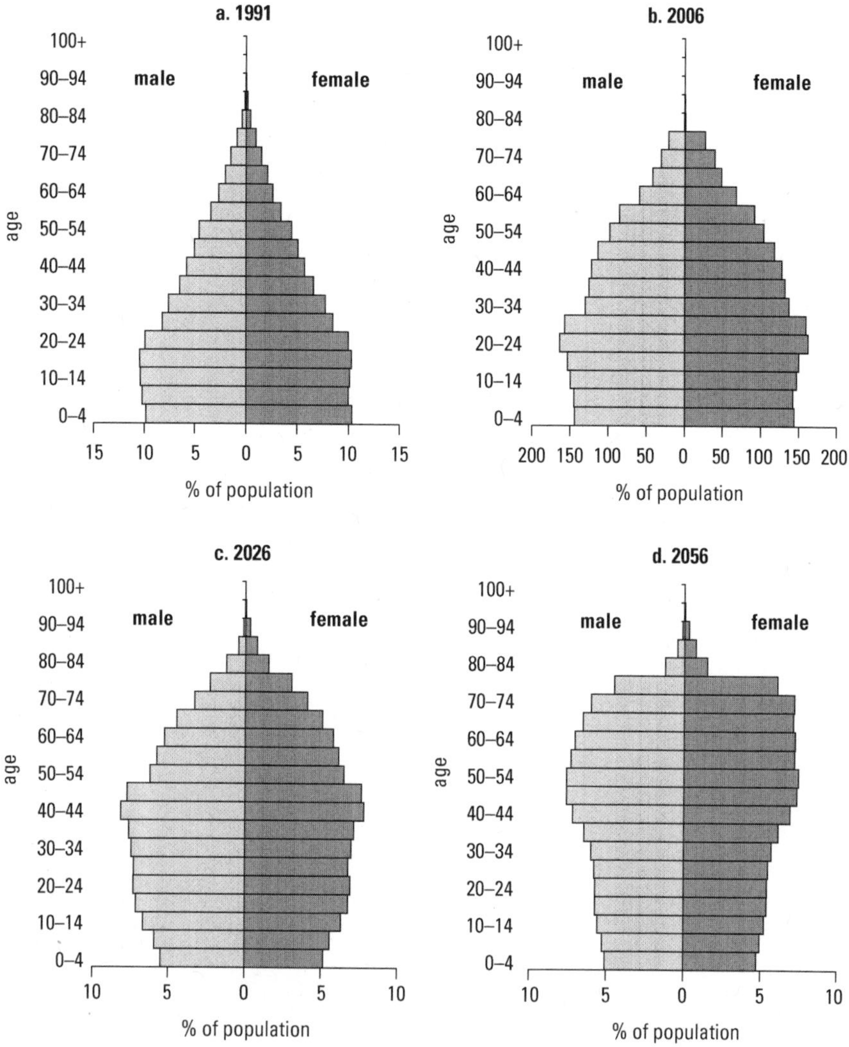

*Source:* Authors' computations using data from De Silva 2007.

## Government and Politics

Sri Lanka consists administratively of nine provinces[1] and 24 districts. The central government is responsible for national policy, and for tertiary and specialized services. In health and education, the provincial governments are responsible for operation of primary and secondary services. The provincial governments are

**Table 11.4    Sri Lanka: Leading Causes of Mortality, 2001**

| Rank order | Cause | Percent of all deaths |
|---|---|---|
| 1 | Ischemic heart disease | 8.5 |
| 2 | Other nervous system diseases | 6.9 |
| 3 | Other heart diseases | 6.1 |
| 4 | Intentional self-harm | 4.2 |
| 5 | Liver diseases | 4.2 |
| 6 | All other external causes | 4.1 |
| 7 | Chronic lower respiratory diseases | 3.8 |
| 8 | Hypertensive diseases | 3.7 |
| 9 | Remainder of malignant neoplasm | 3.2 |
| 10 | Cerebrovascular diseases | 3.1 |

*Source:* Computed by authors from data kindly provided by Registrar Generals Department.

*Note:* Deaths classified with no clear diagnosis are excluded, but accounted for 24.9 percent of all recorded deaths.

**Table 11.5    Sri Lanka: Patient Morbidity, Inpatients and Outpatients**

| Inpatient morbidity Cause | % | Outpatient morbidity Problem | % |
|---|---|---|---|
| Traumatic injuries | 16.7 | Viral fever | 15.6 |
| Respiratory disease | 10.8 | Asthma | 6.3 |
| Symptoms, signs, and abnormal clinical and laboratory findings not elsewhere classified | 7.6 | Upper respiratory tract infection | 5.2 |
| Viral diseases | 6.3 | Hypertension | 4.8 |
| Gastrointestinal tract disease | 6.3 | Respiratory infection | 4.2 |
| Direct and indirect obstetric causes | 4.7 | Gastritis | 3.2 |
| Urinary system disease | 4.1 | Gastroenteritis | 2.8 |
| Intestinal infectious diseases | 3.8 | Lower respiratory tract infection | 2.2 |
| Diseases of musculoskeletal system and connective tissue | 3.6 | Urinary tract infection | 2.0 |
| Skin and subcutaneous tissue diseases | 3.5 | Muscle pains | 2.0 |

*Sources:* Inpatient morbidity statistics from unpublished data for 2003 kindly provided by Medical Statistician, Ministry of Health. Outpatient morbidity statistics from Rannan-Eliya et al. 2003.

elected and report to provincial legislatures, although in practice politics remains centralized.

Democracy has been the primary explanation for Sri Lanka's health achievements. Since 1931, Sri Lanka has always had a democratic government, elected through the ballot box, despite many challenges, including an attempted military coup in the 1960s, two Maoist insurgencies in 1971 and 1987–89, and a separatist conflict since 1972, when the precursors of the Liberation Tigers of Tamil Eelam (LTTE) terrorist organization first took up arms against the government. During this time, several developments have shaped the political system. First, initial electoral competition between a dominant conservative political establishment and Marxist-Trotskyite challengers gave way in the 1950s to a two-party model. Since the 1950s, two dominant political parties—the right-of-center United National Party (UNP) and the left-of-center Sri Lanka Freedom Party (SLFP)—have competed for power. Since 1956, most incumbent governments have lost elections, and political leaders have become extremely sensitive to voter concerns. In health care, this has encouraged bipartisan consensus on major policy features such as an emphasis on universal access, no user fees, and continuing public sector predominance in delivery. Second, the British-inherited constitution was replaced in the 1970s by a presidential system, with an executive president directly elected by a single-transferable vote and a legislature elected through proportional representation. These changes make it harder for governments to introduce radical changes in policy where there is a strong preexisting consensus, and have made coalition politics the norm. Third, as a result of international exhortations to solve the separatist conflict, extensive devolution of government to the provincial level was introduced in 1988, although it has failed to stop the conflict.

## Health Financing and Coverage

This section presents an overview of the financing of Sri Lanka's health system, key historical trends, and its performance in terms of equity and efficiency.

### Health Expenditures

Total expenditure on health in Sri Lanka was close to Rs. 100 billion (US$1 billion) during 2005 (annex table 11A.1), equivalent to 4.2 percent of GDP (Institute for Health Policy, forthcoming). Total health expenditure, driven mostly by private spending, has increased since the early 1990s. Government spending accounts for 46 percent, and private financing for the rest (annex table 11A.2). In per capita terms, expenditure in 2005 represented US$50 per capita at official exchange rates, and government spending was equivalent to US$23 per capita. Health services account for 8 percent of government budgetary spending. Private financing is mostly out-of-pocket spending by households, with smaller contributions from employers and insurance. Spending by nongovernmental organizations (NGOs) is small.

*Use of expenditures.* Health spending reflects the structure of what is a public hospital–dominated health care system. Government expenditures have concentrated on hospitals since the health reforms of the 1930s, directed primarily at increasing equity in access and improving risk protection, both of which required substantial increases in hospital coverage. Hospital spending accounted for about

**Table 11.6   Sri Lanka: Trends in Health Care Spending, 1953–2005**

| Spending/source | 1953 | 1980 | 1990 | 2000 | 2005 |
|---|---|---|---|---|---|
| Health expenditures (GDP) | | | | | |
| Total | 3.3 | 3.1 | 3.3 | 3.5 | 4.2 |
| Government | 2.1 | 1.7 | 1.7 | 1.7 | 1.9 |
| Government as of budget | 8.4 | 4.1 | 5.6 | 6.5 | 7.8 |
| National expenditure (%) | | | | | |
| Public | 62 | 57 | 46 | 50 | 46 |
| Private | 38 | 43 | 54 | 50 | 54 |
| Out-of-pocket | 33 | 41 | 42 | 43 | 48 |
| Hospital composition, by source of expenditures (%) | | | | | |
| Total | 47 | 45 | 41 | 43 | 43 |
| Public spending | 72 | 70 | 78 | 69 | 71 |
| Private spending | 4 | 12 | 11 | 17 | 19 |
| Hospital expenditure, by source of financing (%) | | | | | |
| Public | 96 | 87 | 93 | 80 | 76 |
| Private | 4 | 13 | 7 | 20 | 24 |
| Nonhospital expenditure, by source of financing (%) | | | | | |
| Public | 33 | 31 | 17 | 19 | 23 |
| Private | 66 | 69 | 83 | 81 | 77 |

*Sources:* Rannan-Eliya and de Mel 1997; IHP Sri Lanka Health Accounts database (January 2007 revision).

70 percent of government recurrent spending in the 1950s, and the share has changed little since then (table 11.6). Government hospitals have been the primary mode by which modern medical treatment has been made available to people in rural areas, and the prioritization of these facilities in budgetary spending has ensured that the health ministry was able to cover all Sri Lankans for most services. In contrast, most private spending is for outpatient care and for purchasing medicines, but the share of hospital spending in private outlays has increased. This is partly because of expanded delivery of outpatient services by private hospitals and partly because of the increased availability of private insurance. As a consequence, until recently more than 85 percent of hospital spending was by government, while more than 80 percent of nonhospital and outpatient care spending was financed privately.

*Benefit-incidence of government health expenditures.* Government health expenditures have reached the poor effectively since at least the 1950s, after the health reforms expanded government health services into rural areas. Estimates of the actual incidence of government health spending are available for only the late 1970s and beyond. Although these estimates are not strictly comparable, because they were computed by different authors using different methods, they suggest that the targeting of government health spending was quite pro-poor in the late 1970s, then became less so during the 1980s to 1990s (table 11.7). In 2003/04 the poorest quintile received 20 percent of government health spending; the richest quintile, 15 percent.

**Table 11.7    Sri Lanka: Incidence of Public Health Expenditures, 1979–2004**

| Year | Share of government health expenditure received by poorest household quintile (%) | Share of government health expenditure received by richest household quintile (%) |
|------|-------------------------------------------------------------------------------------|------------------------------------------------------------------------------------|
| 1979 | 30 | 9 |
| 1992 | 24 | 15 |
| 1996/97 | 22 | 18 |
| 2003/04 | 20 | 15 |

*Sources:* Alailima and Mohideen 1983; estimations by authors and Aparnaa Somanathan of IHP.

Government outpatient spending is the most pro-poor (27 percent went to the poorest quintile in 2003/04 versus 11 percent to the richest quintile), and inpatient spending is more evenly distributed (18 percent versus 16 percent). Because Sri Lanka does not means test access to public services, the main reasons for the pro-poor targeting of government health subsidies are: a dense network of health facilities that makes government health services physically accessible to the poor, lack of user charges, and the voluntary opting-out of the rich into the private sector (Rannan-Eliya 2001).

In effect, what Sri Lanka does is guarantee its poor effective access to free health services, especially hospital care, and then relies on differentials in consumer quality in services to persuade the richer patients to voluntarily opt to use and pay for private delivery. The role of these consumer differentials is discussed later. This approach resembles closely those of two other Asian health systems, Malaysia and Hong Kong (China), where government-operated hospital services also effectively reach the poor. Together with these cases, Sri Lanka differs as a result in the income gradients in use of public and private hospital services. Throughout Asia, the rich use private hospital services more than the poor, and this is generally true for public services, but in Sri Lanka and the other two cases, the gradient is reversed for public hospitals. Why Sri Lanka, and other countries like it, are able to achieve this, when most countries do not, has not yet been fully explained.[2]

*Incidence of financing.* The health financing system is close to progressive and, in comparative terms, does better than developed countries in Asia, but not as well as some countries such as Thailand and Philippines (table 11.8). The burden of paying for the half of total health expenditures that come from general revenues falls mostly on the richer households. Indirect taxation is neither progressive nor regressive, but direct taxes are very progressive. Spending from private sources is mostly out of pocket, and these payments are very progressive, because the rich are more likely than the poor to seek private care. To improve the progressivity of its health care financing, Sri Lanka would need to increase the share of direct taxation in overall government revenues, as well as modify its system of indirect taxes to place a heavier burden on goods and services used more by the rich than the poor.

**Table 11.8   Sri Lanka: Progressivity in Health Financing Compared with Selected Asian Countries**

| Country (year) | Direct taxes | Indirect taxes | Social insurance | Private insurance | Direct payments | Total |
|---|---|---|---|---|---|---|
| Bangladesh (1999/2000) | 0.552 | 0.111 | n.a. | n.a. | 0.219 | 0.214 |
| China (2000) | 0.152 | 0.040 | 0.235 | n.a. | −0.017 | 0.040 |
| Hong Kong (China) (1999/2000) | 0.386 | 0.119 | n.a. | 0.040 | 0.011 | 0.166 |
| Japan (1998) | 0.095 | −0.223 | −0.041 | n.a. | −0.269 | −0.069 |
| South Korea (2000) | 0.268 | 0.038 | −0.163 | n.a. | 0.012 | −0.024 |
| Kyrgyz Republic (2000) | 0.074 | −0.096 | −0.034 | n.a. | 0.264 | 0.125 |
| Nepal (1995/96) | 0.144 | 0.114 | n.a. | n.a. | 0.053 | 0.063 |
| Philippines (1999) | 0.381 | 0.002 | 0.205 | 0.120 | 0.139 | 0.163 |
| Sri Lanka (1996/97) | 0.569 | −0.010 | n.a. | n.a. | 0.069 | 0.085 |
| Thailand (2000) | 0.510 | 0.182 | 0.180 | 0.004 | 0.091 | 0.197 |

*Source:* Excerpted results of the Equitap study as published in Rannan-Eliya and Somanathan 2006.

*Note:* The *Kakwani Index* is a numerical index of the distribution of payments in relation to ability to pay. It is calculated graphically by looking at the distribution curve of overall tax payments made by poor to rich households, and comparing this distribution with the distribution of overall consumption across the same households, with the index computed as twice the size of the area between the two curves. A positive number implies that the share of payments by richer households is greater than their share of overall consumption. A negative number implies the reverse. For further details of these methods, see the World Bank's technical notes for quantitative techniques for health equity analysis at http://web.worldbank.org/WBSITE/EXTERNAL/TOPICS/EXTHEALTHNUTRITIONANDPOPULATION/EXTPAH/0,,contentMDK:20216933~menuPK:400482~pagePK:148956~piPK:216618~theSitePK:400476,00.html.

n.a. = not applicable.

*Protection against catastrophic risk.* Sri Lanka's health system performs very well in protecting the poor against catastrophic financial risks associated with illness. The Equitap study of equity in Asian health systems found that Sri Lanka is one of a small group of Asian countries where few people are pushed into poverty as a result of medical spending (van Doorslaer et al. 2006). Only 0.3 percent of Sri Lankan households are pushed below the PPP$1.08 international poverty line as a result of health expenditure (table 11.9).

## Benefits Package

All government health services, with few exceptions, are available free to all citizens, including all inpatient, outpatient, and community health services. Free services range from antiretrovirals for HIV/AIDS patients to coronary bypass surgery. Access to all services is reinforced by a policy of permitting patients to visit any hospital in the country without restriction, and with no enforcement of a referral system. The government is able to do this because of a high level of technical efficiency in its delivery system, which keeps costs low, and the implicit strategy of encouraging the richer patients not to burden the government health system by voluntarily opting to use private providers.

**Table 11.9   Sri Lanka: Proportion of Population Pushed below the PPP$1.08 Poverty Line by Household Health Spending, Compared with Selected Asian Countries**

| Country (year) | Prepayment headcount (%) | Postpayment headcount (%) | Change in poverty headcount (%) |
|---|---|---|---|
| Bangladesh (1999/2000) | 22.5 | 26.3 | 3.8 |
| India (1999/2000) | 31.1 | 34.8 | 3.7 |
| China (2000) | 13.7 | 16.2 | 2.6 |
| Nepal (1995/6) | 39.3 | 41.6 | 2.2 |
| Vietnam (1998) | 3.6 | 4.7 | 1.1 |
| Indonesia (2001) | 7.9 | 8.6 | 0.7 |
| Philippines (1999) | 15.8 | 16.4 | 0.6 |
| Kyrgyz Republic (2000/01) | 2.2 | 2.7 | 0.5 |
| Sri Lanka (1996/97) | 3.8 | 4.1 | 0.3 |
| Thailand (2002) | 2.1 | 2.3 | 0.2 |
| Malaysia (1998/99) | 1.0 | 1.1 | 0.1 |

*Source:* van Doorslaer et al. 2006.

The first exception to free care consists of family planning commodities. Condoms and oral contraceptive pills are made available through government primary care facilities at cost, but at much lower prices than private sector alternatives. The second exception consists of private paying-wards in less than a dozen government hospitals. These offer the same treatment as in the main hospital wards, but greater privacy. However, in practice these beds are underused and account for less than 1 percent of all Ministry of Health(MOH) inpatients. The third exception is the Sri Jayewardenapura General Hospital, an autonomous, tertiary care, 1,000-bed hospital constructed with Japanese development assistance. Probably for ideological reasons and poor economic analysis, the Japanese stipulated that user fees be charged at this facility. The hospital maintains three classes of wards, with different fee schedules based on a means test, although in no case are the fees sufficient to cover full costs. In practice, even though the general hospital's subsidy per bed is greater than in any other government hospital, it cannot generate sufficient fees and operates at a loss.

Nevertheless, there is implicit rationing of care. This occurs in a number of ways. First, through internal purchasing controls and investment decisions, the MOH can and does restrict the availability of services it considers too expensive. For example, government hospitals are prohibited from, or limited in, buying individual drugs or certain high-technology equipment. Second, using administrative controls, the central ministry can restrict the supply of specific services to only certain government hospitals. This can be done by controls such as the placement of specialists or through the lists of drugs approved for different levels of hospital. Even basic equipment is rationed; for example, most lower-level MOH facilities lack X-ray machines. However, although services may be restricted to certain facilities, all patients still have the right to travel to those facilities, and many do. Although these decisions often have some rational basis, most are taken implicitly and without public debate. While this process lacks transparency, it does prevent much public opposition. Third, it has been official policy that, if medicines are not available in hospital stocks, patients may be asked to buy drugs themselves from private pharmacies. This results in extensive self-purchasing by patients, because the medicines budget is inadequate. However, there is evidence that MOH personnel protect the poor to some extent by using discretion to reserve limited drug stocks for the poor and by being more likely to encourage richer patients to self-purchase.

### Financing and Payment

Public sector health spending is financed exclusively from general tax revenue, with a small contribution from international development assistance (less than 5 percent). There is no social insurance. Government health spending is mostly by the central government (62 percent of public) and provincial governments (36 percent), with small contributions from local governments at municipality and village levels. However, financing for provincial and local government health budgets comes principally from the central government. Provincial governments have the authority to raise their own tax revenues, but owing to inherent economic limitations, they raise less than 5 percent of overall government tax revenues, and most of these are raised in Western Province. This is because most provinces are essentially rural and direct income taxation is limited. The most buoyant domestic tax mechanism is the value-added tax, which can practically be levied only at the national level, given the small size of the island. In addition, 50 percent of the country's economic output, and an even greater share of its formal sector, is located in Western Province. There is a modest contribution from international donor assistance (4 to 6 percent of public financing). User charges and miscellaneous income account for the rest (less than 2 percent).

Private health services are funded principally from out-of-pocket spending by households. Private doctors either dispense and charge only for their medicines, or charge separately for consultation and for drugs (Rannan-Eliya, Jayawardhane, and Karunaratne 2003). Most private doctors are actually government medical officers who are allowed to undertake private practice in their off-duty hours. Private hospitals typically charge by item for cost of services, except for the fees of attending physicians, who may bill the patient separately.

A fifth of private financing is from employer spending on medical benefit schemes for their employees and on group medical insurance schemes, plus a smaller amount from individually purchased medical insurance (Institute for Health Policy, forthcoming). Most of this spending pays for private hospital services and benefits mostly the top income quintile. Typically, all these schemes reimburse the patient for their expenses, so patients must first pay out of pocket,

**Figure 11.2   Sri Lanka: Government Recurrent Health Spending, 1927–2005**

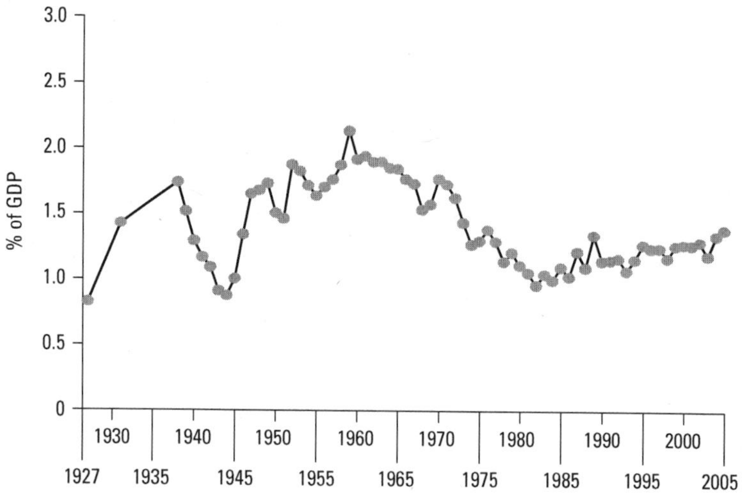

*Source:* Adapted from Rannan-Eliya and de Mel 1997. Estimates for 1990 to 2005 were derived by modifying estimates for central MOH and provincial council health department expenditures as compiled in the IHP Sri Lanka Health Accounts database to fit earlier definitions of recurrent departmental spending.

and then claim reimbursement. The amounts reimbursed vary with the specific rules of their insurance or employer policy, but most medical insurance in Sri Lanka is indemnity insurance, reimbursing up to a fixed maximum. The contribution of nonprofit institutions to health care financing is about 1 percent (Annex table 11A).

## Development of Health Financing

Before the health reforms of the 1930s, the government took a noninterventionist role in health, and health services and financing were treated as a private responsibility. The government's involvements were limited to funding urban hospitals to look after European residents and its own civil and military personnel, and to making regulations to ensure medical services for the important plantation workforce. However, during the reforms in the 1930s to 1940s, government expenditure on health increased substantially. By the mid-1950s, national health spending was between 3.2 and 3.5 percent of GDP, of which the public share was about 60 percent (Rannan-Eliya and de Mel 1997). From the early 1960s, spending fell, as the government faced stringent fiscal constraints, and has remained in the range of 1.3 to 1.8 percent of GDP until 2005 (figure 11.2). During these years, private spending has gradually increased its share of total financing to more than half.

## Equity—Health Indicators, Outcomes, and Their Distribution

Prior to the 19th century, there is no evidence of significant differentials in health outcomes. However, as in Britain, urbanization and growth of the formal economy

**Table 11.10    Sri Lanka: Infant Mortality Rates in Different Social Groups, 1920–22**

| Ethnic group and district | Proxy for social group | Males | Females |
|---|---|---|---|
| Sinhalese in Kalutara | Rural villagers | 114 | 101 |
| Tamils in Nuwara Eliya | Plantation workers | 248 | 210 |
| Tamils, Moor, and Malays in Colombo | Urban poor | 341 | 320 |
| Burghers and Eurasians in Colombo | Middle class | 144 | 158 |

*Source:* Computed from data of Registrar General of Ceylon in Meegama 1986.

in the 19th century brought deterioration in health conditions and health inequalities. In Colombo, an urban proletariat emerged, crowded into a large poor quarter. Living there under unhygienic conditions, with no basic sanitation, they were prey to epidemics. Dense population settlement in poor and unsanitary housing conditions was also found in the plantation sector, where indentured labor was imported from India. Two significant differentials in health status arose. First, health conditions in urban areas were worse than in rural areas. The urban middle classes enjoyed better health than their poor neighbors, but their mortality rates were no lower than those in rural areas and, for infants were worse. Second, the worst health was among poor urban and plantation sector workers (Meegama 1986). Evidence for this comes from analysis of death registration data by ethnic group and district, which are reasonable proxies for socioeconomic status (table 11.10).

It was in the context of these large health disparities that the introduction of democracy made a difference. Full democracy did not exist until 1931, but municipal governments, elected by residents under limited franchise, were introduced into most Sri Lankan towns during the 19th century. These local governments intervened over several decades to enforce basic standards for sanitation, to provide maternal and child health services, and to construct public sewerage and water systems. These interventions succeeded in reducing urban mortality rates and by the early 1930s had eliminated the urban-rural differentials in mortality rates. By then, the major mortality differentials were between the malarial and nonmalarial areas of the country.

With the advent of democracy in 1931, the government, under electoral pressures, expanded the rural network of medical facilities throughout Sri Lanka, and most substantially in the previously underserved malarial districts (Rannan-Eliya and de Mel 1997; Langford 1996). Sri Lanka is an example of how democratic politics can provide a means of government accountability for services to the poor (World Bank 2003). The small size of electorates encouraged a form of "parish pump politics," in which national politicians, some elected by as few as 5,000 voters (Wriggins 1960), competed to ensure that the government built dispensaries and later hospitals in their home constituencies.

The health impact of this expansion did not, however, show up until after World War II. Between 1945 and 1952, mortality rates in Sri Lanka across all demographic groups were halved, and life expectancy increased 12 years. For many

**Table 11.11  Sri Lanka: Infant Mortality Rate, Selected Districts, 1921–2000**

| Year | Colombo | Anuradhapura | Kandy | Hambantota |
|------|---------|--------------|-------|------------|
| 1921 | 161 | 366 | 196 | 293 |
| 1931 | 139 | 266 | 167 | 189 |
| 1951 | 94 | 69 | 89 | 62 |
| 1971 | 41 | 34 | 61 | 37 |
| 1991 | 26 | 21 | 23 | 6 |
| 2000 | 18 | 16 | 20 | 4 |

*Source:* Data from Registrar General's Department and Annual Health Bulletin of MOH.

decades this progress was attributed to the introduction of DDT-spraying against the malaria vector, but the most recent assessments demonstrate that malaria control played only a minor role: mortality reductions occurred in both malarial and nonmalarial areas. The critical intervention was expanded access to curative facilities in rural areas, plus the improved supply of antibiotics, other drugs, and staff that became possible after 1945 (Langford 1996). Table 11.11 shows this has substantially reduced and even reversed interdistrict inequalities in health outcomes.

With consolidation of the health system in the 1960s, physical access to basic health services within close proximity became the reality for almost the entire population. High coverage has been the key to reducing mortality rates (Caldwell et al. 1989; De Silva et al. 2001; Langford 1996; Rannan-Eliya 2001) and has led to continuous improvement in health indicators for rich and poor. Continuing expansions in access at the margin benefit primarily the poor, once the richer households are served. This is illustrated by using asset indices to disaggregate data collected in the Sri Lanka Demographic and Health Survey (DHS). Infant mortality rates declined in all income groups, and the absolute difference between the richest and poorest quintiles substantially narrowed during the 1990s (figure 11.3). The role of universal access in this performance is demonstrated by trends in access to qualified medical care at childbirth. People in the poorest quintile were the major beneficiaries of marginal improvements in access to such care in the 1990s (figure 11.4). Moreover, access of the poor to services is such that when demand is greater among the poor, actual uptake of services can be more than in rich, as shown by trends in use of modern contraception where the poorest quintile has higher use (figure 11.5).

*Targeting and equity implications of reforms.* Central to Sri Lanka's health reforms has been the concept of universalism and its link to citizenship. From their inception, Sri Lanka's health reforms were driven by the close connection between citizenship and political rights and government obligations to the people. The government does not explicitly target services to specific groups and does not accommodate different systems of care to different groups—so much so that pilot

**Figure 11.3    Sri Lanka: Differentials in Infant Mortality Rate, by Asset Quintile, 1987–2000**

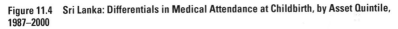

*Source:* IHP estimates from the Sri Lanka Demographic and Health Surveys for relevant years.

**Figure 11.4    Sri Lanka: Differentials in Medical Attendance at Childbirth, by Asset Quintile, 1987–2000**

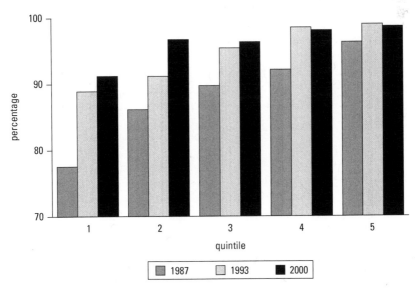

*Source:* IHP estimates from the Sri Lanka Demographic and Health Surveys for relevant years.

**Figure 11.5   Sri Lanka: Differentials in Use of Modern Methods of Contraception by Currently Married Women, 1987–2000**

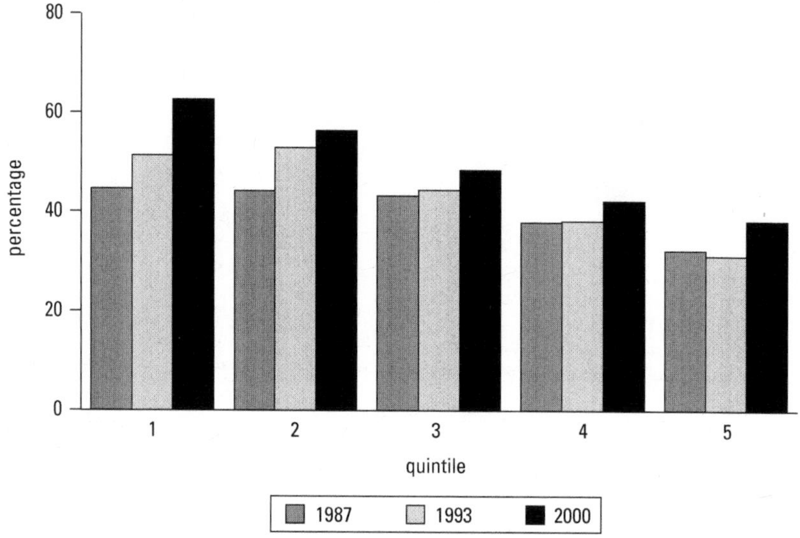

Source: IHP estimates from the Sri Lanka Demographic and Health Surveys for relevant years.

projects to test different approaches to health care delivery in small areas have not flourished. Access to health care is treated as a fundamental social right and thus not subject to arbitration. The symbolic commitment to the principle of free universal care to all citizens is taken so seriously that, despite more than a quarter of a century of war against the terrorist group LTTE, successive governments have consistently refused to restrict the right to free care that LTTE members have by virtue of their citizenship. Hospitals in LTTE-controlled areas continue to be funded, supplied, and staffed at government expense, and injured LTTE rebels continue to be treated in these facilities.

This attitude, which may seem impractical given resource limitations, has been a critical success factor. First, government services continue to be used by and accountable to all in society, including the influential middle classes and urban elite who have remained political supporters of good quality government services. Furthermore, expansion has not been at the cost of reductions in clinical quality of services, although it has been at the cost of accepting lower consumer quality in amenities. Moreover, with a universalist approach, once the rich and middle-income classes are provided for, marginal increases in provision inevitably favor the poor.

There has been one defect in this approach. If individuals do not have citizenship, they often fail to benefit. This link was most obvious in the case of the Tamil-speaking plantation workers of Indian origin. As noted elsewhere, they were the first beneficiaries of state action to expand access to medical services, and by the 1940s, their health indicators were better than those for the rest of the rural population. However, just before independence, legislative changes deprived most of them of Sri Lankan citizenship and, thus voting rights. After 1948, they had no electoral representation, and the government left responsibility for their social service provision to the British and U.S. private plantation companies. The results of this natural experiment to compare private and public provision are evident. The private sector failed to match the improvements in public service provision that came about through government intervention in rural areas from the 1950s through the 1970s, even though such efforts would have improved labor productivity. Health improvements in the estate population began to lag those of the rest of the population. By 1970, their mortality rates were much higher than the rest of the population's. Then two important changes occurred. First, the government nationalized the plantations in the early 1970s and thus indirectly became responsible for providing the estate workers with health care. Second, the CWC (Ceylon Workers Congress), the trade union cum political party representing the estate workers, joined the government in 1978. Once in government, this party lobbied for enhanced state social service provision to its community and, in the 1980s, persuaded the government to restore first voting rights and then citizenship. The impact of the restoration of voting rights was immediate and led to concerted government efforts to improve health services in the estates. In the 1990s, the plantations were effectively privatized, but, at the urging of the CWC, the government agreed to nationalize the plantation health care facilities and to integrate them into the MOH network.

The impact of these changes in citizenship and voting rights on health indicators in the estate population has been dramatic (figure 11.6). Prior to the 1940s, government-legislated employer mandates were successful in eliminating and, eventually, reversing the mortality disadvantage of the estate population. In the four decades that followed disenfranchisement, the community missed out on the national health reforms. The health services provided to them by the private plantation companies could not match those in the public sector, and a significant disparity again appeared, with the infant mortality rate (IMR) reaching almost double the national average. Within two years after the CWC joined government, rapid improvements in mortality began to take place. Now, 30 years later, there are good signs that the disparity in health outcomes will be eliminated in the future. This performance in reducing these ethnic differentials compares favorably with that of countries such as the United States, which have conspicuously failed to narrow historical ethnic disparities in mortality.

## *Efficiency*

There are two different types of efficiency—technical efficiency and allocational efficiency, and these can be considered either from a system or "macro" perspective

**Figure 11.6    Sri Lanka: Trends in Infant Mortality Rates, Country and Nuwara Eliya District, 1920–2003**

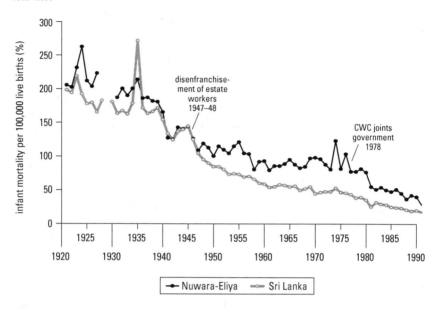

*Source:* Based on data from Registrar General's Department.

*Note:* The population of Nuwara Eliya district is predominantly Indian-origin estate Tamil, and so its IMR rate provides a good proxy for health conditions in the plantation community.

or from a provider or "micro" perspective. Although Sri Lanka's health system does not meet conventional expectations, it can be considered highly efficient.

Efficiency has been an important and critical element in Sri Lanka's success in extending coverage. It enabled it to use a limited health budget to reach the poor. In other countries, increasing access to services often leads to such increases in patient demand that the public sector must ration access to care to match available resources to apparent patient needs. However, Sri Lankan health care managers were denied this response, and were, instead, forced to pursue continuous gains in efficiency. This approach made it possible to financially sustain Sri Lanka's policies of universal access to health services (Rannan-Eliya 2001; Rannan-Eliya and de Mel 1997). In fact, Sri Lanka managed to expand access to health services while reducing government health spending as a share of GDP after 1960.

*Technical efficiency at the macrolevel.* From a macrolevel perspective, the Sri Lankan health system is a global outlier. It spends less in absolute and relative terms than comparable low-income developing countries but achieves better health indicators than some European countries and does so by providing levels of access to medical services comparable to a developed country (table 11.12). For

**Table 11.12  Sri Lanka: Health Services Use and Spending, Compared with Selected Comparable Countries**

| Country | Year | Physician visits (per capita per year) | Inpatient admissions (per 100 people per year) | Total health expenditure (GDP) |
|---|---|---|---|---|
| Bangladesh | 2001 | 1 | 2 | 3.2 |
| Egypt, Arab Rep. of | 1996 | 4 | 3 | 3.7 |
| Indonesia | 2001 | 1 | 1 | 4.2 |
| Sri Lanka | 2003 | 5 | 22 | 3.6 |
| Thailand | 1993 | 2 | 8 | 3.6 |

*Source:* Estimated by authors from various sources.

five decades after 1950, Sri Lanka was a low-income developing country, with a per capita GDP less than US$350. Overall national health spending was only 3.0 to 3.6 percent of GDP throughout, equivalent to less than US$10 per capita, well below the US$13 per capita cost of the minimum cost-effective package of services proposed by the World Bank (1993).[3] Of this, only half was public spending, which averaged between US$4 and US$6 per capita between 1950 and 1990. Most of Sri Lanka's health transition was achieved with less national and government health spending in per capita terms than in the majority of Sub-Saharan African countries in 1990: according to the World Development Report, 24 out of 30 spent more than US$5 per capita (World Bank 1993).

*Technical efficiency at the microlevel.* The OECD suggests three low-level indicators for assessing technical efficiency at the microlevel (Hurst and Jee-Hughes 2001): unit costs, length of stay, and ratios of day cases to all surgery. Sri Lankan data available for the first two indicators show that its public sector services are highly efficient in their use of available human and financial resources. Sri Lankan public hospitals deliver inpatient admissions and outpatient visits at a far lower ratio of cost to per capita GDP than the average developing country and, in many instances, at lower costs than any other country for which data are available (table 11.13). This is achieved by high patient throughput, reflected in bed-turnover rates and short average length of stay (ALOS), and high labor productivity with government doctors and nurses seeing, on average, more patients in both inpatient and outpatient settings than is the norm in other developing countries (Rannan-Eliya 2001).

How these high levels of technical efficiency came about is not well understood. Yet it does appear that they are the result of incremental productivity improvements since the early 1950s or earlier. Research on productivity trends in public sector health services in developing countries has been almost nonexistent (Hensher 2001). Recent research by Sri Lankan researchers suggests that such trends can

Table 11.13   Sri Lanka: Technical Efficiency in Public Hospitals, Compared with Selected Countries

| Country | Year | Cost per admission (ratio of per capita daily GDP) | Cost per outpatient visit (ratio of per capita daily GDP) | Bed turnover rate | Average length of stay (days) |
|---|---|---|---|---|---|
| **Complex hospitals** | | | | | |
| Sri Lanka | 1997 | 7 | 1.0 | 65 | 5 |
| Bangladesh | 1997 | 26 | 0.8 | 47 | 11 |
| Colombia | 1978 | 25 | 0.8 | 38 | 7 |
| Indonesia | 1985 | 26 | 0.7 | 29 | 9 |
| Jamaica | 1985–86 | 40 | 1.5 | 35 | 8 |
| China | 1989 | 76 | 0.8 | 14 | 25 |
| **Basic and intermediate hospitals** | | | | | |
| Sri Lanka | 1997 | 5 | 0.1 | 57 | 3 |
| Bangladesh | 1997 | 14 | 0.5 | 77 | 4 |
| Indonesia | 1987 | 6 | 0.6 | 33 | 6 |
| Jamaica | 1985–86 | 18 | 1.1 | 32 | 8 |
| Malawi | 1987–88 | 17 | 0.4 | 47 | 9 |
| China | 1986 | 30 | 0.5 | 21 | 16 |

*Sources:* Excerpted from Rannan-Eliya 2001; Rannan-Eliya and Somanathan 2003.

be positive over long periods of time in many countries and that the rates of improvement in Sri Lanka historically have been greater than in the average developing country (Rannan-Eliya 2006). Specific empirical analysis of why Sri Lanka has performed so well in this area is lacking, but possible explanations include: a strong public service ethos established in the MOH by the 1950s; strong centralized control of budgets, inputs, and operating procedures, which minimized input prices and constantly forced health workers to meet increasing demand through efficiency savings instead of relying on more resources; and low administrative overheads associated with a civil service–run, command-and-control management system (Hsiao and Associates 2001).

*Allocational efficiency. Allocational efficiency* refers to the correct allocation of available resources to different treatment or service interventions. This may refer to the allocation of expenditures by disease according to cost-effectiveness criteria or to the allocation of resources by service type, or both. With respect to the former, the question is moot, because Sri Lankan health service managers have never allocated budgets by disease using cost-effectiveness criteria. Nor have they had the capacity to do so because budgets are not managed this way.

With respect to allocation by service type, Sri Lanka has consistently followed a strategy of allocating the largest share of its budget to hospitals (between 75 and

**Table 11.14  Sri Lanka: Proportion of MOH Expenditures Devoted to Hospitals (percent)**

| Year | Recurrent expenditures | Capital expenditures | Total expenditures |
|------|------------------------|----------------------|--------------------|
| 1958 | 75 | — | — |
| 1973 | — | — | 65 |
| 1986 | 77 | 59 | 75 |
| 1991 | 78 | 86 | 80 |
| 1996 | 74 | — | — |
| 2005 | — | — | 71 |

*Sources:* Derived by authors from various sources cited in Rannan-Eliya and de Mel 1997, and Sri Lanka Health Accounts database maintained at Institute for Health Policy.

*Note:* — = not available.

85 percent), and within that to inpatient care (table 11.14). Preventive and public health spending has averaged 25 percent or less of the budget and less than 12 percent during the past decade. The hospital emphasis has been a feature of the system since the 1950s, and from a regional perspective is surpassed only by Hong Kong (China) (Rannan-Eliya and de Mel 1997). It is much higher than the share of between 30 and 60 percent in other Asian developing countries. Although this strategy runs counter to standard prescriptions, in the Sri Lankan situation it made sense for two reasons. First, a key goal of health policy, and one benefiting the poor the most, has been protection against catastrophic risk. For this, a high hospital subsidy makes sense, considering that many patients are more able to pay for private outpatient services. Second, Sri Lanka has found that well-run government hospitals are an efficient way of delivering primary care, owing to economies of scale. Most government hospitals have only minimal capital investment and treat only simple illnesses but are more cost-efficient than smaller outpatient facilities (Somanathan et al. 2000).

## Health Delivery System

Sri Lankans benefit from extensive and organized health services, consisting of parallel public and private sectors.

### Health Services Organization

Public services, financed and provided in an integrated fashion by the Ministry of Health and eight provincial Departments of Health, span the full range from preventive and basic primary care activities to complex hospital-provided tertiary care. The public sector network ranges from teaching hospitals with specialized services to small dispensaries that provide only outpatient services. Medical Officers of Health units (MOOHs) provide most preventive and public health services

**Table 11.15   Sri Lanka: Provision of Health Service Inputs and Activities, 2003**

| Resource | Public sector | Private sector | Total | Population ratio |
|---|---|---|---|---|
| Physicians | ~7,000 | ~1,000 | ~8,000 | 0.4 per 1,000 |
| Nurses | ~6,000 | ~5,000 | ~11,000 | 0.6 per 1,000 |
| Hospital beds | 59.262 | ~3,000 | 62,000 | 3.2 per 1,000 |
| Inpatient admissions | 4.1 million | 0.3 million | 4.4 million | 22 per 100 |
| Outpatient visits | 45 million | ~50 million | 95 million | 4.8 per capita |

*Source:* Computed by authors from data provided by Medical Statistician, Ministry of Health and IHP databases.

*Note:* ~ denotes approximation.

**Table 11.16   Sri Lanka: Trends in Treatment Sources Used by Sick Persons, 1978–2004 (percent)**

| Source of treatment | 1978/79 | 1981/82 | 1986/87 | 1996/97 | 2003/04 |
|---|---|---|---|---|---|
| Western government sector | 42.6 | 45.6 | 44.1 | 50.7 | 43.5 |
| Ayurvedic government sector | 1.9 | 2.2 | 1.9 | 2.0 | 1.2 |
| Western private sector | 34.3 | 34.2 | 37.2 | 38.1 | 45.1 |
| Ayurvedic private sector | 16.1 | 12.1 | 12.9 | 7.6 | 5.0 |
| Others | 5.1 | 6.0 | 3.8 | 1.7 | 1.6 |

*Source:* Central Bank Consumer Finance Surveys, based on published reports and analysis by authors.

*Note:* The percentages are for individuals who reported falling ill during a 14-day reference period and used any source of treatment. Western private includes private clinics, private hospitals, and pharmacies.

through teams of doctors, community midwives, and others. Their organizational model was developed in the 1920s and expanded in the 1930s and 1940s.

MOH facilities form a dense, integrated network with more than a thousand institutions. Most Sri Lankans live within 3 kilometers of a public facility. Although there is a formal referral system with patients expected to use primary-level services as the first point of contact, this is not enforced for reasons of equity. Patients can seek care in the medical institution of their choice, recognizing the reality of service quality variations and the lack of organized general practitioner services to act as gatekeeper for accessing hospital services.

The largest part of private provision is ambulatory, with most outpatient services provided by government medical officers working in their off-duty hours. A smaller number (estimated to be a thousand) full-time private doctors are concentrated in urban areas. This is supplemented by a private hospital sector, concentrated in the Colombo district and providing inpatient and tertiary services. The overall use of health services in Sri Lanka is high relative to comparable countries, and the overall cost of the health system is low (table 11.15). The public sector predominates inpatient provision (more than 95 percent), but shares the outpatient load with the increasingly important private sector (table 11.16).

## Growth of Health Service Provision

Before the 1930s, modern medical care was limited to government, missionary, and private hospitals in urban areas and estate-company provision for the plantation workforce. In rural areas, demand and purchasing power were insufficient to make private sector investment feasible. The reforms starting in the 1930s changed this. Although there was significant construction of rural facilities in the 1930s, difficult economic conditions then and during World War II constrained expansion, which just kept up with population growth. After the end of the war and the economic recovery, the hospital-building program took off, and provision grew much faster than the population. The number of government hospital beds increased from 1.9 per 100 before 1945 to just over 3.1 by 1960 (figure 11.7). Since then hospital expansion has continued, but only enough as to keep up with population growth.

Without the reforms, rural people would not have had equitable access to basic medical services. Today, although higher-level facilities and services are located only in urban areas, they are still accessible to the rural population, owing to the short distances in Sri Lanka between town and countryside and cheap public transport. Consequently, urban–rural differentials in service accessibility are minimal. The differences that do remain relate more to quality differentials and the increased travel costs that rural people encounter in accessing tertiary care.

## Medical Education and Regulation

The public universities operate the medical schools and have been graduating a thousand new physicians a year for the past decade. Admission is based strictly on

**Figure 11.7   Sri Lanka: Government Hospital Provision, 1920–2000**

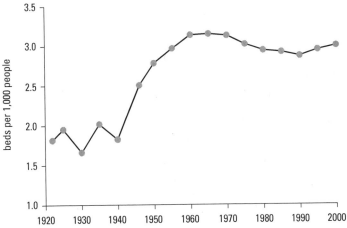

*Source:* Estimated by authors from health ministry statistics.

grades in the school-leaving examinations, and tuition is free (as are all public university courses). The medical school curriculum, a five-year course, is based on the British system. All medical graduates must complete a two-year internship in a public hospital before they can receive a full license to practice. Placement in an internship is by merit, and the lower ranked are placed in rural areas. Refusing the assigned internship debars a medical graduate from ever obtaining a license, so compliance is good. Sri Lankans who have obtained medical degrees abroad are given last preference. Further training to become a specialist requires both formal postgraduate examinations and clinical work to obtain expertise. This postgraduate training, including government-funded placements overseas, is available only in the public sector and is a major incentive for doctors to stay in the public sector.

Once fully licensed, a doctor may practice indefinitely. The Sri Lanka Medical Council, a statutory body, regulates physicians and has the ultimate power to remove the license. However, this power is almost never exercised. Although the law does allow for cases to be brought against physicians on the grounds of professional negligence, they are rare owing to the difficulty of proving these cases in court and lack of patient awareness of their legal rights.

In the private sector, Sri Lanka follows a laissez-faire policy of light regulation. Private doctors can practice as they wish, as long as they have the basic license. Private hospitals are barely regulated, and government did not even require these institutions to register centrally until 2008. Nor does government attempt to control prices in any way. For more than a decade, the MOH has been proposing a price-control statute, but no draft has made it out of the parliament. The small private medical insurance market is not subject to specific regulation, although it is regulated as part of the overall insurance and financial services sector.

## Pharmaceuticals and Medical Technology

Sri Lanka's public sector–initiated policies for the control and management of medicines in government hospitals as early as the 1950s, several decades before WHO adopted the concept of the rational use of drugs. To control medical technology, there is no policy other than a basic registration requirement.

*Pharmaceutical supply and regulation.* Pharmaceutical supply and regulation policies include a national formulary of drugs approved for use in government hospitals, a policy of purchasing public sector drugs only through international tender and bulk purchasing, the use of only generic medicines in the public sector, and the adoption of a national essential drugs list. Most government drugs are bought centrally for distribution to medical facilities and the provinces. The existence of these policies does not limit the range of medicines available in the public sector. The health ministry's essential drug list contains several thousand products, and the MOH purchased almost 3,000 different drugs and medical items in 2005. Nevertheless, not every medicine is available in every hospital. For cost control reasons, the number of drugs lower-level hospitals can stock is controlled through administrative procedures, based on an assessment of how essential a drug is, and the more expensive drugs are restricted to tertiary facilities.

The private sector may import any drug that is registered with national authorities. In practice, any drug that registered in the United States or Europe will be registered in Sri Lanka upon application. Until 2002, prices of imported drugs were controlled by setting the retail price at a maximum of 165 percent of the import price.

*Medical technology.* Despite the lack of a formal policy, adoption and purchase of expensive high technologies are tightly controlled in the health ministry using managerial procedures. For example, the purchase of CAT scanners and MRI scanners was long delayed in the public sector, despite pressure from medical specialists, and only small numbers have been purchased. The private sector may import any registered medical technology, but until recently the implications of this were limited, since tertiary medical care was effectively a public sector monopoly. However, in the past decade, with growth in investor-financed private tertiary private hospitals in Colombo, the private sector has begun to import the more expensive high-technology devices, such as MRI scanners.

## Strengths and Weaknesses

The main strengths of Sri Lanka's system are its equity, high system efficiency, good health outcomes, and relatively low costs for government and households (Hsiao and Associates 2001). The system affords the poor effective protection against financial risk of illness and ensures their access to basic medical services. The incidence of government spending is not pro-rich, as it is in many developing countries. In addition, the general revenue–based system of financing is progressive, and most out-of-pocket spending falls, by choice, on the richer households.

The main weaknesses of the system result primarily from underfunding; the government cannot increase the budget because it has not raised taxes sufficiently (Hsiao and Associates 2001). Underfunding means that hospital services do not meet the demands for services and amenities of richer households, which have been turning increasingly to the private sector. The risk is recognized that the continued shift of patients out of the public system may destabilize the health system as a whole and undermine political support for government health services. The system has also failed to adopt modern methods for management and treatment of chronic, noncommunicable diseases such as ischemic heart disease. This is a growing challenge owing to the stagnation in male adult life expectancy. But, lack of funding precludes a reorientation.

A related problem is the increase in consumer nonhealth expectations for better amenities in government hospitals and a more consumer-oriented approach by staff. Again, the organizational changes and flexibility that the system needs to respond to cannot currently be implemented until the financing gap is resolved.

Table 11.17   Sri Lanka: The Chronology of Scaling-Up Health Reforms

| Year | Event or Reform | Government expenditure (GDP) | Inpatient admissions/ 100 capita | IMR |
|------|-----------------|----------------------------|----------------------------------|-----|
| 1858 | Establishment of first government medical department | < 0.5 | < 1.0 | n.a. |
| 1931 | Democracy: First national elections by universal franchise and transfer of power to elected Sri Lankan leaders | 1.4 | 3.3 | 158 |
| 1934–35 | Rural economies ravaged by Ceylon malaria epidemic | 1.5 | 4.3 | 263 |
| 1936–47 | Expansion of government medical services into rural areas | 0.9–1.7 | 5.5–7.9 | 120 |
| 1948 | Commission on Social Services rejects introduction of social health insurance, recognizing that direct government hospital provision is a form of insurance | 1.7 | 9.3 | 101 |
| 1951 | User fees ended at government hospitals | 1.5 | 11.0 | 82 |
| 1959 | End of increases in health budget | 2.1 | 14.0 | 58 |

*Source:* Statistics for government expenditure, admissions and IMR from official data.

## Health Coverage Reforms

The good and equitable health outcomes in Sri Lanka result from health care reforms (table 11.17). They are not an inevitable outcome of culture and history. Prior to reform, health conditions in the island were no better and mortality rates were higher than the South Asian average (Langford and Storey 1993). The subsequent health achievements of Sri Lanka are chiefly due to the role of its health services in reducing mortality and morbidity and the success in expanding coverage of its health system. The main scaling-up phase of reforms (1931–59) put in place all the key features of the current system, including high coverage of the poor. The core elements have not been disturbed by subsequent, incremental developments. A look at the formative 1930s through 1950s reveals how Sri Lanka reformed its health system; the years before that tell why.

### The Precursors to Sri Lanka's Health Reforms

History facilitated Sri Lanka's health reforms. An ancient history of public provision of health care meant that public services were not necessarily alien. Exposure to western medicine during the colonial era and the development of an extensive physical and social infrastructure funded from exports provided a conducive environment. Ultimately, precipitating and critical events played their role, principally the advent of democracy in 1931 with the transfer of power by the British to a representative government elected through universal suffrage and lessons about health market failure, driven home by the Ceylon Malaria Epidemic.

*A history of state intervention.* Public financing of health services in Sri Lanka dates back at least 2,300 years. In the premodern era, Sri Lankan kings opened public hospitals and funded them from government revenues. The rulers were motivated by the prospect of merit, which Buddhism taught would accrue to the builder, and by the high value placed by Buddhism on the alleviation of human suffering (Rannan-Eliya and de Mel 1997). This was in a context, where the Theravada strand of Buddhism, which is dominant in Sri Lanka, encouraged a close nexus between religion and state action. Unlike in premodern Europe, most hospitals were built in Sri Lanka not through private charitable action, but as state initiatives. Records date the earliest such facilities to the fourth century BC (Uragoda 1987).

State financing of health services collapsed in the 13th century, with internal conflict and foreign invasion, and the resulting collapse of the public revenue collection system. Although the period from then until the end of the colonial period represents a clear discontinuity in social policy development, contemporary public attitudes in Sri Lanka, which assign to the state primary responsibility for providing health care, echo these earlier traditions and find support in contemporary religious thought.

*Exposure to western medicine.* During the colonial era, the Dutch and British occupiers opened a few urban hospitals for the benefit of colonial officials and European residents. They were financed by a mix of user fees and general revenues and were beyond the reach of rural Sri Lankans. For them, the only option was treatment by traditional doctors who, in accordance with Buddhist tradition, charged fees only for dispensing medicines, and not directly for diagnosis. Nevertheless, the colonial medical services were important in introducing the concepts of modern scientific medicine. Sri Lankan culture, much as in Japan and Kerala, proved receptive to the western biomedical model, as it blended easily into a context where individuals would look for signs of illness and doctors would treat with medicines (Caldwell et al. 1989). This ready cultural acceptance of scientific medicine partly explains the alacrity with which Sri Lanka's rural people later welcomed expansion of health services.

In the 19th century, the British occupation authorities tried to extend health services by introducing, in 1880, a scheme for the plantation companies to provide basic medical services to their workers, to be financed by reimbursements of a cess on exports. This was motivated not by humanitarian reasons, but because of the importance of these workers to the plantation economy and pressure from the Indian government. By the 1930s, the estate workers enjoyed better health services than the rural population, and better health indicators. After 1931, these plantation services became a model for the rural population to aspire to.

*The colonial state and introduction of democracy.* The British occupation was marked by the development of the plantation economy. Plantation exports, easily taxed, provided the authorities with a ready source of revenues. In 1848, the British defeated the last armed rebellion against occupation. This event was an important milestone. First, the rebellion was essentially a peasant revolt and marked the start of a transition in Sri Lankan society between leadership by feudal elites to one based on the support of ordinary people. Second, the occupation authorities no longer faced internal threats requiring maintenance of a large military, and tax revenues were invested in building physical and social infrastructure servicing the plantation sector and an administrative structure that was more sophisticated and substantial than in the rest of South Asia. One indicator is that by the 1930s, Sri Lanka had a functioning vital registration system recording most births and deaths.

The relatively advanced state of institutions in the island led the British in 1928 to embark on a major experiment in social engineering, by granting Sri Lankans self-rule under a representative government elected through universal suffrage. This transfer of power, not to the local elites but directly to the majority of the population, was opposed by the leading Sri Lankan politicians. Its radical nature is evident, considering that only in 1929 were the first elections by universal suffrage held in the United Kingdom.

In introducing democratic government, there was an explicit recognition that democratic accountability to voters would promote health conditions and reduce mortality:

> We have given serious consideration to the question of women's franchise. Apart from the familiar arguments in its favour, and the general principle of sex equality, we have been impressed by the high infantile mortality in the Island, and the need for better housing, and for the development of child welfare, midwifery and ante-natal services, all providing problems in the solution of which women's interest and help would be of special value, It is true that though the position of women in the East has not, till recent years, been suitable for the exercise of political power, that position is rapidly changing and the demand for the vote was put to us by a large and representative deputation of Ceylonese ladies' (Government of Ceylon 1928).

The first legislature selected through universal franchise was elected in 1931. British civil servants ceded all responsibility for domestic policy to Sri Lankan politicians until independence in 1948, when the new Sri Lankan government took over responsibility for foreign and security affairs. Competitive electoral politics during the following two decades would drive all major changes in social policy, including the introduction of the personal income tax (1932), the expansion of government health services to rural areas (1931–40), the introduction of free education (1930s and 1940s), and the abolition of user fees for health services (1951).

***The lessons of market failure in the health sector.*** The period leading up to 1931 created the preconditions for Sri Lanka's health reforms: a population receptive to modern medical services, a model of health care provision in the plantations that the rural population could aspire to, a fiscal base adequate to support significant public expenditures, and a political mechanism to translate social preferences into actual policy. The missing element was the understanding by policy makers of the need for reform of the existing health system. This came about as a result of an unprecedented health crisis, the Ceylon Malaria Epidemic (Rannan-Eliya and de Mel 1997).

In 1934–35, owing to unusual climatic conditions, a major epidemic of malaria spread to every part of the island, hitting most severely normally nonmalarial areas, where people had no natural immunity. Most of the population was infected, and a significant fraction died. When this hit, the politically conservative, newly elected Sri Lankan government left the response to market forces, primarily charitable action. This proved totally inadequate in face of the disaster, which followed a deep rural crisis induced by the impact of the global recession of the early 1930s. Other than direct morbidity, the epidemic economically devastated rural areas, because farmers were too ill to cultivate their crops, and their family members, burdened by the responsibility of caring for the sick, could not attend to their normal work. In the absence of state intervention, the Marxist opposition parties made much political capital by organizing missions to assist the afflicted rural poor. Although these missions were not that effective, they created political alarm among the elite.

After the epidemic, an official government inquiry observed that the health crisis had forced rural households into poverty and that relying on charitable and market actions was totally inadequate to deal with the challenge. It concluded that direct state intervention was needed through provision of hospitals that could treat and feed the sick, so as to help the affected families survive such events. This series of events, through official reports recognizing the financial impoverishment created by ill-health in rural areas, increased political pressure to expand health services. It is almost identical to the sequence of events in Japan in the early 1930s that led the Japanese government to embark on the eventually successful effort to extend health insurance coverage to all its people (Hasegawa 2005).

In effect, Sri Lankan state and other policy makers realized early that health was not just an individual matter and that health policy was more than just curing disease. Although there was little effective treatment for malaria at the time, they understood that ill health had economic implications and was linked to poverty, that the market would not provide effective health insurance against catastrophic risks, and that the public sector had a crucial role to play in providing it. They also realized that failure to address the market failure would carry significant political risks in the new political environment where the poor had a vote. The recognition that direct public provision of hospital services was a form of social insurance would be later explicitly stated by the influential Commission on Social Services (1947).

## Health System Reforms

From the early 1930s, the government launched an expansion of free health services in rural areas, primarily through building and staffing hospitals and dispensaries. The immediate impact of this expansion was obscured by financial constraints during World War II. When the economy returned to normal after 1945, there was an immediate increase in the quality of services at the new facilities as staffing and the supply of the new antibiotics improved. This fed directly into the jump in life expectancy in postwar years (Langford 1996).

The initial expansion of the service network chiefly involved the building of new health ministry facilities in places where there had been none. At first they were simple dispensaries and unsophisticated rural hospitals, but they brought most Sri Lankans within a short distance of some treatment point and encouraged them to try modern medicine instead of traditional care. The construction program was promoted by the lobbying of the health ministry by individual members of parliament, which, in effect, ensured that all electorates ended up with at least some health services. This lobbying was biased in favor of rural areas, because rural electorates had fewer voters on average than urban electorates, and thus were overrepresented in parliament. In addition, until the late 1940s, party political organization was weak, and most legislators competed for election not on the basis of a party platform, but on their ability to bring their constituents benefits such as hospitals, schools, and roads (Wriggins 1960). By 1945, the health ministry was operating more than a thousand hospitals and dispensaries for a population of only 7 million. Later, after the network was in place, further expansion shifted to upgrading and expanding existing facilities, a process that continues today. By the 1950s, Sri Lanka thus ended up with the far-flung facility network that minimized distance, which is so important for reaching the poor. As more contemporary analyses have found, distance is as important a factor as quality in the demand for health services in developing countries (Lavy and Quigley 1983). By building so many facilities, the distance that the poor have to travel to obtain care was reduced, and a key barrier to access was removed.

*Abolition of user fees.* In common with most British colonies, government hospitals charged user fees prior to the 1930s. However, a means-tested exemption was provided to those considered poor, and the income limit was set so high that most rural patients did not pay. Yet in the electoral scenario that emerged after 1931, even these limited fees were considered unreasonable. User fees were abolished in 1951 by the UNP government in power at the time but were reintroduced in 1971 by a Trotskyite finance minister. Demand for health services, especially by the poor, immediately plummeted, and the fees were again abolished by the next UNP government in 1977. Consequently, in Sri Lanka user charges have never been a barrier to access by the poor, and the national policy of free care has been firmly supported by all major political parties and, in fact, was instigated by the most promarket of them.

*The emphasis on hospitals.* The health reforms, from the beginning, relied heavily on hospitals in extending coverage. Unlike in many developing countries today, Sri Lankan health planners early recognized not only the insurance function of a hospital, but also the fact that most illnesses could not be prevented and thus needed to be treated through curative interventions. They thus believed that hospitals had to play the lead role in combating illness and allocated budgetary resources accordingly. The prioritization of hospitals in the health ministry budget was thus an important feature of official health policy from the 1930s and marked a major change from British colonial policy, which had concentrated on preventive, sanitation, and quarantine measures for the rural population.

*Indigenization of medical department.* The health ministry that executed these reforms was distinctively different from other ministries. In the latter part of the British occupation, government departments were no longer the preserve of British civil servants, and Sri Lankans were progressively recruited into them. This process of indigenization had most advanced in the case of the medical department, regarded by the British as the least important or prestigious. Not only were almost all its personnel Sri Lankan by 1930, but it was also the first department in which the most senior civil service position could be filled by a local. This departmental history was important. It imbued the ministry with a distinctive pro-poor attitude: its personnel took pride in the fact that it was the first to be controlled by Sri Lankans, which encouraged an ethos that saw the mission of the ministry as "serving the masses." This contrasts with neighboring India, where the Indian Medical Service was seen as an agent of the occupiers (Jeffery 1988).

*Tradeoff of quality versus access.* As rural access to services improved in the 1940s, the health ministry was met with sustained and wholly unanticipated surges in patient demand. For example, in 1948 total inpatient numbers increased by 22 percent; outpatients, by 30 percent. Government hospitals were filled beyond their design capacity, and average bed-occupancy rates of more than 200 percent were common. In this situation, medical personnel and planners often pushed for measures to restrict demand, including closing hospitals when bed-occupancy breached the official limit of 200 percent, because further admissions would damage treatment quality. However, political pressures not to restrict access made it impossible for the health ministry to accede. In several instances, doctors were dismissed from service for implementing departmental rules on overcrowding, after patients refused admittance complained to their legislators, who then complained to the health minister. In this situation, an implicit tradeoff was made to prioritize access to services over service quality. Although it had the perverse result of making overcrowding inevitable, it benefited the poor, because any measures that might have restricted demand would have affected the poor inevitably more than the rich.

*Productivity improvement.* The ambitious expansion of health services that was planned and achieved was expensive. After the mid-1950s, fiscal constraints made it impossible for the government to increase the health budget, and subsequently health spending fell as a share of national income. Despite this, political leaders would not accept any reductions in services by the MOH or any policies to restrict demand. Faced with these conflicting pressures, the ministry responded by searching relentlessly for productivity increases and pushing its staff to work harder. To do this it had to rely largely on administrative and managerial measures, ranging from simple changes such as reducing the minimum distance allowed between hospital beds to changing the pension regulations, so that doctors were compensated adequately for working longer hours. Over time this created an organizational culture that has promoted continuous productivity increases.

*Compulsory posting and dual medical practice.*  An important pre-1930s reform concerning private practice has facilitated expansion of coverage to rural areas. When the health department was first established, medical officers were not permitted to engage in private business, consistent with general civil service regulations. However, the department discovered that it was hard to recruit medical officers from the United Kingdom to work in Sri Lanka owing to the difficult working conditions and low pay. It was therefore decided to allow medical officers to supplement their official salary by doing private practice outside official work hours and off government premises. This enabled the department to recruit and retain medical staff. This policy was in effect in the 1930s, by when most new recruits were local graduates. It has supported expansion of coverage into rural areas, because the health ministry cannot afford to pay market wages to entice doctors, but doctors can substantially raise their incomes by private practice. In rural areas where the government medical officers are usually the only physicians, private practice can be lucrative. In 1970–77, when private practice was abolished, the distribution of government doctors to rural areas suffered, as did overall retention of medical officers in the health ministry.

The health ministry has adopted another policy to improve availability of medical personnel in rural areas: rotating all junior doctors—on a regular basis and compulsorily—posting many of them to rural areas. This policy has been enforced by firing doctors who refuse to comply, a significant disincentive because junior doctors cannot obtain specialist training outside the public sector. Through the carrot of specialist training and seniority, which are necessary for doctors to earn the highest private practice incomes, doctors are persuaded to accept lower than market wages during the early part of their careers.

## Evaluation of Reforms

Between 1931 and 1951, Sri Lanka expanded access to health services by using direct government provision and building a highly dispersed health facility network in rural areas. The reforms fundamentally altered the health system. They changed it from one in which the urban rich used modern medical services and rural people relied on traditional providers, to one in which the whole population had easy access to and used modern medical services. This involved not only increases in coverage, but also a change in health-seeking behavior as rural Sri

**Table 11.18    Sri Lanka: Expansion of Health Service Coverage, 1931–51**

| Item | 1927 | 1931 | 1936 | 1946 | 1951 |
|---|---|---|---|---|---|
| Inpatient admissions (per 100 capita) | 3.7 | 3.3 | 6.0 | 7.5 | 11.0 |
| Outpatient visits (per capita) | 0.5 | 0.6 | 1.0 | 1.1 | 1.5 |
| Government health expenditure (GDP) | 0.8 | 1.4 | 1.7 | 1.3 | 1.5 |

*Source:* IHP databases and official statistics.

*Note:* Data are given for 1927 to provide an indication of the prereform trends. Other years selected are based on availability of data, which are incomplete for the 1939–45 time period owing to wartime censorship of government administrative data.

Lankans were persuaded to switch from traditional to modern medical care. So effective was the expansion in coverage that by 1951 Sri Lanka was able to achieve quantitative levels of health service access comparable to many middle-income developing countries today and substantially equalize use of modern medical treatment between rich and poor. In addition, this expansion of coverage involved access to not only primary care services, but also to general hospital services, including inpatient treatment. The aggregate increase in population coverage was between 200 and 300 percent during the 20-year period (table 11.18).

There is an important aspect to this expansion in coverage. Since the initial reforms in the 1930s, a major implicit goal of health care provision has not been to improve health outcomes, but to protect households against the catastrophic economic impacts of severe illness. The reforms have not only increased access to services but have also extended insurance protection to the poor in the form of hospital services. This has been possible because the public sector has allocated the largest share of the budget to hospital services, and has implicitly accepted the role of the health services in providing insurance against the catastrophic financial risks of illness.

*Institutional change.* To achieve this expansion in coverage, Sri Lanka transformed its government health ministry's mission from serving the workforce of the occupation authorities to serving the rural people. Moreover, the expansion created a management culture focused on productivity improvement as the means of expanding coverage within limited resources. This was done without changing the civil service structure or regulations and relied primarily on organizational ethos and culture.

*Health outcomes.* The expansion in coverage enabled Sri Lanka to rapidly reap the advances in medical technology that had been made globally in the previous half century and substantially reduce mortality in all areas and in every population subgroup. Not only were health indicators dramatically improved after 1945 as a result of the better access to medical treatment, but a process was also started that substantially reduced health inequalities between urban and rural and rich and poor Sri Lankans. The health reforms started a process of rapid and continuing mortality decline that has enabled Sri Lanka to complete its mortality transition in less than a half century.

*Cost implications of scaling up and targeting.* The expansion in services during the scaling-up phase of the reforms involved large increases in government outlays in funding. After the 1950s, however, the government could not continue to increase funding to keep up with the increases in patient demand manifest since the early 1930s. At the end of the scaling-up phase, the reforms could easily have imploded, because increased demand so outstripped financing capacity as to endanger the principle and practice of universal access. That this did not happen can be attributed to two factors: technical efficiency gains in the public sector substituted substantially for the lack of additional funding, and implicit targeting was achieved by interaction with private sector supply.

As noted, more than half the increase in service volume was achieved through productivity increases. By the 1950s, the government was able to start reducing health spending as a share of GDP, while still continuing to expand and improve services.

The other contribution to meeting the financing gap involved in committing to universal coverage has come from the dynamics of demand for public and private services. As noted, the health ministry has permitted dual practice by its medical officers since the 19th century and takes a laissez-faire attitude to the private sector. Consequently, in all areas some private medical services are available, and in rural areas almost all outpatient services are provided on a fee-for-service basis by government medical officers. Even in urban areas, where there is significant private inpatient provision, the attending physicians are usually government specialists, or they are full-time private GPs, most of whom, for many years, worked in the public sector (Rannan-Eliya, Jayawardhane, and Karunaratne 2003). Consequently, there is little difference in the technical quality of medical services in the public and private sectors. The only reason that patients choose to pay for private services, when they can, in theory, see the same doctors for free in government hospitals, is that in the private sector the hotel amenities are better, the facilities are less crowded and the queues shorter, the opening times can be more convenient, patients can choose their doctor, and the doctors and staff will spend a little more time with the patient and are perhaps more polite and courteous. In this context, the richer patients, who have a higher opportunity cost of waiting and a greater preference for the consumer aspects of quality, voluntarily choose to use the private sector. This choice is reflected in a strong prorich gradient in the use of private outpatient services and a propoor gradient in the use of public outpatient services. For inpatient services, for which few Sri Lankans without insurance can afford to pay out of pocket, the gradients are less obvious. This situation allows the government—without having to identify rich and poor directly—to effectively target its spending to the poor and maintain its explicit commitment to universalism, while relying on the rich to reveal their own preferences by voluntarily opting out.

*Politics and sustainability.* There is no evidence to suggest that Sri Lankan politicians are significantly more altruistic and concerned for the poor than those in any other country. When the malaria epidemic of 1934–35 struck, most politicians stood by and left the population to fend for itself. However, the political system, where political power must be obtained though the ballot box and where the voters are not disinclined to throw out incumbents, taught political leaders to be highly sensitive to the demands and preferences of the people, including the rural poor. Thus, the political leadership embarked on health reforms that invested significant public funds in expanding access to free health services and subsequently ensuring that this system was maintained and improved. This sensitivity to social preferences has also been behind the prioritization of budgetary resources for hospitals. Because the political rationale still exists for governments to maintain the system, as long as the population favors it, the current health care system is sustainable. At the same time, the political system has been effective in transmitting its concerns about financial costs to the health ministry, so overall government health expenditures in Sri Lanka have never been high by international standards.

## Key Conditions

The key conditions for Sri Lanka's success in expanding access were as follows:

- *Democracy.* A competitive electoral process has ensured that the political elite must take into account the preferences and needs of the poor and forced policy makers to build an accessible health system in every part of the country.
- *Taxes.* The early availability of a ready tax base in the form of export taxes on tea, rubber, and coconut enabled the government to provide the public financing to pay for service expansions for the rural poor.
- *A committed and efficient public sector.* Sri Lanka still faced the challenge of how to expand services within limited budgetary resources. It succeeded primarily because its centralized civil service management of health care services gave it an efficient means of expanding services through continuous productivity gains.
- *A pragmatic approach to targeting.* The approach involves adopting an explicit commitment of universal access but implicitly allowing the rich to opt out and use private services, thus allowing government spending to be focused on the poor.
- *The existence of models.* At various points, Sri Lankans were able to copy, emulate, or aspire to introduce models of health care delivery. These provided them with a template for transformation and reduced the need to experiment. The models included Western biomedicine introduced by the European occupiers, the free health care provided to estate workers and civil servants, and the British health ministry organization that took root in colonial times.

## Lessons for Other Countries

Sri Lanka offers many lessons for broadening access to basic health services to the poor in developing countries.

*Democratic accountability can ensure that health systems are responsive to the needs of the poor.* For health systems to be responsive to the needs and preferences of the poor requires that the political system itself be responsive to their wishes. A democratic political system in which the poor are given voice through regular, free, and fair elections can be an effective mechanism for achieving this, although the scale and level of electoral representation are important mediating factors. Democratic accountability should not be confused with community participation or cost sharing or political decentralization. Sri Lanka has had little success with community participation in local government or in running individual facilities, but the most basic decisions about the health system are not made locally, but nationally. It is at the national level that the poor have had a voice.

In fact, the most important issue for the poor—the redistribution of resources from the wealthiest parts of the country to the poorest—can be resolved only through central government action. But well-meaning technocratic intentions will not permanently guarantee attention to the poor. Only when a political system has incentives to consider the interests of the poor will it actually do so, and continue to do so. Political considerations frequently override technical concerns, and Sri Lanka's history provides numerous examples of public choices superior in welfare terms to choices by experts. At the same time, for a health system to be able to act on the preferences of the poor it must not emasculate its capability to do so. Building and maintaining efficient systems for public revenue collection and public production of health services are integral to making democratic accountability real in poor countries.

*Fair access for all should be a priority goal of health systems.* Equity of access to services must be a priority goal if health gains are to reach the poor. All health systems operate under resource constraints. Inevitably, some attempt will be made to match supply and demand, but almost all rationing mechanisms have negative implications for the poor. Unless fair access is the highest priority, choices about rationing will be made that will shortchange the poor. Sri Lanka's democratic political system ensured that fair access was the priority goal. This led to the disavowal of user fees and other financial barriers to accessing health services, the building of a highly dispersed government health care system that reduced nonfinancial barriers to access such as travel costs, the imposition of incentives for government providers to accept all patients regardless of cost and quality implications, and the outranking of concerns for rational referrals by the principle of free choice of providers.

*Health systems must provide the poor with insurance against catastrophic illness.* Independent of the impact on health status, health systems make an important contribution to the welfare of the poor when they provide insurance against the economic costs of severe illness. This has been one of the most important objectives of Sri Lankan health policy, recognized as early as 1935. Its importance is reflected in the highest priority given to inpatient services in government budgetary allocations. The economic costs of illness include not only the cost of medical treatment, but also the care and feeding of the patient, and the loss of income as household members must divert time from their normal household and other activities to tend the sick. Catastrophe insurance cannot be provided by charity or by private markets in any country. Only public action can provide it either through free inpatient services or some other method of social insurance.

*Efficiency in health service production is more important than resource mobilization in overcoming resource constraints.* Fair access in resource-constrained environments requires that health services be efficient producers. Sri Lanka did not respond to its budget constraints by limiting service delivery, but expanding services by using efficiency gains of 1 to 4 percent every year in its public sector. Sri Lanka was better able to achieve efficiency gains to mobilize additional resources than spend more money. The potential for such efficiency gains in health systems should throw into question the assumption that tight resources pose insuperable barriers to ensuring better health for the poor. Sri Lanka completed its health transition and achieved access to health services similar to OECD economies while spending less than 50 percent of the World Bank–stipulated "minimum cost-effective package"—and without resorting to user fees, community financing, or insurance.

*Pessimism about the relative inefficiency of public sector health service production is as unwarranted empirically as it is theoretically.* Sri Lanka's experience is unusual, but it should not be assumed that the public sector is inherently incapable of efficient service delivery or necessarily the worst of possible alternatives. Sri Lanka's government hospital system has been effective both in achieving high efficiency and in generating continuous efficiency gains. This was done without giving autonomy to individual hospitals, without decentralization, and without changing civil service conditions of employment, despite the existence of strong health sector unions. More attention by researchers and by policy makers needs to be given to understanding the determinants of efficient performance by public sector providers, and perhaps more than is now given to maximizing efficiency in private delivery. Experience in Sri Lanka (and several countries with similar health departments; e.g., Malaysia, Hong Kong [China], and Mauritius) suggests that within the spectrum of public sector organization patterns, unobserved and poorly understood possibilities remain for excellence in public sector delivery. Since Sri Lanka neither pays its health personnel well nor uses performance-related financial incentives, the evidence indicates that nonfinancial incentives and organizational culture can be more important determinants of performance.

*Cost-effectiveness of interventions and a disease-focused approach to allocational efficiency are irrational and inefficient guides to resource allocation and may lead to erroneous use of resources.* Sri Lanka never relied upon cost-effectiveness or disease focus as a guide to allocating resources. Allocating resources according to specific diseases and interventions would have been mostly impossible inasmuch as resources were budgeted by facility and input type, and physicians make decisions about treatment at the lowest level. As to cost-effectiveness decisions, Sri Lanka never had the data or expertise to make the necessary calculations. The Sri Lankan experience fundamentally contradicts the basic conclusions of most cost-effectiveness analysis. Sri Lanka, influenced by its political process, has placed government resources where they would have the greatest marginal welfare benefits in the context of social inequality and dual public and private markets. Inpatient care has been favored not because of its health impact, but because of underlying welfare gains in terms of risk protection, and the inability of private markets to ensure adequate supply. Routine primary care receives a lower share of government budgetary resources, because many households are likely to be able to pay for adequate care themselves from private sources.

*Use of consumer quality differentials in a dual public-private system can be a more effective mechanism of targeting health subsidies than explicit targeting.* Sri Lanka found that targeting any subsidy to the poor faces the informational constraint that governments lack sufficient information to distinguish accurately between the poor and the rich. This is the same information constraint that prevents poor countries from relying on income taxation as the main source of general revenue. Consistent with the insight from the theory of optimal income taxation that tax and subsidy systems should be incentive compatible, a health system can efficiently target health subsidies by enforcing universal access and relying on differentials in consumer quality to persuade richer individuals to self-select private services. Such a system, as in Sri Lanka, is politically sustainable as long as sufficient people continue to use the public service. That this is a general attribute of the health system is demonstrated by similar outcomes in several other ex-British dependent territories with similar health systems, such as Jamaica, Barbados, Mauritius, Malaysia, Hong Kong (China), and Ireland.

**Annex table 11A.1   Sri Lanka: Total Health Expenditures, 1993–2005**

| | 1993 | 1994 | 1995 | 1996 | 1997 | 1998 | 1999 | 2000 | 2001 | 2002 | 2003 | 2004 | 2005 |
|---|---|---|---|---|---|---|---|---|---|---|---|---|---|
| **Total expenditures on health** | | | | | | | | | | | | | |
| Rs. million | 17,263 | 20,346 | 24,372 | 28,485 | 31,964 | 38,224 | 42,694 | 48,457 | 55,724 | 62,828 | 72,108 | 86,893 | 100,115 |
| US$million | 358 | 412 | 476 | 515 | 542 | 592 | 607 | 640 | 624 | 657 | 747 | 859 | 996 |
| **Ratios** | | | | | | | | | | | | | |
| Share of GDP (%) | 3.5 | 3.5 | 3.6 | 3.7 | 3.6 | 3.8 | 3.9 | 3.9 | 4.0 | 4.0 | 4.1 | 4.3 | 4.2 |
| Per capita (US$) | 21 | 24 | 27 | 29 | 31 | 33 | 33 | 35 | 33 | 35 | 39 | 44 | 51 |
| Population (million) | 16.3 | 16.4 | 16.6 | 16.9 | 17.1 | 17.3 | 17.5 | 17.7 | 17.9 | 18.2 | 18.5 | 18.7 | 19.0 |

*Source:* Institute for Health Policy (IHP) Sri Lanka Health Accounts database.

**Annex table 11A.2   Sri Lanka: Health Expenditures, by Source, 1993–2005 (percent of total)**

| | 1993 | 1994 | 1995 | 1996 | 1997 | 1998 | 1999 | 2000 | 2001 | 2002 | 2003 | 2004 | 2005 |
|---|---|---|---|---|---|---|---|---|---|---|---|---|---|
| General government | 44 | 45 | 47 | 47 | 47 | 49 | 48 | 49 | 47 | 47 | 45 | 47 | 47 |
| Central government | 27 | 26 | 30 | 30 | 31 | 33 | 32 | 33 | 31 | 31 | 30 | 32 | 31 |
| Provincial government | 14 | 16 | 15 | 15 | 14 | 14 | 14 | 15 | 14 | 14 | 13 | 13 | 15 |
| Local government | 2 | 2 | 2 | 2 | 2 | 2 | 2 | 2 | 2 | 2 | 2 | 2 | 2 |
| Private sector | 56 | 55 | 53 | 53 | 53 | 51 | 52 | 51 | 53 | 53 | 55 | 53 | 53 |
| Household out-of-pocket | 51 | 51 | 48 | 48 | 49 | 48 | 47 | 46 | 48 | 49 | 50 | 49 | 49 |
| Private insurance | 1 | 1 | 1 | 1 | 1 | 1 | 1 | 1 | 1 | 1 | 1 | 1 | 2 |
| Employers | 3 | 3 | 3 | 4 | 2 | 1 | 3 | 2 | 3 | 2 | 3 | 1 | 1 |
| Nonprofit institutions | 1 | 1 | 1 | 1 | 1 | 1 | 1 | 1 | 1 | 1 | 1 | 1 | 1 |

*Source:* IHP Sri Lanka Health Accounts database.

**Annex table 11A.3    Sri Lanka: Health Expenditures, by Provider, 1993–2005 (percentage of total)**

|  | 1993 | 1994 | 1995 | 1996 | 1997 | 1998 | 1999 | 2000 | 2001 | 2002 | 2003 | 2004 | 2005 |
|---|---|---|---|---|---|---|---|---|---|---|---|---|---|
| Hospitals | 33 | 34 | 37 | 36 | 37 | 38 | 38 | 38 | 37 | 39 | 39 | 42 | 43 |
| Ambulatory care providers | 32 | 31 | 29 | 30 | 28 | 26 | 27 | 27 | 27 | 26 | 27 | 26 | 27 |
| Retailers of medical goods | 22 | 22 | 20 | 20 | 21 | 21 | 21 | 20 | 22 | 23 | 22 | 21 | 20 |
| Providers of public health services | 7 | 6 | 6 | 5 | 6 | 6 | 4 | 4 | 4 | 3 | 3 | 3 | 4 |
| General health administration | 4 | 4 | 5 | 6 | 5 | 7 | 8 | 8 | 8 | 6 | 5 | 6 | 4 |
| Others | 2 | 2 | 2 | 2 | 2 | 2 | 2 | 2 | 2 | 2 | 3 | 2 | 2 |
| Rest of the world | 0 | 0 | 0 | 0 | 0 | 0 | 0 | 0 | 0 | 0 | 0 | 0 | 0 |

*Source:* IHP Sri Lanka Health Accounts database.

## Endnotes

*Note:* Any opinions expressed, or recommendations made in this report are those of the authors alone, and not necessarily those of the Institute for Health Policy or the World Bank. The editing of the first draft by Neluka Silva is gratefully acknowledged.

1. Two of provinces were merged in 1987, but in late 2006, Sri Lanka's Supreme Court declared the merger illegal as the required referendum of their voters had not been held.

2. The intensive empirical research this would take has not been a priority for most research-funding agencies.

3. For the sake of comparison the U.S. dollar per capita spending levels given in this and the following paragraphs are in constant 1990 U.S. dollars, to permit direct comparison with the spending estimates published in World Bank (1993).

## References

Alailima, Patricia J., and Faiz Mohideen. 1983. "Health Sector Commodity Requirements and Expenditure Flows." Colombo: National Planning Department.

Bruton, Henry J. 1992. "Sri Lanka and Malaysia." In *The Political Economy of Poverty, Equity and Growth*, ed. D. Lal and H. Myint. New York: Oxford University Press.

Caldwell, J.C. 1986. "Routes to Low Mortality in Poor Countries." *Population and Development Review* 12 (2): 171–220.

Caldwell, John, Indra Gajanayake, Pat Caldwell, and Indrani Peiris. 1989. "Sensitization to Illness and the Risk of Death: An Explanation for Sri Lanka's Approach to Good Health for All." *Social Science and Medicine* 28 (4): 365–79.

Central Bank of Sri Lanka. 2006. *Annual Report 2005.* Colombo: Central Bank of Sri Lanka.

Commission on Social Services. 1947. *Report of the Commission on Social Services.* Vol. VII, *Sessional Papers.* Colombo: Ceylon Government Press.

De Silva, M.W. Amarasiri, Ananda Wijekoon, Robert Hornik, and Jose Martines. 2001. "Care Seeking in Sri Lanka: One Possible Explanation for Low Childhood Mortality." *Social Science and Medicine* 53: 1363–72.

De Silva, W. Indralal. 2007. *A Population Projection of Sri Lanka for the New Millenium, 2001–2101: Trends and Implications.* Colombo: Institute for Health Policy.

Government of Ceylon. 1928. *Report of the Special Commission on the Constitution.* Colombo: H. Ross Cottle, Government Printer.

Hasegawa, Toshihilko. 2005. "Japan." In *Social Health Insurance: Selected Case Studies from Asia and the Pacific.* New Delhi: WHO Regional Office for South-East Asia and WHO Regional Office for Western Pacific Region.

Hensher, Martin. 2001. *Financing Health Systems through Efficiency Gains.* Vol. Paper No. WG3:2, *CMH Working Paper Series.* Geneva: Commission on Macroeconomics and Health.

Hsiao, William C., and Associates. 2001. "A Preliminary Assessment of Sri Lanka's Health Sector and Steps Forward." Cambridge, MA: Harvard University.

Hurst, Jeremy, and Melissa Jee-Hughes. 2001. "Performance Measurement and Performance Management in OECD Health Systems." Labour Market and Social Policy Occasional Paper No. 47. Paris: OECD.

Institute for Health Policy. Forthcoming. Sri Lanka Health Accounts, 1990–2006. Colombo: Institute for Health Policy.

Jeffery, Roger. 1988. *The Politics of Health in India.* Berkeley: University of California.

Langford, Christopher M. 1996. "Reasons for the Decline in Mortality in Sri Lanka Immediately after the Second World War: a Re-examination of the Evidence." *Health Transition Review* 6 (1): 3–23.

Langford, Christopher, and Pamela Storey. 1993. "Sex Differentials in Mortality Early in the Twentieth Century: Sri Lanka and India Compared." *Population and Development Review* 19 (2): 263–82.

Lavy, V, and J. M. Quigley. 1983. "Willingness to Pay for the Quality and Intensity of Medical Care: Low-Income Households in Ghana." World Bank, Washington, DC.

Meegama, A. 1986. "The Mortality Transition in Sri Lanka." In *Determinants of Mortality Change and Differentials in Developing Countries: The Five-Country Case Study Project.* Population Studies, No. 94; ST/ESA/SER.A/94. New York: United Nations.

Rannan-Eliya, Ravi P. 2001. *Strategies for Improving the Health of the Poor—The Sri Lankan Experience.* Colombo: Institute of Policy Studies Health Policy Programme.

———. 2006. *Productivity Change in Health Services: An Empirical Analysis and Exploration of Institutional Determinants.* Colombo: Institute for Health Policy.

———. 2004. "Towards a Model of Endogenous Mortality Decline: The Dynamic Role of Learning and Productivity in Health Systems." Thesis submitted to the Faculty of the Harvard School of Public Health in partial fulfillment of the requirements for the Degree of Doctor of Public Health, Department of Population and International Health, School of Public Health, Harvard University, Boston, MA.

Rannan-Eliya, Ravi P., and Nishan de Mel. 1997. *Resource Mobilization for the Health Sector in Sri Lanka, Data for Decision Making Publication.* Boston, MA: Harvard School of Public Health.

Rannan-Eliya, Ravi P., and Aparnaa Somanathan. 2003. The Bangladesh Health Facility Efficiency Study. In *Health Policy Research in Asia: Guiding Reforms and Building Capacity*, ed. A.S. Yazbeck and D.H. Peters. Washington, DC: World Bank.

Rannan-Eliya, Ravi P., Prashanthi Jayawardhane, and Leela Karunaratne. 2003. "Private Primary Care Practitioners in Sri Lanka." In *Health Policy Research in Asia: Guiding Reforms and Building Capacity*, ed. A.S. Yazbeck and D.H. Peters. Washington, DC, USA: World Bank.

Snodgrass, Donald R. 1966. *Ceylon: An Export Economy in Transition*. Homewood, IL: Richard D. Irwin.

Somanathan, Aparnaa, Kara Hanson, Tamara Dorabawila, and Bilesha Perera. 2000. "Operating Efficiency in Public Sector Health Facilities in Sri Lanka: Measurement and Institutional Determinants of Performance." Partnerships for Health Reform, Abt Associates Inc. Bethesda, MD.

Uragoda, C. G. 1987. *A History of Medicine in Sri Lanka*. Colombo: Sri Lanka Medical Association.

van Doorslaer, Eddy, Owen O'Donnell, Ravi P. Rannan-Eliya, Aparnaa Somanathan, Shiva Raj Adhikari, Charu C. Garg, Deni Harbianto, Alejandro N. Herrin, Mohammed Nazmul Huq, Shamsia Ibragimova, Anup Karan, Chiu Wan Ng, Badri Raj Pande, Rachel Racelis, Sihai Tao, Keith Tin, Kanjana Tisayaticom, Laksono Trisnantoro, Chitpranee Visasvid, and Yuxin Zhao. 2006. "Effect of Payments for Health Care on Poverty Estimates in 11 Countries in Asia: An Analysis of Household Survey Data. *Lancet* (9544): 1357–64.

World Bank. 1993. *World Development Report: Investing in Health*. New York: Oxford University Press.

———. 2003. *World Development Report 2004: Making Services Work For Poor People*. New York: Oxford University Press.

Wriggins, W. Howard. 1960. *Ceylon: Dilemmas of a New Nation*. Princeton, NJ: Princeton University Press.

# 12

# Thailand: Good Practice in Expanding Health Coverage—Lessons from the Thai Health Care Reforms

*Suwit Wibulpolprasert and Suriwan Thaiprayoon*

## Background

*The Thai health care system is pluralistic, with more than two-thirds of the health resources and three-fourths of service utilization in the public sector. The attempt at universal health coverage started in the era of the Primary Health Care and Health for All movement in the late 1970s. Significant progress was achieved in the past three decades, and 75 percent of the population was covered with some kind of health insurance by 1998. Nevertheless, not until after the 2001 election under the new people's constitution and the new government did universal health insurance and health care coverage become a reality. The policy on universal access to antiretrovirals (ARVs) was adopted in October 2003. Coverage was also expanded to include renal replacement therapy in January 2008 along with seasonal flu vaccination among high-risk groups. This paper tells the story behind the movements, all the contributing factors and actors, the good experiences, and the lessons learned from implementing this universal health care coverage policy in its first six years.*

## The Socioeconomic and Political Context

Thailand is a lower-middle-income developing country located in Southeast Asia with a population of 64.2 million in 2005 (NSO 2006). There are 76 provinces, 876 / 81 districts / subdistrict, 7,255 *tambons* [communes], and 68,839 villages. The Thais are almost universally literate, except for a small fraction of the elderly population.

From 1965 to 1996, the Thai economy grew at a rate of 7.8 percent annually, with double-digit growth in 1986 to 1990 (NESDB 2004). This sustained rapid economic growth allowed the government to pay off the public debt and freed a big portion of the national budget for investments in the social sectors, including education and health. The proportion of the national budget devoted to public debt went down from 24.7 percent in 1987 to 5 percent in 1997 (NESDB 2004). The education and health budgets went up from 18.1 percent and 4.1 percent in 1987 to 24.5 percent and 8 percent in 1998, respectively (Wibulpolprasert 2004). An economic crisis hit Thailand in 1997 when economic growth dramatically declined to –1.7 percent and –10.8 percent in 1997 and 1998, respectively (Wibulpolprasert 2004). This was reflected in a drop in the proportion of the budget devoted to education and health, to 21.8 percent and 7.1 percent, respectively, in 2002. However, the recent economic recovery once again allows more public resources to be devoted to the social sectors, and in 2007, the education and health budget shares rose to 25 percent and 8.3 percent, respectively (Wibulpolprasert 2007).

The Thai political system has been a constitutional monarchy since 1932. Social movements against the military government in the mid-1970s created several generations of young social and political leaders who later played active roles in health care system reform. These leaders are interconnected and scattered throughout the political parties and civil society organizations and hold senior posts in the civil service. The 16th constitution, promulgated in 1997 after major social movements, was claimed to be the best and most people-oriented constitution. It aims at creating a more stable, transparent, and participatory democratic system (Office of the Council State 1997). This constitution allows more direct political involvement of the people—that is, more participatory democracy. For example 50,000 Thai citizens can sign on to sponsor a bill in the parliament and will thus share some influential seats in the parliamentary special commission that considers the detail of a bill after the first reading. This happened in the case of the National Health Security Bill, which has been one of the basic legal structures for health care system reform in Thailand since 2002. Nevertheless, the populist government, amid accusations of corruption, was brought down by the military in September 2006. The new interim government declared a general election, under the 17th constitution, on December 23, 2007. A new democratic government was set up in February 2008.

Internal peace in the last two decades has resulted in a reduction in national security investment. The budgetary share for national security went down from 25.2 percent in 1984 to 13 percent in 2002 (Bureau of the Budget 2002). This also allowed increases in the resources allocated to social sectors like education and health.

Thailand has also been undergoing a demographic transition for the past four decades. The population growth rate dropped from 3.2 percent in 1970 to 0.7 percent in 2005 (Wibulpolprasert 2007). The demographic structure has changed toward a higher proportion of elderly and a lesser of children (figure 12.1). Approximately 35 percent of the total population lives in urban areas, and this trend is increasing (NSO 2006).

## Overview and Evolution of the Health Care Systems

### The Health Situation and Trend

For three decades, Thailand had faced rapid epidemiological transition with an increasing burden of chronic noncommunicable diseases, when the epidemic of

**Figure 12.1   Thailand: Population Pyramids, 2005, 2010, and 2020**

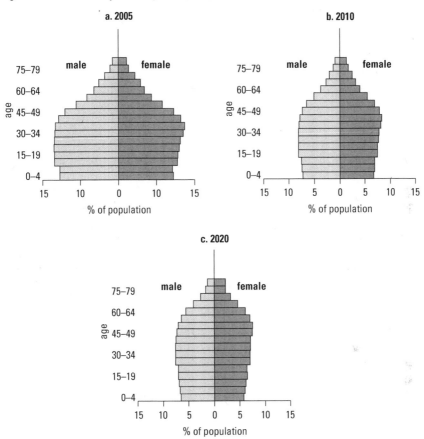

*Sources:* NESDB 2003; Population Projections Bangkok: Office of National Economic and Social Development Board.

HIV/AIDS hit in early 1990s. HIV/AIDS, traffic accidents, noncommunicable diseases, and mental illness are now among the leading causes of the disease burden (table 12.1).

The health status of the Thai people has also significantly improved. Life expectancy at birth gradually increased from 56 and 62 years in 1965 to 70 and 74 years in 2004 for men and women, respectively. The maternal mortality ratio (MMR) declined from 374 per 100,000 live births in 1962 to 15 per 100,000 live births in 2004. In addition, the infant mortality rate (IMR) declined from 84 per 1,000 live births in 1964 to 25 per 1,000 live births in 2004 (Wibulpolprasert 2007).

## Overview of the Health Care Systems

The Thai health care system is pluralistic and dominated by the public sector, particularly in the rural areas, where more than two-thirds of the people live. In 2005,

Table 12.1   Thailand: Top 10 Causes of Disease Burden, by Gender, 2004 (DALYs lost)

| | Males | | | Females | | |
|---|---|---|---|---|---|---|
| Rank | Disease category | DALYs (thousands) | % | Disease category | DALYs (thousands) | % |
| 1 | HIV/AIDS | 645 | 11.3 | Stroke | 313 | 7.4 |
| 2 | Traffic accidents | 584 | 10.2 | HIV/AIDS | 291 | 6.9 |
| 3 | Stroke | 332 | 5.8 | Diabetes | 271 | 6.4 |
| 4 | Alcohol dependence/ harmful use | 332 | 5.8 | Depression | 191 | 4.5 |
| 5 | Liver and bile duct cancer | 280 | 4.9 | Ischemic heart disease | 142 | 3.4 |
| 6 | COPD | 187 | 3.3 | Traffic accidents | 125 | 3.0 |
| 7 | Ischemic heart disease | 184 | 3.2 | Liver and bile conduct cancer | 124 | 3.0 |
| 8 | Diabetes | 175 | 3.1 | Osteoarthritis | 118 | 2.8 |
| 9 | Cirrhosis | 144 | 2.5 | COPD | 115 | 2.7 |
| 10 | Depression | 137 | 2.4 | Cataracts | 111 | 2.6 |

*Source:* Bundhamcharoen 2007.

there were 9,762 rural health centers covering all tambol (communes), 730 community hospitals (10 to 120 beds) covering 91.2 percent of rural districts, 70 general hospitals and 25 regional hospitals covering all provincial cities and big urban districts, 59 military hospitals, 47 specialized hospitals, and 11 medical school hospitals. In total, these public facilities provided 99,590 beds. For the private sector, 344 private hospitals provided 35,806 beds, accounting for more than 25 percent of the total beds in the country. In addition, there were 16,800 private clinics, mainly in the urban centers. More than 15,000 modern drug stores and more than 400,000 rural grocery stores sell drugs (Wibulpolprasert 2007). Around 20 percent of Thais visit private clinics or hospitals when they are sick, more in the urban areas. In addition, medical tourism started to mushroom after the 1997 economic crisis. In 2007, an estimated 2 million foreign patients flocked into Thailand for health services (Pachanee and Wibulpolprasert 2006).

The 2000 census found 22,435 medical doctors, 119,651 nurses, 6,966 dentists, 10,354 pharmacists, and 31,931 rural health workers. The proportion of doctors, nurses, dentists, and pharmacists in the public sectors was 71, 87, 59, and 56 percent, respectively (Thammarangsi 2004). More than 95 percent of human resources are produced by the public institutes, under a heavily subsidized public system (Chunharas, Tangcharoensathien, and Kittidilokkul 1997). At the village level, 829,403 village health volunteers have been trained by health personnel to provide primary health care services (Department of Health Service Support 2007). These volunteers are not remunerated but receive fringe benefits from the local elected government, the responsibility for which was transferred from the Ministry of Public Health since 2003. They have been recruited, trained, replaced, and retrained since the Primary Health Care era (early 1980s) and have been successfully and continuously employed in supporting the delivery of promotive and preventive health care to rural villagers. In the outbreak of SARS and avian influenza, they have played important roles in the extensive public health surveillance and outbreak control system.

## The Evolution of the Health Care System

The evolution of the health system in Thailand can be divided into four eras.

*The era of modernization of medicine (1888–1950).* The first era started in the era of King Rama III when Dr. Dan Beach Bradley, an American Christian missionary, brought the first smallpox vaccination into Thailand in 1882. In the reign of King Rama V, the first modern medical schools were built, and the first provincial dispensary was established in 1888. To expand coverage, the government started building provincial hospitals and health centers, especially in the border areas. Until 1942, there were only 15 provincial hospitals and 343 rural health centers. To support modernization and prevent epidemics, the Ministry of Public Health (MOPH) was established in 1942 (Wibulpolprasert 2004). During this era, hospital care was subsidized by the government, but patients had to buy their own drugs from drug stores outside of the hospitals for their treatment.

*The era of rapid expansion of provincial hospitals (1950–76).* The second era started before the first National Economic Development Plan (1961–1966), supported by the World Bank. There was rapid expansion of infrastructure, including 100 percent coverage of modern provincial hospitals and expansion of coverage for rural health and midwifery centers. The main problem was the shortage and maldistribution of health personnel, especially doctors. Between the mid-1960s and the mid-1970s, a severe external brain-drain of Thai medical doctors occurred, mainly to the United States. More than 1,500 new medical graduates, 25 percent of the total doctors, moved out of the country (Wibulpolprasert 1999). This exodus prompted the government to require new doctors to perform three years' compulsory public work after graduation. In addition, there was extensive training of paramedical personnel to work in rural areas without a doctor or even a graduate nurse. After 1972, private health care providers began to expand their roles in servicing the people. During this period, the public health infrastructure was able to provide health services to only 15 percent of the population while 51 percent of them still practiced self-care and sought care from private providers and traditional healers (Wibulpolprasert 2004). From the beginning of that time, public hospitals were allowed to charge user fees and keep the money for hospital renovation, employment of some staff, and drug replenishment.

**Figure 12.2   Thailand: Shift in Budget Allocations, 1982–89**

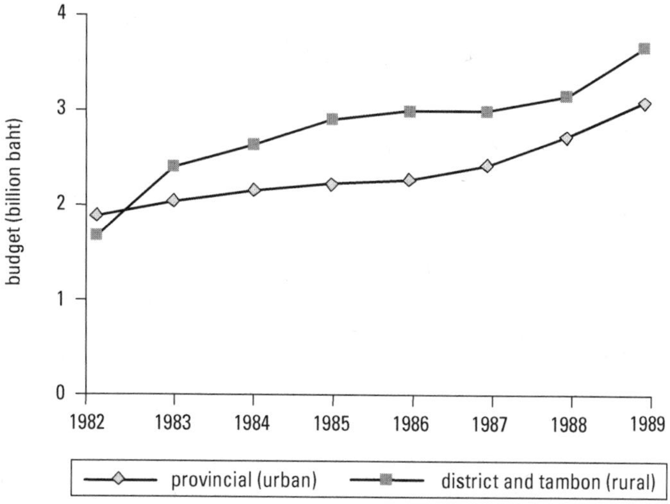

*Source:* Wibulpolprasert 2004.

*The era of Primary Health Care and Health for All and the expansion of rural health care infrastructure and health insurance systems (1977–2001).* The strong political movement against the military government in 1973 resulted in temporary democracy. This political change, together with the global Health for All movements, resulted in a policy for rapid expansion of rural district hospitals and health centers, including the recruitment of village health volunteers and establishment of many community-financing schemes in health, for example, the village drug fund, the sanitary fund, and the nutrition fund. For five years, from 1982 to 1987 while economic growth was low, the public health budget was shifted from the urban provincial hospitals toward the rural district hospitals and health centers (figure 12.2) (Wibulpolprasert 2004). This budget shift was a bold political decision that has resulted in broadened access to essential health services and use of primary health services, as can be seen from the changes in the number and proportion of outpatient visits to rural health centers, rural district hospitals, and urban provincial hospitals from a reverse triangle to the upside one (figure 12.3).

This era also allowed progressive student leaders, who moved against the military government, an opportunity to gain rural public health experience and management skills. They formed the "Rural Doctor Society" in 1978. The leaders of the Rural Doctor Society, scattered throughout the political parties, civil society organizations, business, and civil service, have since played significant leading roles in major health care system reform. During this period, the public health leadership capacity of the country was also built up.

**Figure 12.3  Health Service Delivery Indicators Relative to Income and Spending**

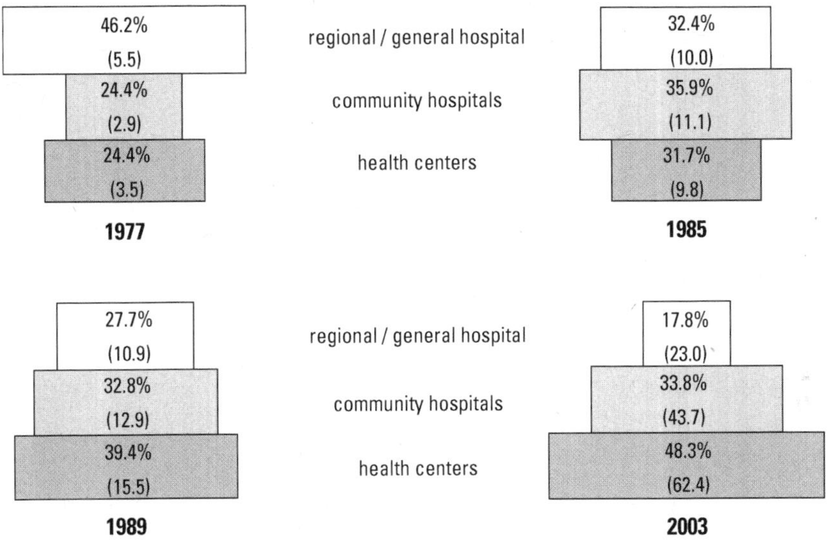

| | regional / general hospital | |
|---|---|---|
| 46.2% (5.5) | | 32.4% (10.0) |
| 24.4% (2.9) | community hospitals | 35.9% (11.1) |
| 24.4% (3.5) | health centers | 31.7% (9.8) |
| **1977** | | **1985** |

| | regional / general hospital | |
|---|---|---|
| 27.7% (10.9) | | 17.8% (23.0) |
| 32.8% (12.9) | community hospitals | 33.8% (43.7) |
| 39.4% (15.5) | health centers | 48.3% (62.4) |
| **1989** | | **2003** |

*Source:* Wibulpolprasert 2004.

*Note:* In parentheses are the numbers of outpatients visits in millions.

During this era, trained village health volunteers and village health communicators were used as the main tool in the primary health care strategy. Their roles were to assist health personnel in delivering basic integrated health care. In spite of the fact that many health personnel failed to understand the role and potential of health volunteers, they have played significant roles in improving access to rural primary health care services (Jongudomsuk 2005).

To mitigate the financial burden for the poor, the Medical Welfare Scheme (MWS), was established in 1975, funded through general taxation. MWS-eligible persons consisted of the poor with monthly incomes of less than B 1,000 (NESDB, 2005). They were offered free medical services from public health facilities. This scheme was later expanded to cover the elderly, children, veterans, disabled, monks, and priests (Pannarunothai 2002). At the same time, two other health insurance schemes without means testing on their income were developed. The first one was the publicly subsidized voluntary health insurance, the "Health Card Scheme." This scheme covered the near-poor population group on a voluntary basis, so there were some problems of selection bias (Srithamrongsawat 2002). The second one was the compulsory Social Security Scheme, started in 1992 and covering all private employees. Since the mid-1990s, all three schemes have required their beneficiaries to register and seek care at certain first-contact health facilities, either a health center or a hospital. Anyone who bypasses this system must pay out of pocket. The systems paid providers based on global budget (for MWS and the Health Card Scheme) and capitation payment system (for the Social Security Scheme).

Civil servants and public employees and their family members were covered by the noncontributory Civil Servant Medical Benefit Scheme (CSMBS), which pays providers based on a fee for service. The CSBMS was fully funded from general tax revenue through the Department of the Comptroller General, Ministry of Finance.

*The era of heath care financing reform and universal coverage of health insurance (2000–present).* Until 2000, all four public health insurance schemes, together with very small fraction of private health insurance, covered around 75 percent of the population (Wibulpolprasert 2004). Several options and movements to establish a universal coverage system were not successful until the election campaign under the 1997 constitution in late 2000. The new Thai-Rak-Thai party proposed a universal health coverage scheme, the "30 Baht treat all diseases" scheme. Their landslide win in the election prompted the government to expand health insurance coverage to all Thais in 2001. The National Health Security Act was promulgated in 2002, with very strong support and influence from civil society and has, since then, been one of the most important social tools for health care system reform in Thailand. Table 12.2 shows the evolution of the coverage of health insurance in Thailand.

## Health Care Financing and Health Insurance

Health care financing in Thailand is based on general taxation paid through the three major public health insurance schemes, out-of-pocket user fees, and some private insurance. The sources of health expenditures is shown in table 12.3.

After three decades of evolution, four main health insurance schemes now cover the entire population (table 12.4).

**Table 12.2   Thailand: Evolution of Health Insurance Coverage**

| | |
|---|---|
| 1963 | Civil servant medical benefits scheme + 9% |
| 1975 | Free medical care for the low income + 20% |
| | **Big gap in progress on coverage; more progress in infrastructures development** |
| 1990 | Voluntary public health insurance (health card) + 13% |
| 1992 | Compulsory Social Security + 11% |
| 1993 | Free medical care for children + 16% |
| 1995 | Free medical care for elderly + 6% |
| **2000** | **Total health insurance = 75%** |
| 2001 | Universal health insurance—US$0.75/visit copayment |
| 2003 | Universal access to ARVs |
| 2006 | Free care for all—no copayment |
| 2008 | Renal replacement therapy and seasonal flu vaccination for high-risk groups |

*Source:* Authors.

**Table 12.3  Thailand: Health Expenditure, by Source, 1995–2005**

| Year | Source of health care financing (% of total) | | | Total health expenditure (% of GDP) |
|------|--------|---------|-------------|--------|
| | Public | Private | External aid | |
| 1995 | 31.17 | 68.79 | 0.04 | 5.43 |
| 1996 | 33.97 | 66.01 | 0.01 | 5.58 |
| 1997 | 37.80 | 62.19 | 0.03 | 5.96 |
| 1998 | 35.98 | 63.99 | 0.03 | 5.97 |
| 1999 | 33.66 | 66.33 | 0.01 | 6.13 |
| 2000 | 32.95 | 67.03 | 0.02 | 6.09 |
| 2001 | 32.91 | 67.03 | 0.06 | 6.26 |
| 2002 | 34.09 | 65.80 | 0.11 | 6.12 |
| 2003 | 34.02 | 65.80 | 0.18 | 6.24 |
| 2004 | 32.00 | 67.60 | 0.40 | 6.05 |
| 2005 | 33.05 | 66.76 | 0.18 | 6.14 |

*Source:* Adapted from Wibulpolprasert 2007.

## The Civil Servant Medical Benefit Scheme

The CSMBS covers civil servants, public employees and their dependants. The scheme is paid totally from general tax revenue, based on a fee-for-service retrospective reimbursement system. Public facilities are the main providers under this scheme.

## The Social Security Scheme

The SSS is a tripartite system, funded by equal-share contributions by employers, employees, and the government. It covers private employees and temporary public employees. The insurees are about equally distributed between public and private facilities. This scheme pays the providers under a contract capitation system.

## Universal Coverage Scheme (UCS or the "30 Baht Scheme")

Universal health insurance coverage, since October 2001, has combined the previous Medical Welfare Scheme and the Voluntary Health Card Scheme, further expanding coverage to 18 million more people. This scheme covers 74.6 percent of the population (NHSO 2007a) with a comprehensive package of care, including both curative and preventive care. It is financed solely from general tax revenue. Public hospitals are the main providers, covering more than 95 percent of the insurees. About 60 private hospitals joined the system and register around 4 percent of the beneficiaries. After the new government assumed office in October 2006, the B 30 copayment was abolished, and the system is now totally free of charge. Since October 2003, the government has also embarked on universal access

**Table 12.4 Thailand: Characteristics of Health Insurance Schemes, 2007**

| Characteristics | UCS | CSMBS | SSS | Private health insurance |
|---|---|---|---|---|
| 1. Scheme nature | Social welfare | Fringe benefit | Compulsory contribution | Voluntary |
| 2. Target group | Every Thai citizen not covered under the CSMBS and the SSS | Government employees, pensioners, and their dependants (spouse, parents, and children) | Private and temporary public employees | Individual and private firms |
| 3. Financing | | | | |
| —Source of funds | General tax revenue | General tax revenue | Tripartite 1.5% of payroll each, up to payroll of B 15,000 (reduced to 1% since 1999) | Out of pocket or employers |
| —Payment mechanism | Mainly capitation | Fee for service | Mainly capitation | Fee for service |
| —Copayment | None, unless using the nonemergency service from nonregistered facilities | Yes, at some inpatient care and at private hospitals | Maternity and emergency services if beyond budget ceiling | Depends on policy |
| 4. Benefit package | | | | |
| —Ambulatory services | Mainly public with some private | Mainly public | Public and private | Public and private |
| —Inpatient services | Mainly public with some private | Public and private (emergency only) | Public and private | Public and private |
| —Choice of provider | Limited and must register with first-line provider in vicinity of residence or workplace | Almost unlimited and can go to any public facility | Moderate limitation, registration required with first-line providers, but with more choices. | High with free choice |
| —Conditions included | Comprehensive package | Comprehensive package | Comprehensive package with nonwork related illnesses | Depends on policy |
| —Conditions excluded | 15 conditions | No | 15 conditions | Depends on policy |
| —Maternity benefit | Yes | Yes | Yes | Depends on policy |
| —Annual physical check up | Yes | Yes | No | Depends on policy |
| —Prevention and health promotion | Yes | Yes | Yes | Usually not |
| —Population coverage | 74.6% | 8.01% | 12.9% | 2.16% |
| —Expense per capita, 2007 baht | 1,899 | 5,000 | 1,900 | n.a. |

*Sources:* Adapted from Tangcharoensathien, Srithamrongswat, and Pitayarangsarit 2002; SSO 2007; NHSO 2007a.

**Figure 12.4  Thailand: The Health Insurance Model, 2007**

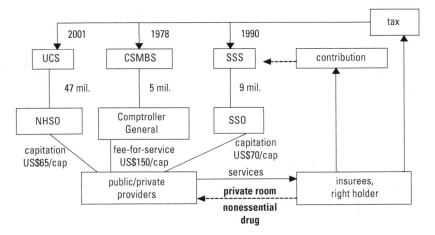

*Source:* Authors.

to antiretroviral drugs (ARVs). Through May 2007, more than 90,000 patients had been registered in the system. These two policies—universal health insurance and universal access to ARVs—have rapidly increased demand for health services in the public sector. The number of outpatient visits in all public hospitals in 2003 increased between 40 and 50 percent (Pachanee and Wibulpolprasert 2006). The decision to expand benefits to include renal replacement therapy from January 2008 will definitely put more burdens on the health care systems. Evidence from cost-benefit analysis showing that the cost of treatment and care for flu patients in high-risk groups is higher than the cost of vaccination has resulted in the decision (2008) to provide seasonal flu vaccination to high-risk groups.

## The Private Health Insurance Scheme

This is a voluntary scheme which usually comes with life insurance. However, some people buy specific health insurance. Their coverage is quite low usually less than 2 percent.

The relationship between the three public schemes, beneficiaries, and provider payment mechanisms is shown in figure 12.4. In addition, the main characteristics of all four schemes are displayed in table 12.4.

## The 2001 Universal Coverage of Health Insurance Policy

### Setting the Agenda

The movements toward universal health insurance were started in the mid-1980s by a few policy elites in the MOPH. These people were the former student leaders against the military in 1970s and the leaders of the Rural Doctor Society. In addition to working to extend health insurance coverage from only the poor to encompass private employees, the elderly, and children, these elites moved in the parliamentary health commission to draft a National Health Insurance Bill in the early 1990s. However, due to political changes, this bill was not considered. The 1996–97 political reform movements, with the promulgation of the new "People's Constitution" in 1997, resulted in strong political movements toward public interest policies. The same group of policy elites in the MOPH, with connections to the leading political party, the Thai Rak Thai (TRT) party, from their past engagement in the social movements against the military government in 1970s and in the Rural Doctor Society movements, was able to push "universal coverage of health insurance" onto the political agenda. This became one of the main populist policies in the campaign for the first general election under the new constitution in early 2001. The TRT party coined the motto "30 Baht[1] treats all diseases" to represent their universal health insurance policy. This motto became extremely popular in the election campaign. The proposed policy was one of the populist policies that won the party a landslide victory in the election.

## Policy Formulation Processes and Social Mobilization

Immediately after the TRT party's landslide victory, with about 40.6 percent of the popular vote (TRT 2005) and the formation of the new government, the plan for implementing the universal health insurance policy was reformulated, based on evidence and experience. After detailed study and discussion, the scheme was modified from the voluntary, publicly subsidized health insurance systems, proposed during the election campaign, to a social welfare, totally tax-based system, with a minimal copayment of B 30 per visit. Two months after setting up the new government, the policy was implemented in six provinces[2] that had experience testing the new systems under the MWS financial reform, supported by the World Bank. Due to political pressure and the leadership of the permanent secretary of the MOPH (who was appointed health minister after the September 2006 coup), the new scheme was rapidly expanded to cover all the other provinces within one year. Evidence from previous research as well as further synthesis of new information were used extensively in the implementation. For example, information from previous costing research and from health care utilization behavior from the Health and Welfare Survey, were used to calculate the capitation figure.[3] Strong social movements to support the National Health Security Bill have been so successful that it was the first draft bill that more than 50,000 people proposed directly to the parliament (as allowed under the new constitution). This movement has made it possible for civil society[4] to gain significant and influential seats on the parliamentary commission to consider this bill. This has resulted in significant and influential seats for civil society organizations on the National Health Security Board, the top decision-making authority for the implementation of the Universal Coverage of Health Insurance System, and has made it difficult for political maneuvering.

**Table 12.5  Thailand: UCS Inclusion and Exclusion List of Expensive Health Care Interventions, 2001**

| Inclusive list | Exclusive list |
|---|---|
| Chemotherapy for cancers | Antiretroviral treatment for HIV[a] |
| Radiation therapy for cancers | Renal replacement therapy including kidney transplants for patients with end-stage renal disease[b] |
| Open heart surgery including prosthetic cardiac valve replacement | |
| Percutaneous transluminal coronary angioplasty (PTCA) | Other organ transplants |
| Coronary artery bypass grafting (CABG) | Cosmetic surgery |
| Stent for treatment of atherosclerotic vessels | Infertility treatment |
| Prosthetic hip replacement therapy | |
| Prosthetic shoulder replacement therapy | |
| Neurosurgery, e.g., craniotomy | |
| Antifungal treatments for cryptococcal meningitis | |

*Source:* NHSO 2001.

a. Included since October 2003.

b. Included since January 2008.

## The Content of the Policy and the Essential Reform Component

*The coverage and the benefit scheme.* The Universal Health Care Coverage Scheme aims at providing universal access to essential health care and reducing catastrophic illnesses from out-of-pocket payments by establishing a tax-based financing system and paying providers on a capitation basis.[5] All Thai citizens are entitled to access to quality[6] health care and a single standard benefit package. The benefit package includes a set of health interventions stipulated in a contract between purchaser and provider at every level of health services. It has been classified into three components: the curative package, the high-cost care package, and the promotive and preventive package. The curative package covers ambulatory and hospitalization services with some exclusions, such as cosmetic surgery, infertility treatments, organ transplants, and the provision of private room and board. Initially ARV treatment for HIV/AIDs and renal replacement therapy were excluded (NHSO 2001) but were included in October 2003 and January 2008, respectively, because of strong social movements. In January 2008, based on a cost-benefit analysis, the NHS Board decided to provide the seasonal flu vaccination to high-risk groups. There was no increase to the budget because it was determined that it costs less to vaccinate for the flu than to treat it. For high-cost care, the UCS has adopted a similar package to the one provided by the SSS in order to standardize the packages across the scheme to minimize inequities in health care services. Thus, substantial high-cost interventions are offered (table 12.5). The UCS preventive package, focused on health promotion and disease prevention, covers immunizations, annual physical checkups, premarital counseling, voluntary HIV counseling and testing, antenatal care and family planning services, as well as other preventive and promotive care. All contracted public and private providers are bound to provide registered beneficiaries with these services (NHSO 2001). The expenses are budgeted under an annual fixed capitation system that includes each facility's labor costs. The rate of capitation payment increased gradually at first and more rapidly since fiscal year 2006 (started October 2005). The additional benefits of ARV and renal replacement therapy were separately budgeted and managed, based on central procurement and payment systems.

*The financial reform toward more equity and efficiency.* The Health Systems Research Institute has reviewed the strengths and weaknesses of the capitation payment under the SSS and diagnosis-related group (DRG) payment of the MWS and suggested two main payment mechanisms for two main split budgets: outpatient and inpatient services (HSRI 2001). Capitation payment has been used for ambulatory care whereas case payment, based on global budget-capped DRGs, was used for inpatient care. Inclusive and exclusive capitations have been proposed as provider payment methods for the UCS. The capitation budgeting systems was expected to increase equity because it depends on the population size in each locality. It was also expected to increase efficiency. Because it includes all costs, and the hospitals must act like an insurer of registered beneficiaries, for financial survival, the hospitals have to improve their efficiency. This is like the health maintenance organization (HMO) systems in the United States.

Inclusive capitation covers the cost of health promotion and preventive and curative care, including primary, secondary, and tertiary care. Exclusive capitation covers the cost of health promotion and preventive and primary health care. It requires a reinsurance system through collection of funds, deducted from the capitation rate, to be managed by provinces to pay for higher-expense inpatient care. Payments are calculated on weighted allocations based on DRGs (Pitayarangsarit et al. 2004).

The payment mechanisms have been gradually modified to include other expenses and using a mixed system of capitation, DRG-based capped global budget, and fixed rate fees for some services (table 12.6).

Regarding resource allocations from the central government to the provinces, budgets were shifted from a historical supply-based to demand-based allocation, according to the number of people registered. In principle, UCS beneficiaries will be free to choose their primary providers. However, because of the underdeveloped registration information system and the limited number of primary providers in rural areas, the beneficiaries were assigned mainly to public primary providers close to their communities or their workplaces.

Initially, the MOPH managed the budget and allowed provinces to choose either inclusive or exclusive capitation (split outpatient and inpatient budgets) to pay providers within their provinces. However, due to the disincentive to pay providers for high-cost care and delays in case referrals resulting from the inclusive

**Table 12.6   Thailand: The 13 Elements for UCS Budget Allocation, 2002–08 (baht)**

| Category | 2002 | 2003 | 2004 | 2005 | 2006 | 2007 | 2008 |
|---|---|---|---|---|---|---|---|
| 1. Outpatient care (OP)[a] | 574.00 | 574.00 | 488.20 | 533.01 | 585.11 | 645.52 | 645.52 |
| 2. Inpatient care (IP)[b] | 303.00 | 303.00 | 418.30 | 435.01 | 460.35 | 513.96 | 868.08 |
| 3. Prevention and promotion services (P&P)[a] | 175.00 | 175.00 | 206.00 | 210.00 | 224.89 | 248.04 | 253.01 |
| 4. Accident and emergency care (A&E)[c] | 25.00 | 25.00 | 19.70 | 24.73 | 52.07 | 51.20 | 44.61 |
| 5. High cost care | 32.00 | 32.00 | 66.30 | 99.48 | 190.00 | 209.56 | 104.65 |
| 6. Ambulance system (EMS) | — | 10.00 | 10.00 | 10.00 | 6.00 | 10.00 | 10.00 |
| 7. Disability | — | — | — | 4.00 | 4.00 | 4.00 | 4.00 |
| 8. Capital replacement | 93.40 | 83.40 | 85.00 | 76.80 | 129.25 | 142.55 | 143.73 |
| 9. Remote area | — | — | 10.00 | 7.07 | 7.00 | 30.00 | 30.00 |
| 10. Patient compensation | — | — | 5.00 | 0.20 | 0.53 | 0.53 | Use remaining budget |
| 11. Provider compensation | — | — | — | — | — | 0.40 | 0.40 |
| 12. Service quality | — | — | — | — | — | 20.00 | — |
| 13. Compensation for noncopayment | — | — | — | — | — | 24.11 | — |
| Total | 1,202.40 | 1,202.40 | 1,308.50 | 1,396.30 | 1,659.20 | 1,899.69 | 2,100.00 |

*Source:* NHSO 2007b.

a. Capitation payment.

b. DRG based capped global budget.

c. Reserved at the NHSO to pay hospitals providing high-cost care to UCS beneficiaries and emergency care in case of services used outside their registered hospital.

capitation employed, the MOPH decided to use a single system of exclusive capitation for all of the provinces since fiscal year 2003 (October 2002) (Pitayarangsarit et al. 2004). Since the shifting of budget management responsibility to the National Health Security Office in 2005, the exclusive payment systems continue.

*The primary care–based systems.* Primary care provider units (PCUs) have been designated as gatekeepers to provide care for UCS beneficiaries. As gatekeepers, PCUs are expected to provide people in their catchment areas with continuous and comprehensive care with a holistic approach. According to the services provided, health facilities under the UCS can be classified into three groups (NHSO 2001):

- *Contracting unit for primary care.* The CUPs are primary health facilities offering curative, promotive, preventive, and rehabilitative services such as ambulatory care, home care, and community care. They can be facilities ranging from community hospitals to tertiary care public or private hospitals. Each CUP has its own catchment area and population.

---

**B O X   12.1**   *Thailand: Minimum CUP Requirements*

**Inputs and Structure**

1. One PCU facility for 10,000—personnel work in CUP more than 75% of population their working time
2. Facility is located close to the registered–available laboratory system for the population (transportation time < 30 minutes) investigation
3. Adequate health personnel–available vehicle for the referral
   —Physician, 1 : 10,000 to 20,000 *Provision of Services*

—Dentist, 1 : 20,000 to 40,000—service available at least 56 hours/week
—Pharmacist, 1: 20,000 to 30,000—able to provide comprehensive primary care
—Registered nurse, 1 : 5,000—able to provide in-house service and
—Health personnel, 1: 1,250—community based services

*Source:* NHSO 2001.

---

- *Contracting unit for secondary care.* The CUSs are health facilities that offer secondary care, mainly in patient health services. They can be facilities ranging from community hospitals to tertiary care public or private hospitals.
- *Contracting unit for tertiary care.* The CUTs provide expensive care and specialized care with high technologies. They can be regional hospitals, university hospitals, or specialized health institutes.

In principle, all CUPs must have at least one PCU for every 10,000 people registered. The prerequisites for a primary care provider to be a main contractor are outlined in box 12.1.

## The Difficulties and Negative Implications

The UCS has increased the demand for health services, as it has reduced the financial barrier to access to health care services.

*Increase in workload and dissatisfaction of health personnel.* This increase in demand for services had implications for health care personnel's workload. More than 70 percent of health personnel surveyed claimed that their workload increased as a result of the UCS (NHSO and ABAC Poll 2007). A comparison of service utilization between 2002 and 2007 revealed that the utilization rate of public health care services increased more than 20 percent for outpatient care and nearly 20 percent for hospital admissions (table 12.7) (NHSO 2007c).

As a result, health care providers' satisfaction with the UCS is not high, just above 50 percent (figure 12.5.). However, there have been significant increases in satisfaction since a significant increase in the amount of the capitation rate in 2005. Furthermore, in comparison with 2001, the number of doctors who resigned from rural public hospitals in 2003 tripled (figure 12.6). Among their reasons for leaving were overwork and poor payment (Srithamrongsawat and Torwatanakitkul 2004). However, this internal brain-drain was also due to the

**Table 12.7　Thailand: Utilization by UCS Beneficiaries, 2002–07**

|  | 2002 | 2003 | 2004 | 2005 | 2006 | 2007 |
|---|---|---|---|---|---|---|
| **Outpatient** | | | | | | |
| Number of visits (millions) | 102.95 | 115.01 | 119.64 | 120.88 | 116.37 | 116.45 |
| Utilization rate (visits/person/year) | 2.27 | 2.52 | 2.54 | 2.56 | 2.45 | 2.75 |
| **Inpatient** | | | | | | |
| Number of utilization (millions of days) | 14.93 | 14.56 | 16.83 | 17.89 | 17.65 | 16.38 |
| Utilization rate (episodes/person/year) | 0.085 | 0.087 | 0.092 | 0.096 | 0.095 | 0.100 |

*Source:* NHSO 2007c.

**Figure 12.5　Thailand: Health Care Providers' Satisfaction with the UCS, 2003–07**

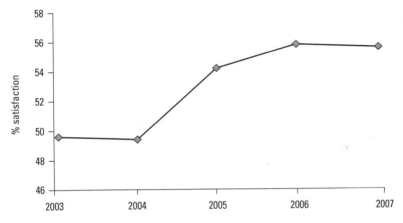

*Source:* NHSO and ABAC Poll, 2003–07.

*Note:* The providers surveyed were doctors, dentists, pharmacists, nurses, and health personnel.

improvement of the economy and the increase in private sector demand from both local Thais and foreign patients.

*Adverse effects of resource allocation reform.* A capitation-based budget, which included staff salary and nonsalary budget to provinces, created much concern and some conflicts. The new budget allocation, shifting from a historical supply-based to a need- or demand-based allocation, aimed to achieve more equitable allocation of budgets. Due to a severe maldistribution of health personnel, however, it has created significant concerns and conflicts. Under a single capitation rate in 2002, affluent but small provinces—especially those not too far from the capital and with a high concentration of health personnel—received inadequate budgets due to the small registered population size. Larger provinces in the Northeast with a low

**Figure 12.6   Thailand: Number of Doctors Who Resigned from MOPH Rural Facilities, 1995–2006**

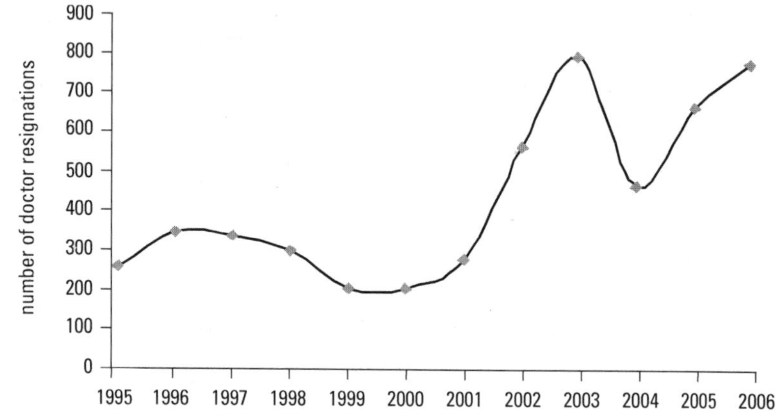

*Source:* Wibulpolprasert 2007.

concentration of health personnel received huge budgets due to a larger registered population (Srithamraongsawat and Torwatanakitkul 2004). This actually helped in the redistribution of personnel. Provinces that used to have less concentration of staff but now receive huge budgets started to recruit more staff. Smaller, more urban provinces that used to receive more budget and now receive less, refused to hire more new staff. If allowed to continue, this situation was expected to improve the distribution of health personnel. Nevertheless, the new allocation system bankrupted some urban provincial hospitals to the point that the MOPH had to set aside some contingency funds to support them on the condition that they extensively reform their management systems (Bureau of Policy and Strategy 2007). This situation has created strong protest and social pressures from the urban hospitals as well as the tertiary care medical schools. The protest was so successful that a new system of resource allocation was started in 2003, based on the same capitation-based budgeting system, using a salary-excluded capitation payment system.

The situation was then reversed and resulted in a new inequity gap in budget allocation. The new payment systems favored the affluent provinces and urban provincial hospitals. The less-affluent provinces and the rural district hospitals, particularly small and remote ones, experienced financial constraints. Strong protests and reactions came from these hospitals, particularly from the Rural Doctor Society. Finally, after lengthy negotiations, another new system of resource allocation was established in 2005, based on both capitation and facility workload. The National Health Security Board (NHSB) also established a specific budget line to support hospitals in remote and hardship areas, which usually have small populations.

Historically, for more than four decades, rural community hospital leaders and urban provincial hospital groups have been in conflict. This battle about the UCS resource allocation system is just one example of such conflict.

Figure 12.7  Thailand: Proposed and Approved Capitation, 2002–08

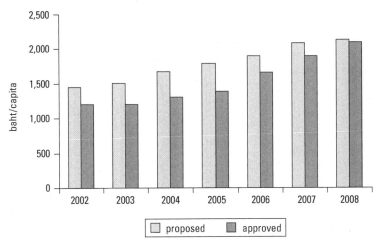

*Source:* NHSO 2007a.

*Financial implications.* In the first year of implementation, the UCS was criticized by health care providers for being underfinanced, particularly for inpatient care. The capitation budget of B 1,202 (US$31.63) per registered person per year was inadequate (Leesmidt et al. 2005). (The real budget allocated was B 1,052 (US$27.68), as B 150.40 (US$3.96) was reserved at the NHSO for high-cost care and emergency care.)[7] The rate was based on the 1996 service utilization rate, which did not take into account the aging population and the increase in inpatient admissions between 1996 and 2001. When using the 2001 service utilization rate and unit cost of services provided in the same years, the per capita budgets for fiscal year 2002 was underestimated by B 212 (US$5.58). A gap between a proposed capitation rate and the approved budgets is depicted in figure 12.7.

Kittikanya (2004) also reported that more than 30 percent of public hospitals under the UCS were in financial trouble, with an accumulated debt of B 1.365 billion (US$35.9 million). In particular, rural community hospitals in the north and northeast were severely affected. The percentage of rural community hospitals in the northeast with financial problems significantly increased from 3 percent in 2002 to 27 percent in 2003. This was also due to the change in the resource allocation system, mentioned earlier. The costs of the rapid expansion of primary care units according to budget gained in the first year could partly explain the problem of these district hospitals when they received lower budgets in the following year. The number of hospitals with financial constraints and receiving extra financial support from the Contingency Fund is shown in figure 12.8.

The inadequate finance and providers' reactions prompted the government to finally increased the capitation budget significantly from fiscal years 2006 to 2008 (table 12.6). The financial situation of most hospitals has thus greatly improved.

**Figure 12.8   Thailand: Number of Financially Constrained Hospitals Receiving Contingency Fund Support, 2002–04**

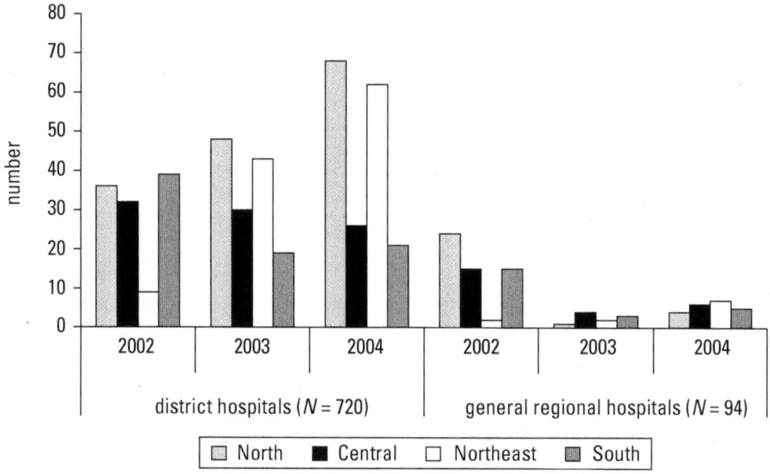

*Source:* Health Financing Office, MOPH 2002–04.

## The Evidence of Success

Evidence that the UCS has succeeded is abundant. Nearly everyone is covered, the number of people facing catastrophic health expenses has decreased, and relief from health care expenses has brought an estimated million people out of poverty. The majority of people are satisfied with the quality of the care provided, and the depth of the benefit package has been improved. Health professionals and managers are being trained, and people have a strong political voice in health policy.

*Near-disappearance of uninsured.* The UCS has achieved very nearly universal coverage. The number of uninsured has dramatically decreased from 20 percent of the total population in 1998 to 2 percent in 2007 (table 12.8) (NHSO 2007a). In principle, coverage can be assumed to be universal. Anyone still uninsured can register at any time. An individual who gets sick or needs health services can appear at a health facility near home, register, and receive free care at the same time. The capitation payment system gives health care providers an incentive to reach out to enroll people in their catchment areas. The more people registered, the higher will be their income. The higher registration rate also increase the "risk-sharing" effect of the insurance system.

*Significant reduction of the catastrophic illnesses and out-of-pocket health expense as well as poverty reduction.* Vasavid et al. (2004) reported that household health expenditures decreased after the UC implementation. In 2002, household savings

**Table 12.8  Thailand: Progress in Health Insurance Coverage (percent coverage)**

| Health insurance scheme | 1991 | 1996 | 1998 | 2001 | 2003 | 2006 | 2007 |
|---|---|---|---|---|---|---|---|
| Universal coverage | — | — | — | — | 74.7 | 74.3 | 74.6 |
| Social welfare | 12.7 | 12.6 | 45.1 | 32.4 | — | — | — |
| Civil servants (CSMBS) | 15.3 | 10.2 | 10.8 | 8.5 | 8.9 | 8.0 | 8.01 |
| Social security | — | 5.6 | 8.5 | 7.2 | 9.6 | 11.4 | 12.9 |
| Voluntary health card | 1.4 | 15.3 | 13.9 | 20.8 | — | — | — |
| Private health insurance | 4.0 | 1.8 | 2.0 | 2.1 | 1.7 | 2.3 | 2.16 |
| Total insured | 33.4 | 45.5 | 80.3 | 71.0 | 94.9 | 96.0 | 97.7 |
| Uninsured | 66.6 | 54.5 | 19.7 | 29.0 | 5.1 | 4.0 | 2.3 |

*Sources:* NSO 2006; NHSO 2007a.

*Note:* — = not available.

on health care services among the previously uninsured and currently insured by the UCS was approximately B 9,650 million (US$253.95 million). A year later, savings gradually increased to B 12,726 million (US$334.89 million). The evidence from three low-income provinces suggested that the UCS would ease the burden on household expenditures only if UC beneficiaries seek care from facilities operated under the UCS (Suraratdecha, Saithanu, and Tangcharoensathien 2005). If they seek care from facilities at which they are not registered, they will have to pay out of pocket. The proportion of people facing catastrophic[8] health expenditures was also been reduced significantly from 5.4 percent in 2000 to 2.0 percent in 2006 (table 12.9) (Tangcharoensathien 2007). The Thailand Development Research Institute reported that the UCS has also brought at least one million Thais out of poverty (Na Ranong, Na Ranong, and Vongmontha 2005).

*Consumer satisfaction.* One public concern about the UCS was quality of services. Successive survey of UCS beneficiaries about their perceptions of the UCS

**Table 12.9  Thailand: Catastrophic Health Care Expenditure by Households, 2000–06**

| Year | All households (%) | | |
|---|---|---|---|
| | Quintile 1 | Quintile 5 | All quintiles |
| 2000 | 4.0 | 5.6 | 5.4 |
| 2002 | 1.7 | 5 | 3.3 |
| 2004 | 1.6 | 4.3 | 2.8 |
| 2006 | 0.9 | 3.3 | 2 |

*Source:* Tangcharoensathien 2007.

Table 12.10   Thailand: Consumer Satisfaction

| Service | Satisfactory (%) | | | | |
| --- | --- | --- | --- | --- | --- |
| | 2003 | 2004 | 2005 | 2006 | 2007 |
| Physician | 92.9 | 92.9 | 93.3 | 92.2 | 90.9 |
| Nurse | 89.4 | 91.2 | 92.0 | 90.5 | 87.6 |
| Other personnel | 89.5 | 91.9 | 92.8 | 91.2 | 88.2 |
| Medicines | 83.3 | 86.6 | 91.1 | 86.8 | 85.9 |
| Medical equipment | 85.8 | 90.4 | 92.9 | 90.2 | 88.5 |

*Sources:* NHSO and ABAC Polls, 2003–07.

were conducted in 34 provinces in 2003 to 2007. More than 85 percent of the respondents expressed satisfaction with service quality (table 12.10) (NHSO and ABAC Polls, 2003–07).

*The expansion of the benefit package.*   Initially, some expensive interventions were not offered (table 12.6). In October 2003, Antiretrovirals for HIV/AIDS treatment were included. In addition, renal replacement therapy, including kidney transplant, continuous peritoneal dialysis, and hemodialysis, was approved by the National Health Security Board and subsequently by the cabinet, in October 2007, to be implemented from January 2008 onward. In January 2008, the NHSB also approved a program to provide flu vaccines to high-risk groups, including those with chronic diseases and the elderly. Furthermore, in 2005 the NHSB also approved coinvesting with the local government at the commune (tambol) level to establish a community health fund. This fund was set up at B 75 (US$2 per capita). Depending on the size of the local government, from 10 percent to 50 percent or from B 7.50 to B 37.50 comes from the local government, the NHSO supports the rest. Around 900 such funds were set up in 2006, these coinvestments will be expanded to cover all the communes in the next few years. Community health funds have both enlisted local governments as active players and mobilized additional resources for the collective health promotion and disease prevention activities in the community.

*The strengthening of the capacity for knowledge generation and management.*   The huge demand for evidence to manage and implement the UCS prompted the Health Systems Research Institute (HSRI) to establish a special program to generate and provide technical support. The Thailand Development Research Institute (TDRI) also played significant technical supportive roles, especially in the evaluation of the UCS and the financial management system. The International Health Policy Program (IHPP), a joint program that originated in the collaboration between the MOPH and the HSRI since 2001, also played significant technical support roles. For example, they collaborated in the calculation of the capitation budget, the estimation of the future financial burden, the formulation of the policy on renal replacement therapy, and seasonal flu vaccinations for high-risk groups, as well as on the study of policy processes in the implementation of the UCS. Technical support to the UCS has provided many health policy graduates with ample material for Master's theses and PhD dissertations. The development of capacity in health policy and health systems research, both within and outside the MOPH, have contributed greatly to the success of the UCS.

*The strong public involvement and support.* The UCS was formulated through civil society involvement and political support. A network of civic groups, mobilized and supported by the MOPH policy elites, waged a campaign for the UC policy since its early phase. These groups began drafting the NHSB and, with more than 50,000 signatories and the new article under the people-oriented 1997 constitution, submitted the bill, in March 2001, to the parliament for its consideration (Chuengsathiansup 2004). This movement allowed them to gain some influential seats in the special parliamentary commission to consider the details of the bill, after its first reading. It also resulted in allocation of some influential seats on the NHSB to civil society organizations. They have become strong advocates for reform of the health care systems using the financial power of the UCS.

## Lessons Learned

Thailand is one of the few developing countries to have struggled to achieve universal coverage of health care policy during an economic recession. Attempts to achieve universal coverage have been ongoing for two decades, but progress was sped up in the past five years. For a lower-middle-income country like Thailand, its 2001 policy of Universal Coverage of Health Insurance was a bold political decision. At the outset, a World Bank analyst suggested to the program director that, due to inadequate funding, the program would likely fail. After five years of implementation, however, the UCS has a record of success and sustainability and has evolved into a system with strong social involvement and ownership, and political commitment. It has affected not only financial reform, but also reform in other components of the health care system. It is a real-life example of evidence-informed decision making. At least three main lessons have been learned from the past two decades of movement toward universal access.

## The Right Strategies: The Strategies of the "Triangle That Moves the Mountain"

The key strategy of health sector reform in Thailand was the "Triangle That Moves the Mountain" (Wasi 2000) (figure 12.9). The Mountain is the symbol of a big and difficult social problem that is usually unmovable due to its multifactoral and complex nature encompassing political, socioeconomic, cultural, environmental, and other aspects.

**Figure 12.9 Thailand: The "Triangle That Moves the Mountain" Strategy**

1. creation of relevant knowledge

2. social movement          3. political involvement

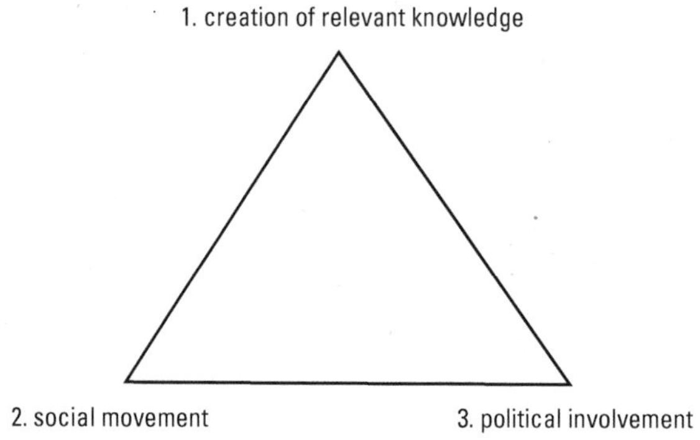

*Source:* Wasi 2000.

The Triangle, depicted in figure 12.9, is the interaction between (1) genera-tion and management of relevant knowledge, (2) strong social movements, and (3) political involvement. Knowledge has been created through health systems research and effectively communicated through some policy elites in the ministry that have close connections with both strong civil society organizations and influ-ential politicians. The digested and relevant knowledge helped policy makers and the civil society network find innovative ways to restructure the health system. The "Mountain" cannot be moved without political involvement because politicians influence resource allocation and utilization and have a significant role in promul-gating laws. Knowledgeable civil society organizations can mobilize public support to influence political decisions. In the process of health system reform in Thailand, the triangle has been applied to restructuring and reforming the health care sys-tem, a hierarchical and sophisticated system, like a mountain.

Another good example is the National Health System Reform Committee (NHSRC), formed in 2000 and chaired by the prime minister. The NHSRC appointed four subcommittees comprised of researchers, civil society leaders, pol-icy makers, and mass media representatives to design a new health system and to draft the National Health Bill (Poolcharoen 2004). The bill was promulgated into the National Health Act in December 2006 with the establishment of a tripartite National Health Commission of 39 members, chaired by the prime minister. One-third of the members each come from the political side (national and local), the professional and academic communities, and civil society organizations. An annual National Health Assembly will be convened to consider significant health policy and health-related public policy issues. These issues will be discussed and formulated by the local health assemblies and issue-specific health assemblies. The outcome will be considered and implemented by relevant authorities. This is a new social system of participatory democracy built and operated under the "Triangle That Moves the Mountain" strategy.

The linkages among the three main strategies forming the triangle are the key to the success of many social reforms in Thailand. These include the movement toward the promulgation of the 1997 people-oriented constitution, strong tobacco and alcohol control, and health systems reform.

## The Tipping Point

In addition to the "Triangle That Moves the Mountain" strategy, some factors helped tip the situation from near-universal toward fully universal coverage. These include the "stickiness" of the issue. The motto "30 Baht treats all diseases" has been so popular that it is embedded in the mind of every Thai. This has resulted in very strong social support for UCS sustainability. Some policy elites and the civic actors who play the role of the "Mavens," the "Connectors," and the "Salesmen" (Gladwell 2000) also helped create strong social movements and political commitment. The health policy researchers, within and outside the MOPH, are like "Mavens" who produced the evidence for the formulation of the universal coverage policy, while policy elites in the ministry played a crucial role connecting the researchers with politicians and civil society organizations. The policy elites also acted as "Salesmen" who persuaded politicians to consider the idea of a universal coverage policy until it was adopted and it became a popular policy in the campaign of the general election in 2001. Thus, the existence and the roles of these powerful people contributed greatly to building up political commitment and social movements. The conducive political, social, and economic environments, especially after the 1997 economic crisis and the strong social demand for social reform, also allowed the acceptance of the universal coverage idea and mobilization of funds to support its implementation.

## The Dos and Don'ts

### (1) The dos

In addition to the triangle strategy, the dos include gradual but determined and progressive reform, flexible implementation, decentralization, transparency and accountability, and appropriate involvement of private providers, civil society organizations, and local government. One of the most important things that needs to move in parallel to the UCS is adequate investment in health care infrastructure for service delivery and management. Thailand started serious investment in this health care infrastructure in the public sector five decades ago and in the private sector two decades ago. Finally, it has to be realized that health personnel are the people who must deliver quality health services and who therefore need to be involved, supported, and nurtured, so as to build enough technical capacity, morale, and spirit to deliver "humane" health services to all.

### (2) The don'ts

The sound policy directions of the Universal Coverage Scheme were undermined by the circumstances of its hasty introduction. Undoubtedly, the policy faced a variety of obstacles. Inadequate health personnel to respond to increasing demand from the UCS, as well as from the improving economy, is one good example. The direction of the scheme was misinterpreted due to inadequate policy communication. Financial sustainability is one of the serious concerns among the policy elites. Funded by tax revenue, there is some instability in the budget. Most important is the ineffective financial and managerial accounting systems and management capacity of the public hospital managers. Even in 2007, few public hospitals are able to computerize their financial and managerial accounting systems and produce an accrual basis of account. Well-trained financial managers are sorely needed.

A copayment of B 30 did not reflect the marginal cost of interventions, but it helped encourage people to utilize health care services at an affordable cost. It was abolished in 2006 for political reasons. Adversely, demand for health services was increased, adding to hospital workloads, which influenced the negative attitude among health care providers, in spite of better financial incentives. Moreover, the problems of being underfinanced and a less than ideally equitable distribution of medical services resulted from inappropriate decisions about resource allocation. Greatly needed is a rethinking of the cofinancing scheme—for example, the proposal for partial or nonsubsidization of medical care costs for beneficiaries who decide to stay in a private room.

The Thai UCS experience informs us that health care system reform based on the universal coverage concept should avoid

- Too rapid expansion of the depth of the coverage without adequate consideration to the financial and health services burden
- Too rapid, aggressive, and inflexible reform
- Too aggressive social marketing, which can create unrealistic expectations and demand among the people
- Underestimating the effect of the growth of the private sector particularly those that cater the urban rich and the foreign patients
- Using mainly financial incentives to solve the problem of human resources for health and neglecting nonfinancial incentives like motivation, social recognition, and fairness in personnel management.

## Endnotes

1. US$0.79 at the exchange rate of B 38 = US$1.
2. Pathumthanee, Samutprakan, Nakornsawan, Payao, Yasothorn, and Yala.
3. B 1,659 (US$48.79) per head in 2006; US$1 = B 34.
4. Civil society refers to active individuals and groups from voluntary associations and informal networks such as the Rural Doctor Society.
5. Demand-based allocation.
6. Quality assurance of health care services has been assessed by the Hospital Accreditation (HA) procedure.
7. Exchange rate of B 38 = US$1.

8. Out-of-pocket payment on health exceeding 10 percent of total consumption, including expenditure on both food and nonfood items.

## References

Bundhamcharoen, K. 2007. "Burden of Disease and Injuries in Thailand 2004." http://ihpp. thaigov.net/bod/index.html.

Bureau of the Budget. 2002. *Thailand's Budget in Brief: Fiscal Year 2002.* Bangkok: Bureau of the Budget, Office of the Prime Minister.

Bureau of Policy and Strategy, Ministry of Public Health. 2007. *Health Policy in Thailand.* Nonthaburi, Thailand: Bureau of Policy and Strategy, Ministry of Public Health.

Chuengsathiansup, K. 2004. *Deliberative Action: Civil Society and Health System Reform in Thailand.* Nonthaburi, Thailand: Health Systems Research Institute.

Chunharas, S., Tangcharoensathien, V., and Kittidilokkul, S. 1997. "The Role of Public and Private Sector in Manpower Production : A Debate." *Human Resources for Health Development Journal* 1(2) :77–98

Department of Health Service Support, Ministry of Public Health. 2006. Village Health Volunteer Database [in Thai]. http://phc.moph.go.th/phc/.

Gladwell, M. 2000. *The Tipping Point: How Little Things Can Make a Big Difference.* New York: Little Brown.

Health Financing Office, Ministry of Public Health 2004. "Number of Hospitals Receiving Contingency Fund Support during 2002–04" [in Thai]. Unpublished report.

HSRI (Health Systems Research Institute). 2001. "Proposal to Achieve Universal Coverage of Health Care" [in Thai]. Nonthaburi, Thailand: Health Systems Research Institute.

Jongudomsuk, P. 2005. "Health Care System in Thailand: Reforms toward Health Promotion." Paper presented at Sixth Global Conference on Health Promotion, Bangkok, August 12–15.

Kittikanya, C. 2004. "Bangkok Post Economic Review 2004: Health." http://www.bangkok post.net/ecoreviewye2004/health.html.

Leesmidt, V., S. Pitayarangsarit, N. Jeegungwal, N. Piravej, N., and M. Burns. 2005. "Assessment of the Purchasing Functions in the Thai Universal Coverage Scheme for Health Care." http://164.115.5.20/ihpp/publi-report.html.

Na Ranong ,V., A. Na Ranong, and S. Vongmontha. 2005. "Impacts of the Universal Health Coverage and the 30 Baht Health Care Scheme on Household Expenditures and Poverty Reduction in Thailand" [in Thai]. Health Systems Research Institute.

NESDB (National Economic and Social Development Board). 2005. *Thailand's Official Poverty Lines.* http://www.nscb.gov.ph/poverty/conference/papers /7_Thai%official%20 poverty.pdf.

———. 2004. *Summary of Economic Growth Rate.* http://www.nesdb.go.th/econSocial/ macro/dev5.htm.

NHSO (National Health Security Office). 2007a. "The Success of the UCS Implementation." [in Thai]. Paper presented at the National Health Security Board meeting, National Health Security Office, Nonthaburi, Thailand, August 29, 2007.

———. 2007b. *The National Health Security Fiscal Year 2007 User Manual* [in Thai]. Nonthaburi, Thailand: National Health Security Office.

————. 2007c. "Utilization of UCS Beneficiaries during 2002–7" [in Thai]. Unpublished.

————. 2001. *The Universal Health Care Coverage Scheme.* http://www.nhso.go.th/30baht_English/index.htm.

NHSO (National Health Security Office) and ABAC Poll Research Center. 2007. *The Perspectives of UC Members and Health Care Providers to UC Program* [in Thai]. Nonthaburi, Thailand: National Health Security Office.

————. 2006. *The Perspectives of UC Members and Health Care Providers to UC Program* [in Thai]. Nonthaburi, Thailand: National Health Security Office.

————. 2005. *The Perspectives of UC Members and Health Care Providers to UC Program* [in Thai]. Nonthaburi, Thailand: National Health Security Office.

————. 2004. *The Perspectives of UC Members and Health Care Providers to UC Program* [in Thai]. Nonthaburi, Thailand: National Health Security Office.

————. 2003. *The Perspectives of UC Members and Health Care Providers to UC Program* [in Thai]. Nonthaburi, Thailand: National Health Security Office.

NSO (National Statistical Office). 2006. *Key Statistics of Thailand 2006.* Database and Statistics Division, National Statistical Office.

Office of the Council of State. 1997. *Constitution of the Kingdom of Thailand.* http://www.krisdika.go.th.

Pachanee, C., and S. Wibulpolprasert. 2006. "Incoherent Policies on Universal Coverage of Health Insurance and Promotion of International Trade in Health Services in Thailand." *Health Policy and Planning* 21(4): 301–18.

Pannarunothai, S. 2002. "Medical Welfare Scheme: Financing and Targeting the Poor." In *Health Insurance Systems in Thailand,* ed. P. Pramualratana and S. Wibulpolprasert, 62–78. Nonthaburi, Thailand.

Pitayaransarit, S., P. Jongudomsak, T. Sakulpanich, S. Singhapan, and P. Homhual. 2004. "Policy Formulation Process." In *From Policy to Implementation: Historical Events during 2001–2004 of Universal Coverage in Thailand,* ed. V. Tangcharoensathien and P. Jongudomsak, 15-32. Nonthaburi , Thailand: National Health Security Office.

Phoolcharoen, W. 2004. *Quantum Leap: The Reform of Thailand's Health System.* Nonthaburi, Thailand: Health System Research Institute.

SSO (Social Security Office) 2007. Statistics of Social Security Scheme Beneficiaries [in Thai]. http://www.sso.go.th.

Srithamrongsawat, S. 2002."The Health Card Scheme: A Subsidized Voluntary Health Insurance Scheme." In *Health Insurance Systems in Thailand,* ed. P. Pramualratana and S. Wibulpolprasert, 62–78. Nonthaburi, Thailand.

Srithamrongsawat, S., and S. Torwatanakitkul. 2004. "Implications of the Universal Coverage Scheme on Health Service Delivery System in Thailand." In *From Policy to Implementation: Historical Events during 2001–2004 of Universal Coverage in Thailand,* ed. V. Tangcharoensathien and P. Jongudomsak, 51–60. Nonthaburi, Thailand: National Health Security Office.

Suraratdecha, C., S. Saithanu, and V. Tangcharoensathien. 2005. "Is Uuniversal Coverage a Solution for Disparities in Health Care? Findings from Three Low-Income Provinces in Thailand." *Health Policy* 73: 272–84.

Tangcharoensathien, V. 2007. "What Do We Expect on Health Care Financing?" Presentation at an International Labour Organization–World Bank–Ministry of Public Health Workshop on Model Development for Sustainable Health Care Financing, Bangkok, June 11.

Tangcharoensathien, V., S. Srithamrongsawat, and S. Pitayarangsarit. 2002. "Overview of Health Insurance Systems." In *Health Insurance Systems in Thailand*, ed. P. Pramualratana and S. Wibulpolprasert, 28–38. Nonthaburi, Thailand: Health Systems Research Institute.

Thammarangsi, T. 2004. *Analysis of Information on Human Resources for Health from 1999 and 2000 Census*. A research report. Nonthaburi, Thailand: International Health Policy Programme.

TRT (Thai Rak Thai Party). 2005. "The General Election 2001." http://www.thairakthai.or.th/infoparty/info-party.html.

Vasavid, C., K. Tisayaticom, W. Patcharanarumol, and V. Tangcharoensathien. 2004. "Impact of Universal Health Care Coverage on the Thai Households." In *From Policy to Implementation: Historical Events During 2001–2004 of Universal Coverage in Thailand*, ed. V. Tangcharoensathien and P. Jongudomsak, 129–49. Nonthaburi, Thailand: National Health Security Office.

Wasi, P. 2000. " 'Triangle That Moves the Mountain' and Health System Reform Movement in Thailand." http://www.moph.go.th/ops/hrdj/hrdj10/pdf10/PRAWES.PDF.

Wibulpolprasert, S., ed. 2007. *Thailand Health Profile 2005–2007*. Nonthaburi, Thailand: Ministry of Public Health.

———. 2004. *Thailand Health Profile 2001–2004*. Nonthaburi, Thailand: Ministry of Public Health.

———. 1999. "Inequitable Distribution of Doctors: Can It Be Solved?" http://www.moph.go.th/ops/hrdj/hrdj6/pdf31/INEQUIT.PDF.

# 13

# Tunisia: "Good Practice" in Expanding Health Care Coverage: Lessons from Reforms in a Country in Transition

*Chokri Arfa and Hédi Achouri*

## Background

*Tunisia, a 163,610 sq. km. north African country on the Mediterranean, is in the Middle East and North Africa (MENA) Region of the World Bank. Its population numbered 9 million in 2004, according to the latest census. Tunisia's health status is among the best in Africa and in the MENA Region. In this regard, Tunisia does better than other countries with similar income levels. This good performance is largely attributable to a healthy economy, progress in alleviating poverty, and social development. Disparities persist between urban and rural areas, as well as between different socioeconomic groups, but they are less pronounced than in other comparable countries, especially in terms of infant mortality and life expectancy.*

*Until the 1980s, Tunisia's health care system, founded in the colonial tradition of a hospital-centered health infrastructure, was concentrated in large urban areas. In the past three decades, Tunisia has progressively put into place a health system that covers nearly the entire population. More than 85 percent of the population has access to health care—through either a health insurance scheme or a medical assistance program. Private sector providers have been increasingly incorporated in the health care delivery system. However, the public sector is still the main provider of health services, hospital beds (85 percent), and medical personnel (more than 55 percent).*

## The Economic Environment

People's living conditions and general well-being have been continuously improving in Tunisia. GDP per capita has increased steadily, and poverty rates have fallen.

In 2004, after an average GDP growth rate of 5.5 percent for 30 years, Tunisia had the most dynamic economy south of the Mediterranean, despite a slow down

**385**

**Table 13.1   Tunisia: Economic Indicators**

| Indicators | 1990 | 1995 | 2000 | 2004 |
|---|---|---|---|---|
| GDP per capita (constant 2000 US$) | 1,502,921 | 1,655,289 | 2,035,696 | 2,336,479 |
| GDP per capita, PPP (current international $) | 3,705,988 | 4,681,146 | 6,251,551 | 7,767,597 |
| GDP growth (annual %) | 7.951 | 2.320 | 4.671 | 5.843 |
| Poverty gap at $1 a day (PPP) (%) | .. | .. | 0,500 | .. |
| Poverty gap at $2 a day (PPP) (%) | .. | .. | 1,328 | .. |
| Revenue, excluding grants (% of GDP) | 30.705 | 30.089 | 29.203 | 29.676 |
| Tax revenue (% of GDP) | 19.953 | 20.534 | 21.279 | 20.664 |
| External debt (% of GDP) | | | 59.6 | 67.8 |
| Aid (% of GNI) | 3.294 | 0.440 | 1.203 | 1.216 |
| Unemployment, total (% of total labor force) | .. | .. | 15.6 | 13.9 |
| Inflation, consumer prices (annual %) | 6.545 | 6.244 | 2.929 | 3.570 |

*Source:* World Bank 2005.

due to structural adjustments in the early 1980s. Besides its Mediterranean climate, proximity to Europe, sociopolitical stability, and well-qualified population, Tunisia owns significant economic assets in spite of its modest natural resources (oil and phosphates). These assets, together with a stable macroeconomic environment and a sound administration, have allowed Tunisia to continuously increase its GDP per capita (US$2,336.5 in 2004, compared to US$1,502.9 in 1990 (table 13.1). Due to sound macroeconomic management, the annual inflation rate has been held to between 2 and 3 percent for the decade 1996–2005.

Beginning in the early 1990s, Tunisia introduced numerous reforms that allowed it to sustain an annual GDP growth rate around or above 5 percent. These reforms also supported significant growth in the private sector, which contributed to investments, exports, job creation, and the subsequent reduction in the unemployment rate.

Tunisia, a member of the Maghreb collaboration area, has concluded commercial agreements with about 60 countries, some involving preferential trade agreements.[1] Tunisia has signed important trade agreements, including the WTO Agreement, a Bilateral Agreement with the European Union, and the Agreement with the League of Arab States. The liberalization of services, including health care, carries high stakes for Tunisia.

## Government-Sponsored Benefits

Government-sponsored benefits are one of the most important instruments for the success of the social dimension of Tunisia's development strategy (table 13.2). These benefits played a decisive role in reinforcing mutual aid among various social groups, supporting the advancement of human resources, and achieving the

**Table 13.2  Tunisia: Government-Sponsored Benefits**

| Benefits | 1986 | 1998 | 2001 |
|---|---|---|---|
| Government-sponsored benefits (million dinars [TD]) | 1,330 | 4,352 | 5,581 |
| Government-sponsored benefits within the state budget (%) | 44.1 | 50.1 | 51.6 |
| Government-sponsored benefits per household per month (TD) | 81 | 194 | 221 |

*Source:* Tunisian Agency for External Communications 2002.

indispensable balance between economic efficacy and social well-being, both urgently needed.

Tunisia's social policy includes social assistance programs benefiting both rural and urban residents. These programs include health care, schooling, housing, and employment benefits for youth and indigent populations, as well as financial assistance for purchases of food and other basic products. The latter benefit has proven a costly way (0.5 to 1 percent of GDP) of combating poverty, because the entire population has access to it (Ghali 2004).

Improving living conditions and alleviating poverty have always been a central priority for Tunisia's public authorities. The government commits more than half of its budget to the social sector, 19 percent of GDP. Government investments in social programs have been growing constantly. Between 1996 and 2005, the amount of government-sponsored benefits doubled. This resulted in TD 275 of additional monthly revenue per household. In addition, the government commits financial and in-kind assistance to certain groups under its aid and social assistance programs.

In addition, the government supports numerous programs for job creation and diversification of revenue sources. Some examples are the National Solidarity Funds (created in 1993), the National Employment Funds (created in 2000), and the Tunisian Solidarity Bank (created in 1997). To promote revenue generation, nongovernmental organizations (NGOs) have set up microcredit programs to help rural people finance investments, especially in agriculture and in arts and crafts.

## Poverty

In Tunisia, financial poverty is captured through the National Statistics Institute's national survey[2] (for household budget and consumption), conducted every five years. Table 13.3 provides information on poverty trends since 1975 (UNDP 2004b). Poverty reduction was most perceptible in the second half of the 1990s, because of more efficient and targeted policies and programs in the fight against poverty and because of steady economic growth. Between 1980 and 2000, the poverty rate was cut by a third. Progress continued into 2004 and 2005, with poverty rates estimated at 4 percent and 3.9 percent, respectively. A significant reduction in financial poverty was achieved in rural areas, but poverty is still an urban phenomenon.

Table 13.3   Tunisia: Poverty Trends, by Area, 1975–2000

| Amounts | 1975 | 1980 | 1985 | 1990 | 1995 | 2000 |
|---|---|---|---|---|---|---|
| **Poverty line, Current TD** | | | | | | |
| Urban areas | 87 | 120 | 190 | 278 | 362 | 428 |
| Rural areas | 43 | 60 | 95 | 139 | 181 | 221 |
| Entire country | 64 | 91 | 147 | 222 | 292 | 351 |
| **Poverty line , constant TD** | | | | | | |
| Urban areas | 272 | 267 | 269 | 278 | 273 | 276 |
| Rural areas | 135 | 134 | 134 | 139 | 137 | 142 |
| Entire country | 200 | 203 | 207 | 222 | 220 | 226 |
| **Poverty rate (%)** | | | | | | |
| Urban areas | 26.5 | 11.8 | 8.4 | 7.3 | 7.1 | 4.9 |
| Rural areas | 18.0 | 14.1 | 7.0 | 5.8 | 4.9 | 2.9 |
| Entire country | 22.0 | 12.9 | 7.7 | 6.7 | 6.2 | 4.2 |

*Sources:* INS 1975–2000; UNDP 2004b.

Concerning the nonmonetary aspects of poverty, significant progress has been made in terms of health and education, as evidenced by Tunisia's latest social indicators.

## Social, Demographic, and Epidemiological Environment

Tunisia is in the midst of a triple transition—socioeconomic, demographic, and health-related.

### Socioeconomic Transition

Four principal social transformations are under way in urbanization, lifestyle, tobacco and other addictive behaviors, and family structure. The urban population living has rapidly increased, from 40.1 percent in 1996, to 64.1 percent in 2004. By 2015, it is projected to reach 67 percent. People are becoming more sedentary, and their eating patterns are beginning to resemble those in richer countries. Around 30 percent of Tunisians (but more than 50 percent of the men) use tobacco. Some other behaviors, such as alcoholism and drug abuse, bear watching but are not yet a major public health problem. The Tunisian family is becoming increasingly mononuclear, composed of the parents and their dependent children.

### Demographic Transition

Among countries in the MENA Region, Tunisia has followed a unique pattern of demographic transition. The abolition of polygamy immediately after the country's independence in 1956, as well as the related family planning policy and significant progress in the health system, explain the transition observed in Tunisia.

**Figure 13.1 Tunisia: Population Pyramids, 1990, 2005, and 2020**

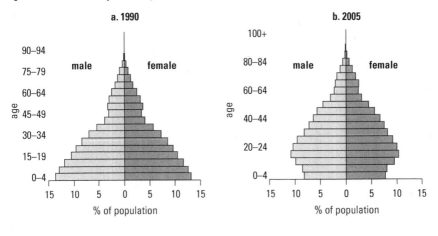

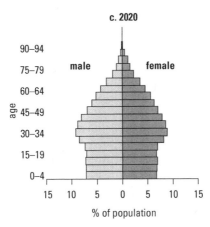

*Source:* UNPD 2004.

The population has more than doubled since independence, from 3.78 billion in 1956 to 9.91 billion in 2004 (INS 2004) and is projected to reach 12.03 million in 2020. The natural growth of the population has been significantly reduced: 3.2 percent in 1966, 2.35 percent (1984–94), and 1.21 percent (1994–2004). This rate will drop to 0.87 percent in 2020–25 (UNPD 2004).

The population's age structure has also changed drastically. Tunisia's population will probably age rapidly (figure 13.1). In 2020, according to United Nations Population Division projections (2004),[3] the number of people older than 60 years will nearly match those younger than 9 years old. The elderly will then make up 12.5 percent of the population, a dramatic difference from 9.5 percent in 2004 and 6.7 percent in 1984).

**Figure 13.2    Tunisia: Trends in Life Expectancy, Men and Women, 1966–2004**

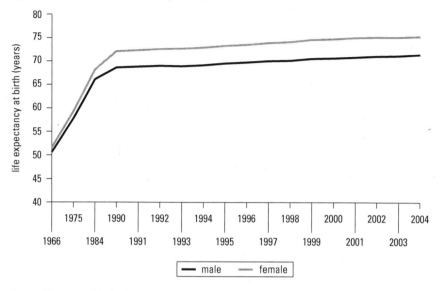

*Sources:* INS reports and databases.

The transition from a high-mortality and high-fertility situation to one characterized by low mortality and low fertility is not occurring at the same time or at the
same pace as in other high-, middle-, or low-income countries. Lambert (2001: 53)
has shown that the demographic transition in developing countries is taking place
faster than in developed countries, and faster still in Tunisia where mortality and
fertility indicators have been reduced more than in other similar countries.

The decrease in infant mortality resulted in an increase of life expectancy at
birth. Life expectancy was 37 years in the late 1940s, 52 years in the late 1960s, and
73 years in 2004 (71.4 for men and 75.3 for women). Between 1956 and 2004, the
Tunisian population gained 26.3 years in life expectancy at birth (figure 13.2).

The infant mortality rate (IMR), close to 200 per thousand in 1956, is now 20.6
per thousand. According to the National Institute of Statistics (INS) projections,
the IMR will further decrease to 10.0 per thousand in 2020 and to 8.0 per thousand in 2030. This spectacular fall in infant mortality is attributable to a close
interaction of three principal strategies: the August 1956 promulgation of a law
prohibiting polygamy; the full-scale implementation of family planning and fertility reduction policy since the early 1960s; and the integration of maternal and
child health and reproductive health into the most important national programs
since 1960 (monitoring of pregnancies, immunizations, postnatal care, and birth
spacing). These strategies have evolved and have been updated periodically, within
an economic environment characterized by the fight against poverty, increased

**Table 13.4  Tunisia: Selected Demographic Indicators**

| Indicators | 1956 | 1966 | 1975 | 1984 | 1990 | 1991 | 1992 | 1993 | 1994 | 1995 | 1996 | 1997 | 1998 | 1999 | 2000 | 2001 | 2002 | 2003 | 2004 |
|---|---|---|---|---|---|---|---|---|---|---|---|---|---|---|---|---|---|---|---|
| Total population (million) | 3.780 | 4.533 | 5.588 | 6.966 | 8.154 | 8.318 | 8.490 | 8.657 | 8.815 | 8.958 | 9.089 | 9.215 | 9.333 | 9.456 | 9.564 | 9.670 | 9.782 | 9.840 | 9.910 |
| Urban population rate (%) | | 40.1 | 47.5 | 52.8 | 58.0 | 58.6 | 59.6 | 60.0 | 61.7 | 61.30 | 61.60 | 61.90 | 62.2 | 62.5 | 62.8 | 63.1 | 63.4 | 63.7 | 64.1 |
| Natural growth rate per year (%) | 3.50 | 3.10 | 2.70 | 2.60 | 2.40 | 2.00 | 2.00 | 2.00 | 1.70 | 1.60 | 1.50 | 1.40 | 1.3 | 1.3 | 1.1 | 1.1 | 1.1 | 1.09 | 1.08 |
| Crude fertility rate (%) | 50.0 | 44.0 | 36.6 | 32.4 | 25.2 | 24.9 | 24.9 | 24.0 | 22.7 | 20.8 | 19.7 | 18.9 | 17.9 | 16.9 | 17.1 | 16.9 | 16.7 | 17.1 | 16.8 |
| Crude mortality rate (%) | 25.0 | 15.0 | 10.0 | 6.5 | 5.6 | 5.6 | 5.6 | 5.7 | 5.5 | 5.8 | 5.5 | 5.6 | 5.6 | 5.6 | 5.6 | 5.5 | 5.8 | 6.1 | 6.0 |
| Crude infant mortality rate (%) | 200 | 120 | 76.9 | 51.4 | 41.0 | | | | 31.8 | 32.0 | 30.0 | 27.6 | 26.6 | 26.2 | 25.0 | | | | 20.6 |
| Total fertility rate (%) | 7.2 | 7.15 | 5.8 | 4.7 | 3.5 | .. | 3.2 | .. | 2.9 | 2.67 | 2.51 | 2.38 | 2.23 | 2.09 | 2.08 | 2.05 | 2.0 | 2.1 | 2.02 |

*Sources:* Reports of Direction of studies and planning (MSP) and Annuals Reports of National Institute of Statistics.

access to mandatory education for females, and a continuous improvement in health care access, in particular regarding childhood infectious diseases.

The continuous drop in fertility is one of the most remarkable aspects of Tunisia's demographic transition. Starting from a level close to that of less-developed countries, Tunisia's fertility rate was 2.02 in 2004, nearing the 1.57 rate of developed countries.

The crude mortality rate was 16.8 per thousand in 2004, compared with 50 per thousand 45 years ago. It is predicted to decrease to 15 per thousand between 2025 and 2030. Thus, because of the slow mortality reduction process post-1950, the consequent rapid decrease in mortality and, in particular, the reduction in fertility, Tunisia can be classified with other countries that have had a delayed demographic transition. Such countries include South Korea, Hong Kong (China), Sri Lanka, and China (Omrane 1983).

## Epidemiologic Transition

A multifaceted epidemiologic transition followed from Tunisia's demographic transition—health-related but also social, economic, and cultural. This transition is inadequately documented in the absence of a reliable information system.

Tunisia's epidemiologic profile has changed since the late 1980s. A decline—occasionally the eradication—has occurred in the "traditional" infectious diseases (malaria, schistosomiasis, trachoma, tuberculosis, infectious diarrhea) and in early childhood diseases (poliomyelitis, neonatal tetanus, diphtheria). In 2002, noncommunicable diseases (NCDs) accounted for 79.7 percent of mortality and 70.8 percent of morbidity (table 13.5). Chronic and degenerative NCDs with multifactorial etiology have emerged, together with high fees for access to treatment. And road traffic accidents have increased, with consequences in terms of mortality and morbidity.

WHO (2004) ranked the top five causes of mortality in Tunisia in 2002 (in descending order): cardiovascular disease, malignant neoplasms, injuries, diges-

**Table 13.5   Tunisia: Global Burden of Disease, 2002 Estimates**

| Disease and injury | Burden of disease by disease category[a] (thousands of estimated total deaths, by cause) | | Burden of Disease by disease category: DALYs (thousands of estimated total DALYs, by cause) | |
|---|---|---|---|---|
| | Value | Percent | Value | Percent |
| Communicable, maternal, perinatal, and nutritional conditions | 5.3 | 9.50 | 217 | 14.10 |
| Noncommunicable diseases | 44.5 | 79.70 | 1,093 | 70.80 |
| Injuries | 6 | 10.80 | 234 | 15.20 |
| Total | 55.8 | 100.00 | 1,544 | 100.00 |

*Source:* WHO 2004.

a. Deaths only.

**Table 13.6    Tunisia: Top Five Burden of Disease Causes, 2002 Estimates**

| | Top five burden of disease[a] causes: deaths only (thousands of estimated total deaths, by cause) | | Top five burden of disease causes: DALYs (thousands of estimated total DALYs, by cause) | |
|---|---|---|---|---|
| Rank | GBD Cause | Value | GBD Cause | Value |
| 1 | Cardiovascular diseases | 26 | Neuropsychiatric conditions | 268 |
| 2 | Malignant neoplasms | 5.5 | Cardiovascular diseases | 237 |
| 3 | Unintentional injuries | 5.4 | Unintentional injuries | 211 |
| 4 | Digestive diseases | 3.3 | Sense organ diseases | 171 |
| 5 | Respiratory diseases | 2.9 | Digestive diseases | 88 |

*Source:* WHO 2004.

a. Deaths only.

tive diseases, and respiratory diseases (table 13.6). When morbidity and disability-adjusted life years (DALYs) are included in the calculations, neuropsychiatric conditions rank second after cardiovascular disease.

Ben Romdhane (2002) shows a disease profile in Tunisia similar to those of western countries. The prevalence of hypertension varies between 15 and 21 percent (Canada: 14 percent). An increase in the prevalence of diabetes is predicted from 3.5 percent in 1976–1977 to 11 percent for urban area and 5 percent in rural areas for 2006. (France: 16.2 percent, Canada: 5 percent). There is a high of tobacco-related cancers in men, with lung cancer at the top of the list. The incidence of cancer (per 100,000 population) is 27.9/17.5 (North/South, respectively). This is much lower than in industrial nations such as France (55.1) or Canada (82.5). The prevalence of mental illnesses (particularly depression) in Tunisia is similar to those reported in the international literature, with a global prevalence of major depression of 8.2 percent and of schizophrenia of 0.57 percent. Overall, the number of disabled individuals has increased by 2.5 in Tunisia since 1975. The global prevalence of disabilities in individuals older than 60 years is four times higher than that of the general population (28 percent versus 6.5 percent).

## The Social and Political Context

Internationally, as part of both the Maghreb and the Mediterranean regions, Tunisia has been dedicated to reinforcing its integration in the Arabic, Muslim, and African environment. It has signed agreements with the World Trade Organization (WTO) and in 1995 became the first country in the MENA Region to reach an Association Agreement with the European Union (EU). Moreover, Tunisia has been the principal leader of initiatives for the revitalization of the Arab Maghreb Union.

Tunisia's economic and social progress has been supported through the coordination of policies and reforms and a competent public administration. Practical macroeconomic policies have created an environment conducive to the growth and development of the private sector. In addition, the constant efforts for sector wide reforms since the early 1990s, as well as determination to integrate Tunisia in the global economy, have created favorable conditions for growth in productivity and economic competition.

In terms of social development, Tunisia's activities have promoted the emergence and expansion of a large middle class that is strongly encouraged to participate in the development process. Tunisia has documented rapid and sustained progress in education and training, and health indicators have also significantly improved.

According to a recent MENA report on governance (World Bank 2003a), Tunisia is given much higher marks than the average lower-middle-income country for the quality of its public administration. This attribute translates into the capacity to formulate and execute sound economic policies, as well as confidence in the institutions that govern relations between the state and its citizens.

## Health Financing and Health Insurance

Health finance sources are often grouped into three major types of financing agencies: the state, Social Security funds (SSF),[4] and households. To that list, must be added: donors and other international organizations,[5] medical services, and in-house medical and occupational health services provided by companies, which contribute about 1 percent.

### Health Care Coverage in Tunisia

The Tunisian health insurance system includes a multitude of schemes, put together over time to meet the needs of certain professional groups. Almost the entire Tunisian population (99 percent) has health care coverage, through various means: mandatory Social Security schemes (66 percent) or free medical services (8 percent free of charge, 25 percent reduced charges). Supplementary insurance schemes (group insurance and mutual insurance companies) have also developed in response to the insufficiencies of the Social Security Fund health insurance schemes (figure 13.3).

*Health care benefits packages.*  The concept of benefits packages has not yet been fully incorporated into the health care and the health insurance systems. Generally speaking, patients have access to all types of health care, without the limitation of a particular benefits package. The only exception lies in the reimbursement option under the mandatory National Pension and Social Protection Fund (NFSPR) discussed below which limits coverage for chronic illnesses (from a predetermined list) and surgical interventions. Nevertheless, all reimbursement schemes set an annual expenditure cap (limit) per household.

*Health insurance mechanisms.*  The health insurance mechanisms vary by social group and financing sources. Preventive and public health activities, individual or collective, are guaranteed at no cost for the entire population. The same model

**Figure 13.3    Tunisia: Coverage Rates by Health Insurance Scheme**

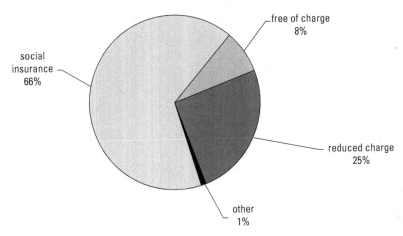

*Source:* Achouri 2005.

applies to individuals with illnesses that qualify them to take part in research studies. Individual costs for preventive services provided privately, however, are a household responsibility. Some professional groups (and their families) receive free health care in primary health care centers and other special schemes, in addition to their social security coverage. In some situations, mutual insurance membership gives some groups[6] access to services from private providers. The members of the resistance movement (participants in Tunisia's liberation movement) and their dependants also receive free health care services through the MSP facilities and military hospitals.

By law,[7] the state guarantees free or subsidized health care services to low-income groups through two public medical aid schemes[8]: the free health care scheme and a reduced-fee plan.

Beneficiaries of the *free health care scheme,* defined according to the poverty line, are target families of a long-term government assistance program. Ruling No. 98-1812 describes the conditions and allocation and distribution mechanisms of the free health care card. The card is issued for five years within national limits and regional quotas.

Beneficiaries of *reduced fees or charges* receive fee-reduction cards according to their annual household income relative to family size. Their income cannot exceed: the minimum wage (*salaire minimum interprofessionnel garanti,* SMIG) for families of two or fewer members; one-and-a-half times the SMIG for a three- to five-member family; and twice the SMIG for families larger than five members. In addition to those conditions, current Social Security affiliates are ineligible for fee reductions. Social agents from the Ministry of Social Affairs, Solidarity, and

Tunisians Abroad (MASSTE) work in the field to make sure the eligibility conditions are met. The fee reduction card is issued for five years, within regional quotas, and must be validated annually through the deposit of TD 10. Cardholders must pay the inclusive contribution for each medical visit.

To better target intervention and support to needy families, the MASSTE has set up a national poverty database. This database includes socioeconomic information on beneficiary families under the National Program of Aid to Poor Families (Programme National d'Aide aux Familles Nécessiteuses, PNAFN). This program's tools for monitoring socioeconomic status are an important resource for various social partners that select the beneficiaries of aid programs (long-term, temporary, free, or reduced charges for health care). They are also useful in the selection of beneficiaries for income generation activities under regional development programs and job creation assistance mechanisms.

Within the framework of the two medical aid programs (free health care and reduced health care charge beneficiaries), access of the poor to health services is not subject to any restrictions, rationing or ceilings. However, public hospitals' budget limitations and drug shortages can be considered an implicit form of service rationing.

In addition, the reform of the public medical aid scheme, introduced in 1998, has helped expand coverage under formal insurance schemes, particularly by appealing to independent individuals, workers in the agricultural and informal sectors. Together with other measures, this program raised the real social coverage rate to 85.5 percent in 2004, and a further rise, to 90 percent, was forecast for 2006 (table 13.7). These formal insurance schemes include Social Security, contracts with private insurance companies and mutual insurance companies, and associations of public and private employees.

*Social Security schemes* are available for employees and employers, both mandated to participate. The funds are pooled within two principal funds: the NFSS

**Table 13.7   Tunisia: CSS Insurance Coverage Rates (percentage of eligible population)**

| Coverage | 1987 | 1997 | 1998 | 2005 | 2006[a] |
|---|---|---|---|---|---|
| Total, private sector (affiliated with NFSS) | 41.6 | 74.6 | 77.0 | 81.0 | |
| Nonagricultural workers | 66.3 | 94.0 | 96.3 | 97.2 | |
| Agricultural workers | 16.9 | 41.7 | 42.8 | 47.0 | |
| Independents | 9.2 | 48.5 | 50.2 | 54.5 | |
| Total, public sector (affiliated with NFPSP) | 100 | 100 | 100 | 100 | 100 |
| Total, eligible beneficiaries | 54.6 | 80.7 | 82.6 | 87.0 | 90.5 |

*Sources:* Achouri 2002; and NHIF 2006.

a. No data are available for 2006.

and the NFPSP. These national funds provide allowances for pensions, family services, and social protection and for industrial accidents and occupational diseases. The NFSS covers private sector workers, while NFPSP covers employees of the state, local public unions, and other public institutions.

Coverage rates vary by sector (table 13.7). All state employees are covered (NFPSP). Coverage of workers in the private sector (NFSS) is gradually increasing for several reasons. Legal allowances for the socially insured and their dependents have grown, reaching more than TD 1,943 million in 2003, equivalent to 30.8 percent of government-sponsored benefits and 6 percent of GDP. Coverage has also been extended to groups not previously covered by Social Security such as homemakers and construction workers, people unable to participate in their respective schemes such as small-scale fishermen, farmers, artisans, craftsmen, and artists.

The health care benefits covered vary by fund organizations. The NFPSP offers two schemes: a mandatory scheme and a facultative (complementary) scheme. The mandatory scheme has two mutually exclusive options:

- The first option offers a "health care card" that gives beneficiaries access to all MSP facilities. Beneficiaries pay a reasonable price.
- The second option is a reimbursement regime that covers only individuals with chronic illnesses and surgical interventions and gives them access to various public and private providers.

The facultative scheme is an extension of the cited second option on providing coverage to all common illnesses.

The NFSS offers its beneficiaries, regardless of which scheme the head of the household belongs to, two means of illness coverage, based on in-kind benefits: (1) within the MSP facilities, the same benefits for the ill as for reduced-fee beneficiaries and (2) within its polyclinics, only ambulatory care services with a copayment at the point of service.

Besides the health care services covered by these schemes, the two Social Security funds finance completely or partially: expenditures for special services, intensive care covered through special agreements with public and private providers, and international health services.

Private and public sector enterprises can contract with private insurance companies to cover their employees. Mutual insurance companies and private and public sector employee associations offer several social services including of health care coverage. In some mutual insurance companies, membership is mandatory. Membership in a mutual insurance company or in an insurance group is parallel to the mandatory affiliation of both the employee and the employer to the SSF. They usually use a fee-for-service reimbursement scheme and put a yearly ceiling on payments to a beneficiary.

Any uninsured patient pays the entire health care cost out of pocket, irrespective of whether care was obtained in the private or public sector.

Table 13.8   Tunisia: Health Expenditure, as a Share of GDP and Per Capita, 1980–2004

| Item | 1980 | 1985 | 1990 | 1995 | 1996 | 1997 | 1998 | 1999 | 2000 | 2001 | 2002 | 2003 | 2004 |
|------|------|------|------|------|------|------|------|------|------|------|------|------|------|
| Health expenditure (TD millions) | 143.0 | 290.3 | 578.0 | 938.0 | 1,160.6 | 1,258.3 | 1,238.0 | 1,367.0 | 1,489.5 | 1,644.0 | 1,673.0 | 1,824.6 | 2,170.0 |
| Expenditure as % of GDP | 3.2 | 4.2 | 5.3 | 5.5 | 5.5 | 5.4 | 5.5 | 5.5 | 5.6 | 5.8 | 5.8 | 5.6 | 5.6 |
| Expenditure per capita (TD) | — | 39 | 72 | 105.5 | 114.5 | 123.4 | 132.7 | 144.5 | 155.8 | 169.9 | 170.4 | 184.5 | 217.5 |

*Source:* MSP 2006.

## Health Expenditure Indicators

Tunisia devotes almost 5.6 percent of GDP to health expenditures, compared with the average of 8 percent in EU member countries. From 1980 to 2004, total health care expenditures increased 15.2 percent, with an average annual increase of 12 percent. Thus, health care expenditures have risen from TD 143 million to TD 2,170 million (table 13.8). Closer analysis shows that expenditures grew only 7.3 percent between 1980 and 1990 but jumped to 9.9 percent between 1990 and 2000, and leveled off at 9.4 percent between 2000 and 2004.

Similarly, the share of GDP committed to health grew from 3.2 percent in 1980 to 5.6 percent in 2004. Health expenditures per capita grew from TD 39 in 1985 to TD 217.5 in 2004, a 5.6 percent overall increase and 9.5 percent average annual growth (table 13.8).

## Trends and Consequences of Public and Private Health Expenditures in Tunisia

Health financing was largely supported by the state budget and the Social Security funds until the end of the 1980s. During this period, public health funding (from fiscal and social contributions) is estimated at 65 percent of total health care financing. The economic and financial crisis during the second half of the 1980s and the subsequent adjustment programs significantly curtailed the state's contribution. The reduction in state aid was made up by increased household expenditure and, later, a reinforcement of Social Security contributions. Between 1995 and 2004, funds for health financing were equally provided from public sources (from the state and Social Security) and private sources (direct payment from households and facultative and/ or private health insurance) (table 13.9).

## Trends in Health Expenditures by Financing Agent

Trends in health expenditures by source for the period between 1980 and 2004 are shown in figure 13.4. Data for household health expenditure are based on a macroeconomic estimate that does not reflect reimbursements from "elective"

**Table 13.9    Tunisia: Health Expenditure Indicators, 1995–2004**

| Indicator | 1995 | 1996 | 1997 | 1998 | 1999 | 2000 | 2001 | 2002 | 2003 | 2004 |
|---|---|---|---|---|---|---|---|---|---|---|
| Public expenditures (PubExp) as percentage of total expenditures (TE) | 49.5 | 52.1 | 47.7 | 49.9 | 51.6 | 48.5 | 51.0 | 50.0 | 47.5 | 48.7 |
| Private expenditures (PrivExp) as percentage of TE | 50.5 | 47.9 | 52.3 | 50.1 | 48.4 | 51.5 | 49.0 | 50.0 | 52.5 | 51.3 |
| PubExp as percentage of total PubExp | 7.1 | 7.2 | 6.7 | 7.1 | 7.6 | 6.9 | 7.9 | 7.6 | 7.7 | 7.7 |
| PubExp financed by external resources as percentage of TE | 0.8 | 0.8 | 0.8 | 0.8 | 0.7 | 0.7 | 0.7 | 0.2 | 0.4 | — |
| Household health expenditures as percentage of PrivExp | 92.5 | 100 | 100 | 92.7 | 83.0 | 81.7 | 82.5 | 83.0 | 82.9 | 82.9 |
| Social Security health expenditures as percentage of PubExp | 28.8 | 31.9 | 24.5 | 24.3 | 24.1 | 26.7 | 22.9 | 22.9 | 23.5 | 23.3 |
| PubExp financed through general taxation as percentage of total health expenditures (THE) | 70.8 | 70.7 | 69.9 | 70.2 | 70.5 | 70.5 | 70.6 | — | — | — |
| THE per capita at current exchange rate (US$) | 111 | 117 | 111 | 116 | 122 | 114 | 120 | 126 | 141 | 163 |

*Sources:* MSP 2005; WHO 2006.

*Note:* — = not available.

group and mutual insurance (although contributions to some mutuals are obligatory in nature). Based on the national health accounts, these reimbursements were estimated at 8.5 percent of all health expenditures in 2000, 7.3 percent in 2004, and 7.1 percent in 2005 (Arfa and Achour 2004). These estimates were made possible through work on the national health accounts recently incorporated in the activities of the National Institute of Public Health. The developments in this area prompt the following conclusions:

*Public expenditures.* State budgetary expenditures on health care grew at the annual average rate of 8.1 percent between 1980 and 2004. Since then, this share has decreased. Financing through contributions to the SSF averaged 13.6 percent annually between 1980 and 2004. This was a significant increase relative to total expenditures.

*Private expenditures.* Private sources of financing include individual expenditures (reimbursed, or not, by private or mutual insurance companies) and occupational health and other expenditures for curative services provided by companies.

**Figure 13.4   Tunisia: Trends in Health Care Spending, by Financing Agent, 1980–2004**

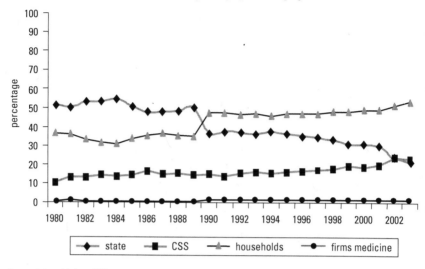

*Source:* Arfa and Achour 2006.

Households continued to bear most of these expenditures. Between 1980 and 2004, private spending grew at an annual average rate of 14.3 percent. There was a significant increase from 36.6 percent in 1980 to 51.3 percent in 2004.

Since 1980, health care financing has been marked by a net decrease in public financing and a significant increase in the direct household contribution due to diminishing incomes and the high prices of health care services and health commodities. Faced with inequity risks through reduced financial access to health care and in the hope of improving the distribution of the health sector's financial burden, the public authorities have initiated reforms in the Social Security health insurance schemes.

Since 1990, the recorded changes have been confirmed by National Health Accounts for 1995, 1997, and 2000. Therefore, some explanations for these developments can be ventured.

The International Monetary Fund (IMF) Structural Adjustment Program resulted in the reduction of the state's social expenditures, especially for health. Because of this contraction in funding, the MSP facilities faced financial difficulties that limited the supply of drugs and other medical commodities, and patients often had to buy their own. Copayments were also raised several times to give the MSP facilities more money. NFPSP reimbursement rates and their annual caps were frozen at their 1980 levels to increase overall financial stability. Yet medical fees and medical commodity prices went on rising. Consequently, copayments also continued to increase.

Health care costs have continued to rise under the double burden of price increases and the demographic transition. They have also been affected by budgetary constraints of public health care facilities and health insurance organizations. Together, these factors have contributed the sharp rise in households' direct health care costs. These trends reduced access to health care and led many households into a vicious circle of illness-caused poverty.

## Financing and Payment

The current financing system, characterized by a diversity of financing sources and payment options, varies by provider category (table 13.10).

### Sources of Financing

In general, government financing is set aside for the MSP facilities. Social Security financing also benefits the MSP facilities. Financing of private sector delivery remains primarily a household responsibility.

*Public sector financing.* Facilities under the auspice of the MSP, are financed by the state, Social Security, and households. Hospital reforms have contributed to a revision of the share of the burden borne by these three agencies. These reforms introduced new payment options through Social Security funds for hospital providers.

The share of Social Security funds increased from 11 percent to 22.2 percent between 1990 and 2003 (figure 13.5). This rise was obtained due to an initiative for priority investments in certain programs and the establishment of a billing system for hospital and ambulatory care through annual agreements between MSP and MASSTE, implemented gradually since 1996 and limited to university and regional hospitals.

Households' share has also risen, from 10 percent in 1990 to 14.2 percent in 2003. This is explained by step-wise modifications in the copayment amounts for public entities, initiated in 1991, 1993, 1994, and 1998; patient contributions to the costs of diagnostic and treatment services (10 percent of the share applied to paying patients) for the socially insured in 1994 and for beneficiaries of reduced tariffs in 1998; an increase in fees for paying patients, initiated successively in 1991, 1993, and 1996; and a revision of the fees associated with classification of medical services in 1996. The state's subsidy to MSP facilities and MSP has increased in value, but its share in public sector financing has decreased by 15.4 percent.

Since 1990, the relative decrease in state subsidies to the public sector was offset by increases in the shares of the SSF (73 percent) and households (27 percent). Public funds remained the principal means of public sector financing. The share of private funds for private sector financing has not surpassed 14.2 percent.

*Private sector financing.* Households bear the greatest share of financing. Insurance groups and mutual insurance companies, in addition to their low coverage, take responsibility for only a small part of these costs. Social Security funds are responsible for health care costs in the private sector under the NFPSP reimbursement schemes and SSF agreements.

**Table 13.10  Tunisia: Health Care Coverage and Financing**

| Affiliated agency | NFSS | NFPSP | | Government assistance | | Supplementary insurance | |
|---|---|---|---|---|---|---|---|
| | | Mandatory scheme (reimbursement) | Optional scheme (reimbursement) | Free health care | Reduced fees | Group insurance | Mutual insurance companies |
| Scheme | General scheme and other schemes | Mandatory scheme (health care card) | Optional scheme (reimbursement) | Free health care | Reduced fees | Group insurance | Mutual insurance companies |
| Financing method | 4.75% for the general scheme, and less for the other schemes | 1% employers + 1% employees | 2.5% employers + 4.0% employees | Complete exemption | TD 10 per year | Monthly premium from 4% to 7%, including both employers and employees | Contribution rates vary from 1% to 7%. For employees, the rates do not exceed 2%. |
| Types of covered health care providers | Public and polyclinics of the NFSS | Public and private | Public and private | Public | Public | Public and private | Public and private |
| Types of coverage | No cap in the public sector, depending on availability. | Reimbursement of 80% of medical fees and all medical services at regular fees (year 1982)<br><br>Complete reimbursement for pharmaceuticals, without a cap. | Reimbursement of 80% of medical fees and of all medical services at regular fees (year 1982)<br><br>Annual cap for reimbursement of pharmaceuticals (TD 200 per year) | All care (ambulatory, hospitalization, emergencies) received in the public sector, depending on availability. | | A cap on total expenditures and some service-specific caps (surgery, dental, drugs) | A cap on total expenditures and some service-specific caps (surgery, dental, drugs) |

*Source:* Adapted from World Bank 2006b.

**Figure 13.5   Tunisia: Shifts in Sources of MSP Financing, 1990–2003**

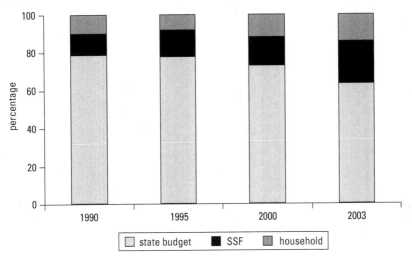

*Source:* MSP 2004.

Table 13.11 provides an overview of health care provider payment options under each health care coverage scheme. Differences in beneficiaries' access to care originate from this situation and are tied to the coverage type. For example, the benefit of free health care and reduced service charges is provided only by the MSP facilities. Access to NFSS polyclinics is reserved for members of this fund. NFSS socially insured cannot be covered for privately provided services (except for extreme cases). This may explain why people buy group insurance that allows coverage of health expenditures in the private sector. Socially insured individuals with NFPSP can seek private care. In addition, they can join professional mutual insurance companies that allow them to use private care as a supplement to the NFPSP mandatory coverage.

This fragmentation in health insurance coverage has arisen from numerous actions taken to improve people's access to health care. These actions have reduced inequities across population groups, the financial difficulties of the Social Security funds (especially NFPSP), and budgetary disequilibrium for the MSP facilities. In this context, the reform of Social Security health insurance schemes were initiated to harmonize access to health care for the insured population, the Tunisian majority.

## Payment Procedures
Payment options and procedures vary by health care scheme: direct patient reimbursement, direct provider reimbursement, payment in-kind, annual lump sum payment, billing, and grants (table 13.11).

**Table 13.11  Tunisia: Health Care Provider Payment Methods, by Type of Coverage**

| Coverage type | Private sector | Public sector | Parastatal sector | |
|---|---|---|---|---|
| | | | NFSS Polyclinics | Military hospitals |
| No coverage | Fee for service | Payment of public fees | n.a. | Payment of specific fees |
| Free health care | n.a. | None | | n.a. |
| Reduced Fees | | Copayment | | |
| NFSS | Negotiated fees for agreed services | Patient pays copayment | Copayment | Patient pays a copayment |
| NFPSP | | | | |
| Mandatory scheme | Negotiated fees for agreed services. Fee for service for long-term illness and surgical interventions | Billing to the funds of charges in university and regional hospitals | n.a. | Billing to the funds of specific conventional charges |
| Optional scheme | Negotiated fees for agreed services | Negotiated fees for agreed services<br>Fee for service (reimbursement) | n.a. | Negotiated fees the agreed services<br>Fee for service (reimbursement) |
| Group insurance and mutual insurance companies | Fee for service (reimbursement) | Fee for service (reimbursement) | n.a. | Fee for service (reimbursement) |

*Source:* Authors.

*Note:* n.a. = not applicable.

Some plans reimburse patients for the fees they pay their public or private providers. Within the framework of the mandatory scheme, CNRPS uses this procedure. Under the optional scheme, group insurers and mutual insurance organizations also use it.

Direct payment to public or private providers is the method used by the two SS under a series of special agreements on intensive care financing. The payments cover all health care costs incurred by the patient according to the tariffs in place at the time of service.

Payment in-kind for certain medical commodities is sometimes used. Under certain conditions, CSSs are required to provide their beneficiaries, in a social action framework, with drugs, prosthetics, and other commodities needed for the patient's complete medical care.

An annual lump-sum payment to the state treasury was the first mechanism used to handle the contribution of the two Social Security funds toward health care costs of the socially insured for services received in public health facilities. This ensured sufficient resources in the Treasury to finance the MSP facilities. This payment is still in effect and has been increased several times, most recently in 2006.

Billing is sometimes used to collect health care charges of people insured by the two Social Security funds. This procedure has become the predominant means of university and regional hospital budget financing. Every year the two Social Security funds allocate a fixed amount for billing services and operations (in addition to the amount that the funds do not cover, but which is provided by the health facilities involved). The MSP distributes this annual amount among the university and regional hospitals, apportioned according to each institution's operating budget projections.

Service fees are negotiated with the funds. A single fee for outpatient services covers the medical visit, any additional medical tests, and prescribed drugs. Fees for medical services in day hospitals are defined according to the pathology and/or therapeutic procedures. Hospitalization charges are set according to length of stay, regardless of the duration, for various medical and surgical specialties.

Finally, the NFSS uses grants to subsidize the polyclinics it owns.

In their encounters with the MSP facilities, and outside the NFPSP reimbursement schemes (table 13.12), the socially insured under both Social Security funds are responsible for copayments for outpatient consultations, for any additional procedures, and for hospitalization. Similar regulations apply to the NFSS socially insured when using polyclinic services (table 13.13).

## Other Considerations Related to Health Care Financing

According to an National Institute of Statistics household survey, hygiene and health care expenditures have risen faster than any other household expenditure (table 13.14). They doubled between 1975 and 2005, from 5.4 percent to 10.3 percent of total expenditures. By income, health expenditures are equal to 4 percent of the family budget for the poorest households, with a monthly income below

**Table 13.12  Tunisia: Provision for NFSPS Affiliates**

| | Mandatory scheme | | Optional scheme |
| --- | --- | --- | --- |
| | Health Care Card | Reimbursement system | Reimbursement system |
| Provision | Coverage of health services provided by government-affiliated hospitals (for health care card holders) | Coverage for surgical interventions and long-term illnesses (common illnesses excluded) | Coverage of common illnesses |
| General consultation | • Copayment[a] TD 1,500 for CSB<br>• Copayment TD 2,000 for HC | 80% of the charge set in the classification of medical services in public and private facilities | • Private: 80% up to TD 3,500 ceiling<br>• Public: 90% of official tariff |
| Medical specialist consultation | • Copayment TD 3 for HR<br>• Copayment TD 4,500 for university hospital centers | 80% of the charge set in the classification of medical services in public and private facilities | • Private: 80% up to TD 5,000 ceiling<br>• Public: 90% of the official tariff |
| Medical services | In public hospitals, the patient pays 20%, not to exceed TD 30 | Long-term illness or surgery: 100% of official tariffs | • Private: 80% official tariffs<br>• Public: 90% of the official tariff<br>With a cap of 50d per beneficiary per year for both provision types |
| Laboratory services | In public hospitals, the patient pays 20%, not to exceed TD 30 | 100% of official tariffs | • Private: 80% official tariffs<br>• Public: 90% of the official tariff<br>With a cap of 50d per beneficiary per year for both provision types |
| Midwifery | In public hospitals, the patient pays 20%, not to exceed TD 30 | 100% of official tariffs | • Private: 80% official tariffs<br>• Public: 90% of the official tariff |
| Speech therapy services | In public hospitals, the patient pays 20%, not to exceed TD 30 | 100% of official tariffs | • Private: 80% official tariffs<br>• Public: 90% of the official tariff |
| Dental surgery services | In public hospitals, the patient pays 20%, not to exceed TD 30<br>• Copayment for consultation<br>• Copayment TD 1,500 for CSB<br>• Copayment TD 2,000 for HC<br>• Copayment TD 3 for HR<br>• Copayment TD 4,500 for university hospital centers | 100% of official tariffs | • Private: 80% official tariffs<br>• Public: 90% of the official tariff<br>With a cap of TD 70 per beneficiary per year for both provision types. |
| Drugs | Provided by public facilities | 100% of related charges | 80 % of related charges, within a limit of TD 200 per family |

*Source:* NFSP (www.cnrps.nat.tn).

a. In the public sector, copayments vary by facility type.

**Table 13.13   Tunisia: Provision for NFSS Affiliates**

| Provision | Coverage provided by MSP facilities and NFSS polyclinics |
|---|---|
| General consultation | • Copayment of TD 1,500 for CSB<br>• Copayment of TD 2,000 for HC |
| Medical specialist consultation | • Copayment of TD 3 for HR<br>• Copayment of TD 4,500 for university hospital centers |
| General practitioner visit in NFSS polyclinic | Copayment of TD 3 |
| Medical specialist visit in NFSS polyclinic | Copayment of TD 4 |
| Medical services | Patient pays:<br>– In public hospitals: 20% of current public sector tariff, up to TD 30 ceiling<br>– In polyclinics: 20% of current public sector tariff. |
| Laboratory services | Patient pays:<br>– In public hospitals: 20% of current public sector tariff, up to TD 30 ceiling<br>– In polyclinics: 20% of current public sector tariff |
| Midwifery | Patient pays:<br>– In public hospitals: 20% of current public sector tariff, up to TD 30 ceiling<br>– In polyclinics: TD 2 |
| Speech therapy | Patient pays:<br>– In public hospitals: 20% of the current public sector tariff, up to TD 30 ceiling<br>– In polyclinics: 20% of the current public sector tariff.. |
| Dental surgery | Patient pays:<br>– In public hospitals: 20% of the current public sector tariff, up to TD 30 ceiling<br>– In polyclinics: 10% of the current public sector tariff |
| Drugs | In NFSS polyclinics, patient pays:<br>– Long-term illness: 15 % of charges<br>– Common illness: 20% of charges<br>In MSP facilities, drugs provided without any patient contribution |

*Source:* NFSS (http://www.cnss.nat.tn).

**Table 13.14   Tunisia: Household Consumption, 1975–2000 (percentage)**

| Function | 1975 | 1980 | 1985 | 1990 | 1995 | 2000 | 2005 |
|---|---|---|---|---|---|---|---|
| Food | 41.7 | 41.7 | 39.0 | 40.0 | 37.7 | 38.0 | 34.8 |
| Housing | 27.9 | 29 | 27.7 | 22 | 22.2 | 21.5 | 22.8 |
| Clothing | 8.8 | 8.5 | 6.0 | 10.2 | 11.9 | 11.1 | 8.8 |
| **Hygiene and health care** | **5.4** | **5.7** | **7.0** | **8.7** | **9.6** | **10.0** | **10.3** |
| Transport and telecommunications | 4.7 | 4.9 | 9.0 | 8.2 | 8.7 | 9.7 | 14.4 |
| Education, culture, and recreation | 8.0 | 7.7 | 8.9 | 8.5 | 8.9 | 8.7 | 8.4 |
| Other expenses | 3.5 | 2.5 | 2.4 | 2.4 | 1.0 | 1.0 | 0.5 |
| Total | 100 | 100 | 100 | 100 | 100 | 100 | 100 |

*Source:* NIS Surveys.

TD 600, and to almost 6 percent for households with monthly incomes ranging between TD 200 and TD 2,400.

The private sector has absorbed a significant portion (87.3 percent) of household health care expenditures in 2000. This can be explained by the subsidization of health care services offered in public (9.9 percent) and parastatal (2.8 percent) facilities (Arfa and Achour 2004).

Household health expenditures represent 55 percent of total "hygiene and health care" expenditures. Drugs and ambulatory medical consultations absorb 79 percent of these expenditures (table 13.15).

Figure 13.6 shows the progression of annual health care expenditures per capita, according to several household surveys. These expenditures, in current dinars,

**Table 13.15   Tunisia: Household Expenditures, by Service Category, 2000**

| Expenditure | Amount (TD) | Percentage |
|---|---|---|
| Pharmaceutical commodities | 33.3 | 47 |
| Ambulatory care | 22.7 | 32 |
| Hospitalization | 9.8 | 14 |
| Additional consultations | 3.7 | 5 |
| Other | 1.4 | 2 |
| Total | 70.9 | 100 |

*Source:* INS 2000.

**Figure 13.6   Tunisia: Annual Health Care Expenditure, per Capita, 1975–2005**

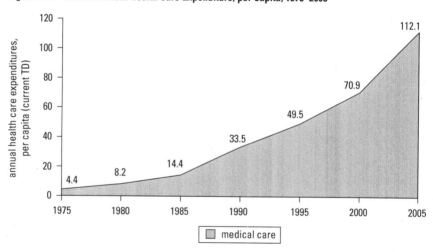

*Source:* INS 1975–2000, 2007.

**Table 13.16   Tunisia: Health Care Provision, by Facility Type, 2004**

| Facility type | | |
|---|---|---|
| **Public (number)** | **Parastatal (number)** | **Private (number)** |
| University hospital centers (22) | NFSS polyclinics (06) | Clinics |
| Regional hospitals (32) | Military hospitals (03) | Multidisciplinary (49) |
| District hospitals (118) | National security force hospitals (01) | Monodisciplinary (32) |
| CSSB (2.067) | | Dialysis centers (99) |
| | | Private physician practices (4.641) |

*Source:* MSP Report 2005.

grew by a factor of 16 between 1975 and 2000, from TD 4.4 to TD 70.9. On the other hand, in 1990 constant dinars, the yearly expenses increased from TD 38.5 in 1995 to TD 48.2 in 2000.

## Health Care Delivery

Health care is delivered through public, parastatal, and private facilities (table 13.16). The facilities are concentrated in the eastern coastal areas. The public sector is predominant, with 87.5 percent of hospital beds and more than 55 percent of all medical personnel. Tertiary health care services are the main public sector providers. Private delivery of health care, especially for hospitalization and basic medical services, has grown rapidly, and private bed capacity has doubled in the past five years.

### Public Sector Trends

The public sector is comprised of parastatal institutions and facilities that report directly to the Ministry of Public Health (table 13.16).

MSP provision of care is organized at three levels. The primary health care centers are the entry point in the public sector (table 13.17). The 2,067 centers, serving 4,500 persons (in 2004), form a decentralized network that responds to the population's most immediate needs. The rural natal care centers and district hospitals (118 hospitals with 2,613 beds) offer medical care, a maternity ward, and basic medical services. The regional hospitals (34 hospitals with 5,479 beds) are located in the administrative centers and are the first referral point for specialized medical services. University hospitals and their related centers (22 facilities with 8,590 beds) are located in the four cities that have medical schools (Tunis, Sousse, Monastir, and Sfax).

The parastatal sector encompasses health facilities that belong to other ministries: three military hospitals and a national security forces hospital. It also has six ambulatory care facilities ("polyclinics"), located in large cities and reserved for NFSS affiliates, and nine health care facilities offering in-house medical services for the personnel of certain companies.

**Table 13.17   Tunisia: Number of Beds in MSP Facilities**

| MSP facilities | 1970 | 1980 | 1989 | 1992 | 1996 | 1998 | 2000 | 2002 | 2004 |
|---|---|---|---|---|---|---|---|---|---|
| University hospital | | | | | | | | | |
| • Number | — | 8 | 22 | 21 | 20 | 22 | 22 | 22 | 22 |
| • Beds | — | — | 7,723 | 7,659 | 7,752 | 7,987 | 7,854 | 7,650 | 8,590 |
| Regional hospitals | | | | | | | | | |
| • Number | 12 | 20 | 24 | 24 | 29 | 31 | 32 | 32 | 34 |
| • Beds | — | — | 4784 | 5,360 | 5,578 | 5,379 | 5,420 | 5,450 | 5,479 |
| District hospitalsa | | | | | | | | | |
| • Number | 54 | 54 | 98 | 109 | 111 | 105 | 118a | 118 | 118 |
| • Beds | — | — | 2,664 | 2,793 | 2,640 | 2,647 | — | — | 2,613 |
| Primary health care centers | 435 | 765 | 1,462 | 1,611 | 1,841 | 1,922 | 2,008 | 2,220 | 2,067 |
| Total public hospitals | | | | | | | | | |
| • Number | — | 82 | 144 | 154 | 160 | 158 | 172 | 172 | 174 |
| • Beds | — | — | 15,407 | 15,812 | 15,970 | 16,013 | 16,659 | — | 16,682 |

*Source:* MSP databases 2005.

*Note:* — = not available.

a. Includes autonomous maternity facilities.

## Private Sector Trends

Medical practice in Tunisia has always been organized around the individual physician's practice. Hospitals are a recent development. With the exception of the St. Augustin clinic, founded in 1930, most other hospitals were created after 1970, especially in the 1990s.

In 2004, 81 private clinics with 2,379 beds were registered, 12.5 percent of the national hospital capacity. The greatest expansion (5.5 percent) has occurred in the number of hemodialysis centers between 1990 and 2004 (table 13.18).

## Increase in Number of Hospital Beds

The reorganization of public and private sector roles in Tunisia can be seen in the sharp rise in the number of private beds since 1992 (table 13.19). Public hospitalization capacity has increased only slightly (and mainly in special services centers and university hospitals). During the same period, private sector capacity has doubled. The combined increases, public and private, has stabilized of the total average number of beds at close to two beds per 1,000 persons (2004).

## Evolution of the Health Sector's Employment Structure

Throughout the 1960s, Tunisia's medical personnel density declined, especially after independence with the departure of many foreign physicians. Since 1985, when there were only four physicians per 10,000 persons, the ratio has almost doubled (table 13.20). This growth has been marked by a much faster increase in specialist physicians (6.9 percent) than in general practitioners (3.7 percent). Growth was also faster in the private sector between 1981 and 2004.

**Table 13.18 Tunisia: Private Health Facilities**

| Facility | 1990 Number | 1990 Beds | 2004 Number | 2004 Beds |
|---|---|---|---|---|
| Clinics | 33 | 1,142 | 81 | 2,379 |
| Multidisciplinary | 25 | 1,060 | 49 | 2,175 |
| Monodisciplinary | 8 | 82 | 32 | 204 |
| Dialysis centers | 18 | 205 | 99 | 986 |

*Source:* MSP databases 2005.

**Table 13.19 Tunisia: Number of Public and Private Hospital Beds, 1985–2004**

| Hospital beds | 1985 | 1989 | 1992 | 1996 | 1997 | 1998 | 2002 | 2004 |
|---|---|---|---|---|---|---|---|---|
| Public sector | 15,000 | 15,400 | 15,845 | 15,792 | 15,943 | 16,013 | 16,182 | 17,269 |
| Private sector | 974 | 950 | 1,638 | 1,974 | 1,894 | 1,944 | 2,000 | 2,379 |
| Total beds | 15,974 | 16,350 | 17,483 | 19,766 | 17,837 | 17,957 | 18,182 | 19,648 |
| Public share (%) | 94 | 94 | 91 | 89 | 89 | 89 | 89 | 88 |

*Source:* MSP databases 2005.

**Table 13.20 Tunisia: The Physician Workforce, 1981–2004**

| Year | General practitioners Public | General practitioners Private | General practitioners Total | Medical specialists Public | Medical specialists Private | Medical specialists Total | Total |
|---|---|---|---|---|---|---|---|
| 1981 | 547 | 380 | 927 | 857 | 294 | 1,151 | 2,078 |
| 1985 | 925 | 670 | 1,595 | 947 | 357 | 1,304 | 2,899 |
| 1991 | 1,524 | 959 | 2,483 | 1,110 | 799 | 1,909 | 4,392 |
| 1995 | 1,767 | 1,468 | 3,235 | 1,425 | 1,305 | 2,730 | 5,965 |
| 1998 | 2,022 | 1,526 | 3,548 | 1,735 | 1,507 | 3,242 | 6,790 |
| 2002 | 1,983 | 1,620 | 3,603 | 2,164 | 1,667 | 3,831 | 7,434 |
| 2003 | 2,552 | 1,620 | 4,667 | 2,115 | 1,677 | 3,297 | 7,469 |
| 2004 | 2,737 | 2,635 | 5,372 | 2,427 | 2,006 | 4,433 | 9,805 |

*Source:* MSP databases 2005.

Tunisia has also invested heavily in paramedical personnel. The number of nurses and midwives has increased at a rate similar to that of physicians, due to intensive recruitment.

The paramedical personnel workforce employed in the private sector increased 10-fold, from 500 in 1998 to 5,000 in 2002. Private clinics are required to maintain 0.3 or 0.4 nurses per bed, depending on the type of care needed. In reality, there are about 0.8 paramedical personnel and 0.3 physicians per bed.

**Figure 13.7  Tunisia: Average Growth in the Number of Physicians, Dentists, Pharmacists, and Paramedical Personnel, Selected Periods**

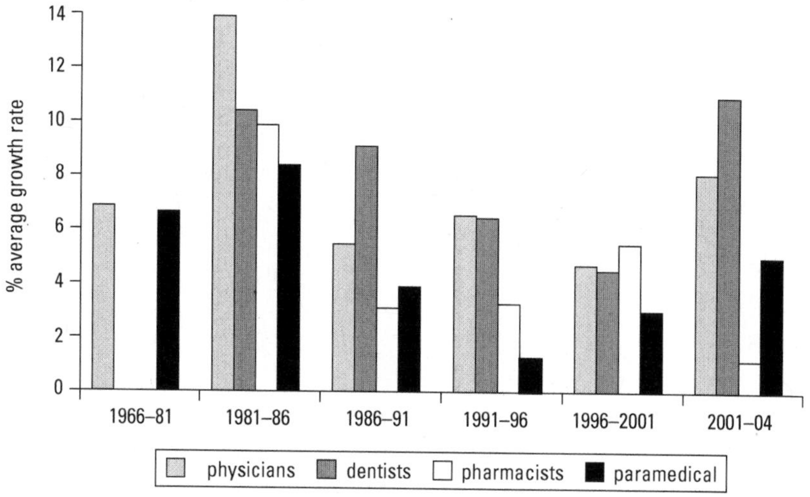

*Source:* MSP databases.

## Human Resources Development

Figure 13.7 shows the growth trends for physicians, dentists, pharmacists, and paramedical personnel for various five-year periods, and table 13.21 shows the most recent numbers. In 1981–86, the highest growth rates were recorded, reflecting both the public sector's need for health professionals and the introduction of certification opportunities. For the other periods, the growth rate remained below 10 percent.

For physicians, growth rates dropped from 14 percent in 1981–86 to 5 percent in 1986–91. Public sector recruitment was reduced for the second period after

**Table 13.21  Tunisia: Number of Medical Personnel, 1990–2004**

| Health professionals | 1981 | 1986 | 1990 | 1995 | 2000 | 2004 |
|---|---|---|---|---|---|---|
| Physicians | 1,800 | 3,450 | 4,424 | 5,965 | 7,444 | 9,805 |
| Dentists | 320 | 525 | 809 | 1,038 | 1,315 | 1,889 |
| Pharmacists | 700 | 1,120 | 1,240 | 1,499 | 1,951 | 2,069 |
| Paramedical staff[a] | 13,570 | 20,300 | 23,743 | 25,874 | 27,392 | 29,584 |
| Population per physician | 3,200 | 2,110 | 1,825 | 1,500 | 1,284 | 1,013 |
| Population per paramedical staff | — | — | 340 | 346 | 340 | 336 |

*Source:* MSP database.

*Note:* — = not available.

a. Technicians, nurses, midwives, and health auxiliaries.

great efforts to satisfy requirements. The adjustments in the economic plan and private sector development also explain the decreased growth in the public sector.

Competitive admission to nursing schools in Tunisia depends solely on the MSP, the major employer of nurses. Nursing employment therefore reflects job availabilities and needs in public facilities as, for example, 4 percent growth in 1991–2004 and a decrease to 1 percent in 1991–96.

Since the second half of the 1990s, Tunisia has been confronted with unemployment among certain health care professionals—general practitioners, technicians, and even some medical specialists. Unemployment is less problematic for pharmacists and dentists.

## Other Components of the Health Care Delivery System

Professional training, pharmaceuticals, and medical technology, all vital inputs to the health system, are available in Tunisia.

*Training of health professionals.* The medical education system consists of 4 medical schools, 1 pharmacy school, 1 dentistry school, 4 Colleges of Science and Health Technology for Medical Technicians (17 sections for midwives, physiotherapists, hygienists, and laboratory technicians), and 19 Professional Schools of Public Health for nurses training.

*Procurement and distribution of pharmaceuticals.* The pharmaceutical sector is characterized by collaboration between public and private actors. The sector is regulated and supervised by the MSP and through its public institutions: the National Pharmaceutical Control Laboratory (Laboratoire National de Contrôle des Médicaments, LNCM), the National Pharmacovigilance Center. (Centre National de Pharmacovigilance, CNPV), the Tunisian Central Medical Store (Pharmacie Centrale de Tunisie, PCT), and the Pasteur Institute in Tunis.

The local pharmaceutical industry has seen significant growth. Consumption of locally produced pharmaceuticals grew from 8 percent in 1987 to almost 45 percent in 2001. Pharmaceutical consumption in Tunisia was estimated at TD 400 million for 2001, less than 0.1 percent of the global market. Pharmaceutical consumption per capita rose from 30 percent in 1995 to 40 percent in 2001, valued at close to TD 42.

The Tunisian Central Medical Store handles drug distribution. Its network of private wholesale dealers covers the entire country. The MSP facilities ensure distribution of pharmaceuticals to patients through a dense network of private pharmacies. The PCT, the only institution authorized to import drugs and vaccines, acts as the central purchasing agency for all national needs.

*The role of medical technology.* The evolution of medical technology is illustrated in table 13.22. MSP regulations maintain a list of medical equipment that needs approval prior to installation. Under these regulations, data are also gathered to determine whether there is a regional need for particular technologies.

**Table 13.22   Tunisia: Amount of Large-Scale Medical Equipment, 1995–2004**

| | 1995 | | 1997 | | 2003 | | 2004 | |
|---|---|---|---|---|---|---|---|---|
| **Equipment** | **Public** | **Private** | **Public** | **Private** | **Public** | **Private** | **Public** | **Private** |
| MRI | 1 | 0 | 2 | 0 | 3 | 5 | 4 | 6 |
| Scanner | 7 | 20 | 8 | 29 | 15 | 54 | 20 | 54 |
| Lithotriptor | 3 | 3 | 3 | 5 | 3 | 12 | 3 | 13 |
| Telecobaltotherapy | 1 | 4 | 2 | 6 | 4 | 5 | 4 | 5 |
| Angiography scanner | — | — | 2 | 9 | 6 | 10 | 6 | 10 |
| Cardiovascular catheterization | 4 | 1 | 7 | 4 | 9 | 10 | 10 | 10 |
| Cardiopulmonary bypass | 4 | — | 4 | 6 | 6 | 12 | 6 | 12 |

*Source:* MSP database.

*Note:* — = not available.

## Health Sector Regulation

Health policy formulation and health care system regulation are ensured by the state government and ministries, professional health organizations, and the Social Security funds.

The regulatory tools are used in health care delivery, and efforts are being made to integrate quality assurance.

## Health Care Provision Regulation

Health care provision policies address productivity factors, professional practice, and financial remuneration for goods and services. During the past 30 years, regulations have been diversified. The current legislation follows the total health supply and its growth for both public and private sectors regarding the certification of health needs which is renewable at least five years.

*Public sector infrastructure.* Infrastructure development is integrated in the five-year plan and the annual budget. "Needs" are defined within the five-year development frameworks that decide infrastructure and equipment projects. The development process is closely associated with the regions, which express their needs to the Ministry of Public Health and to the Ministry of Economic Development (both in charge of planning), as well as to the Ministry of Finance within the annual budget framework.

*Private sector infrastructure.* Private provision of ambulatory health services and hospitalization are not subject to regulations regarding geographic location, but to standard norms for buildings, technical installations, and equipment. Private dialysis centers are the only private health care facilities subject to a prior authorization, based on the regional government's evaluation of the population's needs. The distribution of pharmacists is regulated by quotas.

*Equipment and technology.* The public health organization law defines the large-scale equipment needing authorization prior to installation. The list is defined by a joint decree of the Ministries of Finance, Trade, and Public Health. The MSP defines the population-need indicators for each type of equipment.

*Drugs and other pharmaceutical commodities.* Drugs and pharmaceutical commodities are strictly regulated. The rules cover procurement (state monopoly), manufacturing, distribution, and sale. Drugs distributed in Tunisia are listed under their generic names, in both the public and the private sectors. The pharmaceutical sector is recognized as strategic sector with social implications, so it was subjected to strict rules on retail prices. Pharmaceutical costs are officially recognized and compensated by Tunisian Central Pharmacy.

*Regulation of the medical demography.* Access to medical education, limited by quotas at the four national medical schools, has been limited to around 700 admissions a year since 1994, despite a large increase in the number of bachelor degree holders. Access to medical specialization studies is regulated by annual residency competitions; the number of available places is limited according to the MSP annual budget.

## Demand Regulation

Demand is regulated through user fees. In the public sector, copayments have been in effect since the early 1980s and have been regularly increased. Besides "moderating" health care consumption, they are also believed to channel patient referrals according to various health care needs: copayments are highest in tertiary care facilities and lowest in primary care facilities. All reimbursement schemes, regardless of the insuring institution, have two regulation strategies: user fees and an annual expenditure cap, for which the amounts vary by scheme and by insurance policy.

## Quality Assurance and Control

Since the beginning of the 1990s, quality improvement of health care has become an important component in health facility management. Actions taken to improve the quality of care include: the development of a national strategy for continuous quality improvement, currently in its early implementation stages; awareness-raising and encouragement of practical education in quality management; a system of quality assurance for pharmaceuticals; quality control of laboratory tests; and the execution and acknowledgment of patient satisfaction survey results.

## Other Types of Regulation

Among the other types of medical regulation are a "best practice" guide and medical inspections and controls. Contracting of intensive care services, initially done only for the socially insured, was expanded to routine care in regional and university hospitals under the auspices of the MSP.

## Current Regulation Trends

The latest trends in health system regulation bring together all stakeholders and are reflected in the framework for implementing health insurance reform. In particular, they address contracting and the promotion of medical control procedures.

Health insurance reform is based on a clear-cut distinction between the basic mandatory scheme, administered by the National Health Insurance Fund (NHIF), and the supplementary schemes under private health insurance. To avoid duplication, private insurers are permitted to cover only health care services that supplement services covered by the basic scheme.

Contracting between the NHIF and providers is the only mechanism governing relations between insurers and providers. These agreements allow the definition of specific regulations for medical practice and the setting of health care fees. Medical control procedures monitor the quality of services delivered to the insured against national and international standards.

## The Health Information System

The information system is one of the Tunisian health system's weaknesses. In its present state, the system consists of subsystems for managing the different parts of the health care system. Data from the oldest component, the system for collecting statistical information on health facility activities, are collected by the central administration's statistics division. The national family and population office maintains an efficient information system on family planning, birth rate regulation, and reproductive health mission and activities.

During the 1980s, the accent was placed on basic health care services. Collection methods and data management guidelines were put into place in various domains. Since the 1990s, the hospital system has been the principal interest, sustained by two World Bank projects. One project component involves implementation of a computerized information management system used by the Computer Center of the Ministry of Public Health (Centre d'Informatique du Ministère de la Santé Publique, CIMSP). So far, the system offers only classic management tools and does not integrate patient health care information or data on human resources management.

The information system's current inefficiencies, attributed to its fragmentation and challenges peculiar to the hospital sector, forced the public authorities to commission a comprehensive study. The study objectives are to conceive a new basis for developing and implementing a strategy for a patient-centered information system. This study was submitted to the government within the framework of investment proposals for the 2007–11 development plan.

## Expenditures, Services, and Outcomes

In the absence of quantitative information linking expenditures to services and to outcomes, worsened by a decline in expenditures and revenues, only general information can be provided from comparisons with other countries.

Tunisia is a middle-income country at an average developmental level. Its health care expenditures (5.6 percent) are moderate and comparable with other Middle East and North African countries. With annual expenditures of less than $150 per capita, Tunisia has achieved some remarkable successes in health. One of its most pertinent health-related accomplishments is the significant decrease in the infant mortality rate. Between 1966 and 2004, the Tunisian population's life expectancy at birth increased by 21.8 years (table 13.23). During this period, women gained 23.7 years, men 20.8 years (figure 13.2). Throughout these 44 years, life expectancy at birth has been higher in Tunisia than in other MENA Region countries (World Bank 2006b), a continuing trend that is bringing Tunisia's health status closer to that of OECD countries.

Tunisia has made significant progress in health care coverage (table 13.24) and compares favorably with other middle-income countries and other countries in the MENA Region. In terms of primary health care coverage, the indicators have consistently improved (table 13.24), as indicated by the percentage of the population (95 percent) having access to it and to prenatal care (92 percent). Skilled personnel attend births (90 percent) and render child care (96 percent). Similarly, as a result of immunization policy, more than 98 percent of Tunisian children under 1 year of age are vaccinated against diphtheria, tetanus, pertussis, poliomyelitis, measles, and BCG. Vaccine coverage rates are similar to those in OECD countries.

Tunisia's health outcomes compare favorably with those of other similar countries (table 13.25).

## Equity and Access to Health Care

Under current coverage schemes, access to health care is within the reach of the entire Tunisian population, regardless of household financial capacity. These

**Table 13.23   Tunisia: Life Expectancy and Infant Mortality Compared with MENA Region, 1960–2004**

| | 1960 | | 1980 | | 2000 | | 2004 | |
|---|---|---|---|---|---|---|---|---|
| **Indicators** | **MENA** | **Tunisia** | **MENA** | **Tunisia** | **MENA** | **Tunisia** | **MENA** | **Tunisia** |
| Life expectancy at birth (years) | 47 | 48.6 | 58 | 62.4 | 68 | 72.1 | 68 | 73.3 |
| Infant mortality per 1,000 live births | 262 | 160 | 138 | 60 | 47 | 25 | 45 | 20.6 |

*Sources:* World Bank 2004c; NIS 2005; UNPD 2005.

**Table 13.24    Tunisia: Coverage with Primary Health Care Services, 2005**

| Indicator | Coverage rate (%) |
|---|---|
| Population with access to local health services, total | 95 |
| Contraceptive prevalence rate | 62 |
| Prenatal care coverage | 92[a] |
| Births attended by skilled health personnel | 90[a] |
| Infants attended by trained personnel | 96[b] |
| 1-year-olds immunized in 2005 with BCG | 98 |
| 1-year-olds immunized in 2005 with DPT | 98 |
| 1-year-olds immunized in 2005 with OPV | 98 |
| 1-year-olds immunized in 2005 with measles vaccine | 96 |
| 1-year-olds immunized in 2005 with hepatitis B vaccine | 97 |
| Pregnant women immunized with two or more doses of tetanus toxoid | 88 |

*Source:* WHO (http://www.emro.who.int/emrinfo/index.asp?Ctry=tun).

a. Data for 2004.

b. Data for 2000.

schemes are for social protection, with or without supplementary coverage, in place since the late 1950s and the early 1960s and for medical assistance of the poor not covered by the mandatory health insurance schemes. However, despite nearly universal coverage, household expenditures for health care remain very high in Tunisia. This situation is a source of inequity and a principal driver of health insurance reform. Indeed, Tunisia is confronted by two types of problems that explain this high proportion of household expenditures: underfinancing in the public sector, which prevents it from providing all its users with needed goods and services needed, and low reimbursement rates, especially the CNRPS outdated reimbursement schemes.

The World Health Report (WHO 2000) uses a financial contribution indicator to illustrate inequity. On this measure, Tunisia is similar to other middle-income countries in the MENA Region (table 13.26).

The expansion of public provision has improved access to health care, notably through the development of the primary health sector. A dense network of primary health centers throughout the country is connected to a network of district hospitals that provide primary health, pediatric, and obstetric services. Most of the population (90 percent) can walk to a primary health care center in less than an hour.

Along the same lines, access to specialists' services has gradually improved. The public hospital network, offering various specialist services, is comprised of regional and university hospitals. The government, through financial incentives, encourages access to specialist doctors, especially in underserved areas. Yet

**Table 13.25 Tunisia: Health Outcomes Compared with Similar Countries**

| Indicators | Upper middle-income | | Lower middle-income | | Middle-income | | MENA region | | Tunisia | |
|---|---|---|---|---|---|---|---|---|---|---|
| | 1990 | 2004 | 1990 | 2004 | 1990 | 2004 | 1990 | 2004 | 1990 | 2004 |
| **Reduce child mortality** | | | | | | | | | | |
| Immunization, measles (% of children ages 12–23 months) | 79.7 | 91.2 | 87 | 85.4 | 85.9 | 86.5 | 83.3 | 92 | 93 | 95 |
| Mortality rate, infant (per 1,000 live births) | 33 | 23 | 46 | 33 | 44 | 31 | 60 | 44 | 41 | 21 |
| Mortality rate, under-5 (per 1,000) | 41 | 28 | 62 | 42 | 58 | 39 | 81 | 55 | 52 | 25 |
| **Improve maternal health** | | | | | | | | | | |
| Births attended by skilled health staff (% of total) | — | 94.7 | — | 85.7 | — | 87.3 | 45.6 | 72.3 | 83[a] | 92[b] |
| Maternal mortality ratio (modeled estimate, per 100,000 live births) | — | — | — | — | — | — | — | — | 69[c] | 48[b] |
| **Combat HIV/AIDS, malaria, and other diseases** | | | | | | | | | | |
| Incidence of tuberculosis (per 100,000 people) | 69 | 113.6 | 134 | 114.9 | 120.8 | 114.7 | 66.2 | 53.9 | 33.1 | 22 |
| Prevalence of HIV, total (% of population ages 15–49) | — | 2 | — | 0 | — | 1 | — | 0 | — | 0 |
| Tuberculosis cases detected under DOTS (%) | — | 72.3 | — | 68.4 | — | 69.5 | — | 50.2 | — | 95.5 |
| **Life expectancy, fertility, and literacy** | | | | | | | | | | |
| Fertility rate, total (births per woman) | 2.6 | 1.9 | 2.7 | 2.2 | 2.7 | 2.1 | 4.8 | 3 | 3.5 | 2 |
| Life expectancy at birth, total (years) | 69.2 | 69.2 | 67.3 | 70.2 | 67.6 | 70 | 64.3 | 69.3 | 70.3 | 73.3 |
| Literacy rate, adult total (% of people ages 15 and above) | 91.5 | 93.6 | 78.1 | 89 | 80.7 | 89.8 | 51.8 | 72.1 | 59.1 | 74.3 |

*Source:* World Bank 2006c (www.ddp-ext.worldbank.org).

*Note:* — = not available.

a. Data for 1998.

b. MSP database 2005.

c. Data for 1993.

Table 13.26  Tunisia: Inequity of Financial Contribution Indicators
Compared with Similar Countries

| Country | Rank | Inequity of financial contribution indicators |
|---------|------|-----------------------------------------------|
| Jordan | 49 | 0.958 |
| Iraq | 56 | 0.952 |
| Tunisia | 108 | 0.925 |
| Iran, Islamic Rep. of | 112 | 0.923 |
| Egypt, Arab Rep. of | 125 | 0.915 |
| Morocco | 125 | 0.915 |
| Syrian Arab Rep. | 142 | 0.904 |

*Source:* WHO 2000.

significant disparities persist between urban and rural areas in terms of availability of health services. Hospitals and specialized physicians are concentrated in large urban centers (the capital Tunis, Sousse, Monastir in central Tunisia, and Sfax in southern Tunisia).

Uneven improvement in health indicators coincides with geographic disparities in terms of socioeconomic development. It also affects vulnerable groups, such as women, children, adolescents, and the elderly. Infant mortality rates are much higher in rural than in urban areas, sometimes double. Maternal and neonatal mortality, maternal and infant anemia, diarrhea, and respiratory infections in children under five years (U-5) consistently show higher rates in rural or peri-urban underserved areas, as well as in the western and southern regions. The health indicators published by WHO (2006), though reporting 1998 data for Tunisia (table 13.27), confirm significant differences by residential area (rural or urban), as well as the mother's educational attainment.

## The Health System's Strengths and Weaknesses

Accessibility is the greatest strength of the Tunisian health system. The growing needs of its population and its limited resources are its greatest weaknesses.

### Health System Strengths

Five signs point to the accessibility of the Tunisian health system:

- The system has covered almost the entire population since the late 1950s and early 1960s.
- Its modern public health infrastructure has been expanded, regularly maintained, and updated.
- Different types of health care professionals have been educated in Tunisia since the early 1960s.

**Table 13.27  Tunisia: Health Inequalities Compared with Similar Countries**

| Country | Year | Under-5 mortality rate (per 1,000 live births) | | | | | | Proportion of Under-5 children with delayed growth (%) | | | | | |
| | | Place of residence | | | Mother's educational attainment | | | Place of residency | | | Mother's educational attainment | | |
| | | Rural (1) | Urban (2) | Ratio (1)/(2) | Lowest (1) | Highest (2) | Ratio (1)/(2) | Rural (1) | Urban (2) | Ratio (1)/(2) | Lowest (1) | Highest (2) | Ratio (1)/(2) |
|---|---|---|---|---|---|---|---|---|---|---|---|---|---|
| Egypt, Arab Rep. of | 2000 | 79 | 53 | 1.5 | 89 | 40 | 2.2 | 22 | 14 | 1.6 | 23 | 15 | 1.5 |
| Jordan | 2002 | 36 | 27 | 1.3 | 44 | 26 | 1.7 | 13 | 7 | 1.8 | 20 | 8 | 2.7 |
| Morocco | 2003–04 | 69 | 38 | 1.8 | 63 | 27 | 2.3 | 24 | 13 | 1.8 | 22 | 10 | 2.1 |
| South Africa | 1998 | 71 | 43 | 1.6 | 84 | 46 | 1.8 | ... | ... | ... | ... | ... | ... |
| Tunisia | 1988 | 85 | 62 | 1.4 | 84 | 39 | 2.2 | 25 | 12 | 2.1 | 22 | 5 | 4.6 |
| Yemen | 1997 | 128 | 96 | 1.3 | 126 | 71 | 1.8 | 56 | 40 | 1.4 | 54 | 29 | 1.9 |

| Country | Year | Births attended by skilled health personnel (%) | | | | | | Measles immunization coverage among 1-year-olds (%) | | | | | |
| | | Place of residence | | | Mother's educational attainment | | | Place of residency | | | Mother's educational attainment | | |
| | | Rural (1) | Urban (2) | Ratio (1)/(2) | Lowest (1) | Highest (2) | Ratio (1)/(2) | Rural (1) | Urban (2) | Ratio (1)/(2) | Lowest (1) | Highest (2) | Ratio (1)/(2) |
|---|---|---|---|---|---|---|---|---|---|---|---|---|---|
| Egypt, Arab Rep. of | 2000 | 48 | 81 | 1.7 | 40 | 81 | 2.0 | 98 | 96 | 1.0 | 98 | 95 | 1.0 |
| Jordan | 2002 | 97 | 99 | 1.0 | 91 | 99 | 1.1 | 95 | 94 | 1.0 | 96 | 81 | 1.2 |
| Morocco | 2003–04 | 40 | 85 | 2.2 | 49 | 94 | 1.9 | 94 | 86 | 1.1 | 96 | 88 | 1.1 |
| South Africa | 1998 | 76 | 93 | 1.2 | 60 | 91 | 1.5 | 85 | 79 | 1.1 | 86 | 64 | 1.3 |
| Tunisia | 1988 | 50 | 87 | 1.7 | 54 | 97 | 1.8 | 91 | 77 | 1.2 | 94 | 77 | 1.2 |
| Yemen | 1997 | 14 | 47 | 3.3 | 16 | 63 | 3.8 | 72 | 34 | 2.1 | 74 | 37 | 2.0 |

*Source:* World Health Statistics WHO 2006.

- Tunisia has introduced a primary health care strategy, based on WHO recommendations, responding the population's basic health care needs, including family planning and maternal and child health.
- The coexistence of a public and private health delivery system has largely contributed to the population's overall health status improvement.

## Health System Weaknesses

The growing needs of the population, its evolving demographic and socioeconomic status, costly medical technology innovations, and the scarcity of financial resources allocated for health care are all evidence of systemic weaknesses.

In terms of health care provision, there are regional disparities between the east and the west, in terms of infrastructure, human resources, and large-scale medical equipment. In terms of health care financing, the public sector is underfinanced, especially for primary health care. So, too, is health care consumption, as seen in the large share of household spending on out-of-pocket payments. In terms of governance, the system suffers from the absence of an organized evaluation plan, especially for service quality, and the fragmented information systems poses a major barrier to any evaluation attempts. The referral system is also weak. In terms of continuing medical education, current efforts remain insufficient in their general organization and the means allocated to it.

## The Health System during the Reform

When the health insurance reform was designed, health care was provided mainly in a dense, decentralized public sector. In the private sector, the ambulatory component was decentralizing, and the hospital sector was rapidly gaining importance. Health care providers were concentrated in the large urban centers.

Two financing methods coexisted: the Bismarck mandatory health insurance and the Beveridge system of targeting the poor and those with limited incomes. The mandatory health insurance model has been gradually replacing the Beveridge model since 1995.

Financing from public funds is almost completely reserved for public health care provision, and provision in the private sector is financed mostly from households.

The heavy burden of direct financing on households for health expenditures (51.3 percent) resulted in inequity in health care access and, to a certain extent, the impoverishment of certain vulnerable populations. From a grant-based financing of health care, the system moved gradually toward fee for service: increasingly, "money follows the patient." A new sharing of health care–related financial expenditures is being designed to reduce those of government and households and replace them with a contribution toward a mandatory social health insurance scheme. The CNAM has increased competition among health care providers and health care services, based on quality and price. More and more, it will act like an "informed consumer" of health care providers for its members.

In terms of resource mobilization, Tunisia has developed important capacity for training health care professionals of different types. Nevertheless, the health sector needs to integrate new occupations, especially in management, engineering, and computer sciences.

Newly certified health professionals, especially some types of paramedical personnel and general practitioners, undergo a longer than usual unemployment period. Also, despite a high medical density (one physician per 1,000 people), disparities persist. Specialist physicians are scarce, especially in Tunisia's western regions.

The development of medical technology has encouraged the public authorities to introduce a "health card for large-scale medical equipment" as a mechanism for regulating investment in this type of equipment. At the same time, the rapid development of the private hospital sector has promoted a significant growth in capital investment, without any evaluation of the utilization of such large-scale medical equipment.

Due to current regulations, drug management is satisfactory throughout sector. However, public health facilities, strained by underfinancing, cannot fill all the prescriptions received.

In terms of general administration and governance, Tunisia has introduced a strong legal and regulatory arsenal for the administration of the health sector, especially for its policy component. Meanwhile, the regulation of health care provision in the private sector remains weak because of the near-absence of an operational arm, such as public financing. Increasingly, private sector health professionals promote strategic attitudes, allowing them to better manage social negotiations. And decision making in the public sector remains extremely centralized, in terms of both financial investment and deployment of human resources. Despite of current regulations promoting autonomy in the hospital sector, strategic and operational decisions regarding hospitals are still being made externally.

Three main stakeholders play a role in the health insurance reform process, each with divergent interests and often conflicting goals: the central labor union, the General Union of Tunisian Laborers (Union Générale des Travailleurs Tunisiens, UGTT), professional organizations of private providers, and work-based organizations. The governmental departments involved in reform are the ministries responsible for financing and for health and social affairs (under the auspices of the SSF and the health insurance).

The UGTT has proposed an upgrade of the public sector to meet the same standards as the private sector instead of having the two sectors compete with each other. This idea is motivated by fear of health services privatization and the subsequent risks regarding job security in the public sector. The union also opposes an increase in the employees' contributions to the health insurance schemes, for fear of a chain of unrestricted increases, and calls for a direct government contribution to mandatory health insurance schemes. The union also wants an expansion of the benefits packages, without any increases in contribution rates or copayments, preferring third-party payers (NHIF) to reimbursement systems.

The professional organizations of private providers are seeking reimbursement of charges through third-party payers. They are opposed to "managed care" and endorse health care management by the family doctor chosen by the patient. They are against movements to regulate medical practice and prescriptions and want a reduction in outside procedures for managing the insured's health care.

The work-based organizations are the Tunisian Union for Industry, Trade, and Crafts and the Tunisian Union for Agriculture and Fisheries. These organizations favor enforcement of enterprises' social responsibilities in the areas of national and international competition and employment. They are against job insecurity in the agricultural sector, which they say weakens the contributory capacity of both laborers and enterprises.

## Motivations for Key Health Sector Reforms

The reform of the Tunisian health care system is taking place in three overlapping stages, shaped by the shifting needs of the sector, the national and international environment, and the resulting constraints. The first reforms were motivated by the heavy burden of infectious diseases, malnutrition, and maternal mortality and morbidity. Health care provision was extensively expanded through the development of the public health network. This expansion was financed primarily by the government, which also ensured training and recruitment of most health care professionals. Budgetary pressures impelled the next wave of reforms. Intensive efforts were made to raise efficiency in the public sector by improving resource allocation and service quality.

Now public-private partnerships are being explored for delivery and financing to meet new and growing needs arising from the demographic and the epidemiologic transitions. Unable to respond to all these needs, the public authorities have been forced to reexamine the partitioning of health expenditures and to offer the insured a choice between public and private providers. The rapid development of the private sector and the heavy burden of health expenditures on households also influenced this course of action.

Equity considerations and other underlying societal values have been translated into the promotion of access to health care in all three stages. Different population groups place different values on the quality of health care. The better-off are increasingly seeking care in the private sector, which is more responsive to their demand for more than basic services. Economic efficiency is an idea not yet widely accepted among health professionals and remains a great challenge to health care system management.

## Timeline and Principal Reform Measures

The systemic reforms between 1980 and 2004 addressed delivery and financing of health care services.

Reforms of health care delivery took place in three major periods. From 1980 to 1990, the focus was on the development of primary health care. From 1985 to 1999, new management methods were introduced in the university hospital sector, beginning with the creation of the "public health establishment." During this period, a legal arsenal was introduced to incorporate the private hospital sector, previously regulated by laws dating to the end of the 19th century. Regulations were also introduced for the governance of private paramedical practice. From 1990 to 2004 regional hospitals have benefited, within the framework of a sector-wide project, from a revision of their organization and management, associated to the renewal and the modernization of their medical equipment.

In terms of financing, various paths have been followed. The care of the poor and of those with limited income has been the goal of successive revisions to improve targeting of eligible populations. In 1983, copayments were introduced and integrated into the resources of health care institutions. Health care financing mechanisms in public hospitals through Social Security have undergone several developments. The government's contribution to the treasury has been the primary source of MSP facilities financing. In the late 1980s, agreements for intensive care services were reached with some MSP facilities and have been expanded to private facilities in an attempt to reduce the number of foreign health care services used by the public and to build national capacity. Since 1996, a billing system has been gradually introduced and expanded. Apart from some adjustments in the classification of medical service and medical tariffs and fees, no specific measures regarding financing of service provision have been addressed to the private sector.

Measures regarding the general organization of the sector have been undertaken since the 1990s. The principal ones concern the following:

- A national strategy was adopted for the NHIS and its development from existing subsystems, including plans to obtain previously unavailable information (e.g., surveys, registries, death certificates).
- Organizational measures include the revision of the central organization and administration, revision of the mission, objectives and organization of regional administration, and the revision of public hospital management.
- Quality assurance of service provision has been the goal of the national strategy currently being implemented.

## Evaluation of the Reforms

As a result of the reforms, health care coverage has been extended and access to health care improved. However, under the impact of the socioeconomic, demographic, and epidemiologic transitions, these strategies and actions have generated: inefficiencies that have led to management reforms, centered on public hospitals; the need to mobilize additional financial resources for these institutions; and the need to revise intrainstitutional cost-sharing. Moreover, uneven progress in these reforms has left a fragmented system, and their impact on the sector's performance is difficult to evaluate. The weakness of the information system poses a major obstacle both to evaluation and implementation of the reforms.

Despite these limitations, certain evaluations can be ventured:

- The Tunisian health care system ensures reasonable coverage of the population's health care needs, but its eastern and western regions remain underserved, especially with regard to medical specialists. Rebalancing attempts by introducing financial incentives have not resulted in the desired outcomes.
- The private health care delivery sector has rapidly evolved due to a generally favorable environment and some specific support from government dealing with the investment code implemented on 1992, which includes many incentives rules. It still depends on out-of-pocket payment because health insurance is still only a small part of private financing. The recently created health insurance fund was regarded as a solution of this burden.
- The health care financing measures in the public sector have only minimally improved the financial situation of public hospitals; they are still underfinanced. Nonetheless, the new mechanisms will allow gradual replacement of funds allocated by government with funds from the Social Security funds.
- The reform strategies for management in public institutions have resulted in a modernization of management procedures. However, they have not reached the desired objectives, especially increased autonomy for hospitals, due to delays in reorganizing different levels of health sector management.
- The general regulation of the health sector, especially its private component, is weak, despite the numerous regulatory texts governing it.

Finally, the health sector badly needs to improve its capacity for medium- and long-term strategic planning to anticipate and plan for future trends. Two domains should be given priority: the sector's response to the epidemiologic transition and sustainability of health care financing. Indeed, the health sector is again confronted by new challenges such as: the transformation in the population pyramid, with a pronounced increase in the proportion of the elderly needing expensive, tertiary care; the promotion of financial accessibility to health care through more equitable cost sharing between the government and Social Security; the global trend toward liberalization of all economic activities, including services, and its impact on employment, the role of the public sector and its resources, and access to health care.

## Health Insurance Reform

This section deals with different aspects of Tunisia's health insurance reforms: purpose, objectives, introduction process, lessons learned and associated obstacles.

### The Purpose of the Health Insurance Reform

The health insurance system has managed to achieve reasonable coverage and access to health care, but there are still some insufficiencies. Between 1985 and

2004, health care expenditures escalated, with an increasing proportion falling on households. Fragmentation in the health insurance system has generated inequalities in terms of coverage and contribution rates, and the reimbursement rates for health care delivery charges within the NFPSP schemes are too low.

The situation is complicated by the strong influence exerted by private physicians. Because their revenue depends on their clients' solvency, the physicians are lobbying for the extension of health insurance coverage to the private sector.

## Reform Goals and Objectives

The decision to reform health insurance under the Social Security schemes was announced on May 1, 1995. It was analyzed in a preliminary study, presented to the government on February 16, 1996. This large-scale reform was to be based on

- The implementation of a basic, mandatory, unified scheme, ensuring the necessary health care coverage and managed solely by the Social Security funds.
- The introduction of a complementary insurance scheme for health care services complementary to those under the basic scheme, managed by insurance companies and mutual health insurance organizations (in the future, by CSS).
- The organization of relations between financial institutions and public and private health care providers, based on predetermined agreements.
- The control of health expenditures so that the reform does not put too heavy a burden on public finances, while maintaining competition among enterprises in Tunisia's open economy.

The later decision to combine the management of the Social Security health insurance regime within a single agency—the National Health Insurance Fund (CNAM)—was embodied in Law No. 2004-71 of August 2, 2004. This law mandated the creation of a new health insurance system. Negotiations with various partners since then have been ongoing in an effort to reach agreements, implementation decrees, and a framework agreement to regulate interactions between CNAM and private providers.

## Evaluation of the Reform

Because the important details of the insurance reform are still being worked out, its strengths and potential weaknesses cannot be evaluated (table 13.28). When complete, however, it should improve the current situation, starting by safeguarding of the health systems' accomplishments.

## Scalability of the Reform

No conclusive decision has yet been made about planning the implementation of the health insurance reform. However, the following proposals have been made: the implementation of a reimbursement system, with caps, for common illnesses; the continuation of care in a public health facility for anyone not enrolled in a reimbursement scheme; the introduction of a process to transfer long-term illness

**Table 13.28   Tunisia: Stakeholder Analysis for Health Insurance Reform**

| Stakeholder | Actions | Benefits | Risks | Challenges |
|---|---|---|---|---|
| Socially insured | Increased contribution rates for health insurance (social security) | • Access to higher quality health care services<br>• Access to public and private providers<br>• Reduction of uncovered medical expenditures<br>• Better monitoring of personal health status (individual health files) | • Potential for subsequent increases in contribution rates<br>• The increase in copayments<br>• Additional nonregulated payments<br>• Impact on vested rights and benefits | • Does the distribution of health professionals offer true choice between health providers?<br>• Employees' failure to declare their revenues |
| Employer | Increased contribution rates for health insurance | • Reduction in complementary insurance fees.<br>• Better access to health care for employees (productivity) | • Vested rights<br>• Increased social costs | Competition in the national and international market |
| Private providers of goods and services | Greater access to public financing | Predicted demand and solvency of the insured | • Limitation of the choice of physician?<br>• Fees: amounts and revision methods<br>• Delay in payment of NHIF fees<br>• Monitoriong and evaluation systems<br>• Transparency of revenues | • Many new administrative procedures<br>• Continuing medical education<br>• Health care networks and physician referrals<br>• Litigation management with the CNAM |

| | | | | |
|---|---|---|---|---|
| Public providers of goods and services | Competition with private sector | Reduction in the number of patients to lighten workload | • Reduction in resources<br>• Degradation of quality<br>• Migration of competent professionals toward private sector<br>• Employment impact on sector's health professionals | Underfinancing of public sector and mismatching of its capacity and reach |
| Social Security | Increase in resources | Management of a single mandatory scheme by a single agency | • Increase in administrative costs<br>• Financial equilibrium<br>• Introduction of various versions of basic scheme | • Coordination between NFSS and NFPSP for collection of contributions, with NHIF responsible for managing own resources<br>• Financial and Medical Information System<br>• Sociopolitical consequences |
| Group insurance and mutual health insurance companies | Coverage limitation (only supplementary) | | The drastic reduction in the turnover of "illness" has significant appeal | • Optional enrollment in supplementary insurance schemes<br>• Potential competitions with NHIF |
| Government | • Continue to ensure health care to poor and to low-income groups | • Reduction in health expenditures<br>• Better information about private sector | • Dichotomized health system: public for poor and private for those who can afford it<br>• Training capacity of public sector | • Governance capacity |

costs to third-party payers; and the continuation of coverage for hospital care expenses as currently handled and its gradual expansion to the private sector for certain illnesses or for specialist medical care that cannot be obtained in the public sector. These proposals are, of course, minor compared to the comprehensive priorities in terms of payment methods, health care procedures, and fee schedules.

## Key Conditions for the Reform's Success

The underestimation of the actors' strategic capabilities has lengthened the reform process, and diverted it from the intended objectives. Some key conditions for success of the reform are still missing:

- A realistic assessment of the contribution rate. The proper implementation of a mandatory social health insurance system depends on the contribution rate. Studies on this subject have been strongly recommended, but only one has been done.
- Capacity building in management of NHIF (CNAM) and other agencies involved.
- A complete legal arsenal needed to carry out the reform. Still to be defined are: the contents of the benefits package; the reimbursement rate and annual cap; sectorwide conventions; and the stakeholders' frame of reference, standards, and norms, in terms of quality assurance of services and cost control.
- A clear communication strategy known to all partners. This is needed to forestall unnecessary misunderstandings and disputes.

Nonetheless, a principal condition for the success of the health insurance reform is the promotion of public health care delivery and well-managed resources. This should serve as the reference model for the health system so that it can play its full role in service provision, training, and medical research. The economic and sociocultural environment could bring about many unforeseen threats to the sustainability of a health care system with such a significant private component.

## Lessons Drawn from the Reform Process

Tunisia's reform experience suggests several lessons:
- Conduct the analysis within a multidisciplinary and autonomous framework, departing from a thorough understanding of the national health system and drawing freely on international expertise.
- Involve all health system actors, not just one, and anticipate stakeholders' strategies and any potential resistance to change.
- Analyze all potential consequences of the financing reform on the other components of the system.
- Appeal to political experts who must fully play their role as decision makers regardless of party divisions and multiple alternatives.

**Table 13.29  Tunisia: Contribution Rates for Health Insurance Scheme**

| Scheme | Current rates Employer | Current rates Employee | Target rates Employer | Target rates Employee | Variance Employer | Variance Employee |
|---|---|---|---|---|---|---|
| NFPSP | | | | | | |
| – Mandatory | 1 | 1 | 4 | 2.75 | +3 | +1.75 |
| – Mandatory and optional | 2.5 | 4 | 4 | 2.75 | +1.5 | −1.25 |
| NFSS | | | | | | |
| – RSNA | 3.43 | 1.32 | 3.98 | 2.77 | +0.55 | +1.45 |
| – RSA | 0.68 | 0.23 | 3.98 | 2.77 | +3.3 | +2.45 |
| – RSAA | 1.52 | 0.76 | 4 | 2.75 | +2.48 | +1.99 |
| RNS | 3.04 | | 6.75 | | + 3.71 | |
| Pensioners | | | | | | |
| NFPSP mandatory | | 1 | | 3 | | +2 |
| NFPSP mandatory and optional | | 3 | | 3 | | +0 |
| NFSS | | 0 | | 3 | | +3 |

*Source:* Khaled 2001.

- Estimate the missing information through timely studies in order to allow for informed decision making.
- Be well informed about international experiences with health care reform.
- Aim to reach the ideal contribution rate gradually in order to avoid mistakes and mitigate negative repercussions of any increases. In Tunisia, the ideal contribution rate is 6.75 percent which will be reached during a three-year period. The transition period could be prolonged to a five years for low-income populations (table 13.29):

## Implementation Challenges

A number of unanswered questions continue to delay the implementation of the health insurance reform, particularly regarding payment methods and health care networks. These issues continue to be the subject of stakeholder negotiations.

Fee for service has been retained as the payment method for ambulatory care. This called for a revision of the general classification for medical services (realized in 2006) and for setting standard fees for each category (currently in negotiation). For the coverage of fees, the two options foreseen are being discussed among various stakeholders: CNAM reimbursement of fees paid by the insured or third-party payment with copayment by the insured.

For hospital care, the current system promotes a single inclusive fee, dependant on the public sector's costs and, a previously determined fixed fee for pathologic and specialized services. The NHIF (CNAM) will pay health facilities directly for these inclusive tariffs. This method assumes the availability of calculations for various combinations of price and quantity and the preliminary identification of the medical fees included therein.

In line with the cost-control objective, the formation of a health care network allows supervision and guidance of patients' care-seeking behavior. Negotiations continue on this subject, especially on the role of general practitioners as gatekeepers to specialized services. Meanwhile, medical organizations, especially medical specialists, do not favor this proposed system, fearing dichotomization of the medical profession and overconsumption of health services.

Other significant unanswered questions concern: the use of referrals as a method of medical control; the management of drug procurement according to the financial levels used in their classifications (vital, essential, nonessential); the substitution, by the pharmacist, of drugs prescribed by the physician; and the dental care benefits package.

The architects of the reform were able to define the direction of reform and integrate it in the social protection strategy. They also recognized that lengthy negotiations and political discussions would be needed to reach the desired consensus, integrating all the medical, socioeconomic, and political aspects of reform. This situation will require the management of ideological differences, contradictory approaches to preserving the system's gains, and conflicting stakeholder interests.

## Conclusions

The first part of this chapter traced Tunisia's economic and social performance since the end of the 1980s. For a long time, Tunisia has followed an approach based on the indivisibility of the economic and social dimensions of development. Numerous reforms and programs to improve the performance of Tunisian companies have accompanied the country's march toward liberalization and integration in the global economy. They have encouraged foreign investment and diversification of the Tunisian economy. Social policy during the last decade has furthered the general improvement in the quality of life and poverty reduction.

The second part of the chapter, devoted to analysis of the Tunisian health system and health insurance, shows that the system has performed well overall in expanding health care coverage:

- During the past three decades, Tunisia has introduced a health care system that covers almost its entire population, and it compares favorably with those of other middle-income countries. This health care system has developed in a transitional context, where the demographic, socioeconomic, and health status of the population has profoundly changed. This triple transition presents the system with multiple challenges.

- The health status of the Tunisian population continues to improve, with the expansion of preventive and curative health care services and the decrease in the birth rate. Tunisia demonstrates better health outcomes than other average middle-income countries, in particular in terms of life expectancy, infant mortality, malnutrition, and reproductive health.

- The public sector is the main health care service provider, supplying about 85 percent of total hospital beds and more than 55 percent of medical personnel. However, the private sector has developed rapidly, doubling its bed capacity in the past decade and approaching the public sector in the number of external consultations (outpatient care).
- In terms of health financing, the expansion of health care coverage has been accompanied by growth in household contributions, a decrease in government contribution, and a slight increase in the social health insurance contribution in the 16-years period, 1990–2006.

From this review of Tunisia's health policy and reforms since the late 1980s, it is clear that the country has set its course for universal health care coverage. Before the 1980s, the health care system was rooted in the colonial tradition of hospital-centered health infrastructure, concentrated in large urban areas. The public authorities have opted to improve health care provision and coverage, by giving priority to

- Preventive programs (individual and collective) in the fight against illness, financed completely by the government. This allowed the eradication of some infectious diseases and significant reductions in the incidence of others.
- The expansion of geographic coverage of the population through primary health facilities, financially accessible to the entire population.
- Local training of physicians and paramedical personnel, combined with a welcoming policy toward the foreign health workforce in order to meet the needs of the population.
- The gradual development of a hospital infrastructure with the capacity for specialized care.
- The early introduction of mandatory health insurance for a large part of the population (civil servants and formal sector employees), which was gradually extended to additional groups.
- The existence of the private health care sector, which efficiently bolstered the public sector's efforts.

Since 1990, the public authorities have embarked on a new era of health sector development. The strategy includes: continued expansion of primary health care through a delivery-consolidation program; improvements in hospital care through structural and institutional reform of university hospitals; and legislative reform regarding private health care provision.

In terms of public-private partnerships, there have been two main periods. Until the late 1980s, health care delivery was almost entirely public. The private ambulatory sector coexisted and provided services to only a small part of the population. Since the end of the 1980s, the private sector has developed rapidly in terms of the number of both providers and health care categories. Private hospitalization, especially for surgery, has strongly developed, making another form of hospital provision available. One of the current challenges of health insurance reform is to develop efficient public-private partnerships.

The extensive growth of the private sector, associated with quantitative and qualitative changes in health care demand, has contributed to a significant growth in household health expenditures. Out-of-pocket household spending on health care is an increasingly important source of financing for the health care system. Aware of the concerns generated by this situation, the public authorities have reformed the health insurance schemes to lighten the burden on households.

In the current context of health system evolution and ongoing reforms, regulation is one pillar of good governance, but it faces serious challenges. These arise both from the system's progress after a decade of reforms and from the evolution of its macroeconomic and social environments.

The following points summarize key factors in the successful expansion of health care coverage and some lessons from the Tunisian experience:

- Human resource development is a vital part of a modern social policy: "The Tunisians are Tunisia's main natural resource."
- The first success came in the public sector—government-regulated, planned in detail to satisfy community health priorities, and compliant with standardization in geographic expansion as well as with its missions, mandated by law.
- Nearly universal "health insurance" has been achieved. All Tunisians can access health care services in the public sector through Social Security (Bismarkian) or government-managed schemes (Beveridgian). This coverage has been maintained and updated to ensure its adaptation to the socioeconomic conditions of the people it serves.
- Training of human resources in the health sector, especially nurses, has been decentralized.
- A strong commitment was made to primary health care at a time when the cost of more intensive hospital care and new medical technologies is growing.
- The government maintains complete control over drug policy: procurement, distribution, prices, and, more recently, manufacturing and quality control.
- The need for information systems for the health sector is growing, and health care providers and financing institutions, such as NHIF, must be prepared to meet it. The classic data collection and analysis techniques must be enhanced by the integration of health care demand and provision forecasts and the subsequent expenditures and quality concerns.

The dimensions of a large-scale mandatory health insurance reform must not be underestimated. Reform is complicated and comes with high financial risks. Therefore, it is vital to pay special attention to subsystems that must consequently be adapted. The following are priorities:

- The development of public hospitals' management capacity and the promotion of participatory management. Both will lead to an improvement in hospital performance and their capacity to produce the necessary information for cost calculations and quality-driven resource allocation and management.
- The adaptation of public health facilities' leadership to the new system's objectives to improve economic performances and quality of health services. The current system evolved into centralized decision making, and global budget rules provides few or no incentives to promote performance or health care quality.
- The promotion of effective regulation of private practitioners, particularly in matters of medical competency.

Investment in health, a durable public good, promotes economic growth. The time when health expenditures could be considered an uneconomic investment is long gone.

## Endnotes

1. See the Ministry of Trade Web site for a list of most of Tunisia's trade agreements (Ministry of Trade, Information online; http://www.infocommerce.gov.tn/ indexfr.htm.)

2. Eight surveys have been carried out since independence; 1967, 1975, 1980, 1985, 1990, 1995, 2000, and 2005. Only preliminary results, without detailed poverty data, have been published.

3. Data from United Nations Population Division, World Population Prospects the 2004 Revision Population Database: http://esa.un.org/unpp/index.asp.

4. Social Security funds (caisses de sécurité sociales) encompasses the National Pension and Social Protection Fund [Caisse Nationale de Retraite et de Prévoyance Sociale, CNRPS] and the National Social Security Fund (Caisse Nationale de Sécurité Sociale). CNAM is the recently implemented National Health Insurance Fund (Caisse Nationale d'Assurance Maladie). Before CNAM, health insurance (social and mandatory) was managed by CNSS (for private employers) and CNRPS (for public employers).

5. In Tunisia their contribution has never surpassed 1 percent of total health care expenditures, and it was not integrated as a component of financing.

6. These groups are the military, national security forces, customs agents, and health care professionals.

7. Article 35 of Law No. 91-63 July 29, 1991, the public health organization law.

8. In 1998, there was a reform of this health assistance scheme. Eligibility for the health care card was revised, mainly to better target the needy families counted by the MASSTE, and service fees were reduced for persons with limited incomes, who cannot enroll in one of the Social Security funds.

## References

ATCE (Agence Tunisien de Communication Extérieure). 2002. "Principaux indicateurs économiques et sociaux de la Tunisie 1978–2002." ATCE, Tunis.

Arfa, C., and N. Achour. 2006. "Report on Financing Health Care in Tunisia." National Institute of Public Health, Tunis.

————. Achour. 2004. "National Health Accounts Tunisia 2000." Report of the National Institute of Public Health, MSP, Tunis. http://who.int/nha.

Achouri, H. 2005. "Health Insurance Reform: Challenges in Tunisia." Paper presented at the international conference on social health insurance in developing countries, Berlin, Germany, November 21–23. http://www.shi-conference.de/downl/achouri.pdf.

————. 2002. "L'assurance maladie en Tunisie." In *La couverture du risque Maladie: états des lieux et perspectives (cas de l'Algérie, du Maroc et de la Tunisie),"* 103–61, Actes de consultation organisée par le réseau des économistes des systèmes de santé du Maghreb Arabe, l'Institut National de la Santé Publique, Tunisie.

Ben Romdhane, H., R. Khaldi, A. Oueslati, and H. Skhiri. 2002. "Transition épidémiologique et transition alimentaire et nutritionnelle en Tunisie." Options méditerranéennes, série B: Etudes et recherches 41, International Center for Advanced Mediterranean Agronomic Studies, Montpellier, France.

BCT (Banque Centrale de la Tunisie). 2004. *Rapport annuel 2003.* Tunis: BCT.

Ghali, S. 2004. "The Tunisian Path to Development: 1961–2001, A Case Study from Scaling Up Poverty Reduction: A Global Learning Process and Conference." Shanghai, May 25–27, 2004. http://www.worldbank.org/wbi/reducingpoverty/case-Tunisia-Path-Development.html.

Hsairi, M., T. Nacef, N. Achour, and B. Zouari. 2002. "Economie et Santé: Evaluation et Stratégies de mise en oeuvre des interventions." Training manual, Institut National de la Santé, Tunis.

IMF (International Monetary Fund). 1999. "Rapport expérimental du FMI sur l'observation des normes et des codes: Tunisie." http://www.imf.org/external/np/rosc/tun/fre/.

INS (Institut National de la Statistique). 2007. "Note des premiers résultats de l'enquête nationale sur le budget et la consommation des ménages 2005." INS, Tunis. http://www.ins.nat.tn.

————. 2005. "Annuaire statistique de la Tunisie 2005." Publication 47, INS, Tunis.

————. 1975–2000. "Enquêtes nationales sur le budget et la consommation des ménages." Série de Rapports, INS, Tunis.

————. 1966–2004. "Recensement général des ménages et de la population, caractéristiques économiques." Série de rapports, Tunis.

Khaled, M.K. 2001. "Financement des dépenses de santé et perspectives de la réforme de l'assurance maladie en Tunisie." Paper presented at a seminar of the réseau des économistes des systèmes de santé du Maghreb Arabe. Marrakech, Morocco.

Lambert D. C. 2001. *Santé, clé du développement économique: Europe de l'Est et Tiers Monde.* <<**no city**>>, France: Harmattan.

MSP (Ministère de la Santé Publique). 1976–1996. "Série des bulletins épidémiologiques." MSP, Tunis.

————. 1986. "1956–1986 Trente ans au service de la santé: un engagement, une éthique." MSP, Tunis.

NHIF (National Health Insurance Fund). 2006. Informal data. NHIF, Tunis.

Omrane, A. R. 1983. "The Epidemiologic Transition, A Theory: Preliminary Update " *Journal of Tropical Pediatrics* 9: 305–17.

UNDP (United Nations Development Program) 2004a. "World Population Prospects: The 2004 Revision." Population database. http://esa.un.org/unpp/index.asp.

———. 2004b. "Stratégie du phénomène de la pauvreté en Tunisie." Etudes et rapports sur le développement, <<**no city**>>, July 2004.

UNPD (United Nation of Population Division). *World Mortality Report 2005.* New York: UNPD, Department of Economic and Social Affairs.

———. 2001. *Human Development Report.* Brussels: Ed. De Boek.

———. 1999. "World Urbanization Prospects: The 1999 Revision." New York: UNPD.

WBI (World Bank Institute). 2004. "Public Health in the Middle East and North Africa: Meeting the Challenges of the Twenty-First Century." Learning Resource Series Publication 29163, WBI, Washington, DC.

WHO (World Health Organization). 2006. "World Health Statistics." http://www.who.int/whosis/whostat2006/en.index/html.

———. 2004. Department of Measurement and Health Information, December. http://www.who.int/healthinfo/bodestimates/en/index. htm.

———. 2000. *The World Health Report 2000—Health Systems: Improving Performance.* Geneva: WHO.

World Bank. 2006a. *World Development Report: Equity and Development.* Washington, DC.

———. 2006b. "Etude du secteur de la santé en Tunisie." Human Development Department, Middle East and North Africa Region, Washington, DC.

———. 2006c. "World Development Indicators." http://www.ddp-ext.worldbank.org.

———. 2005. "World Development Indicators." http://www.ddp-ext.worldbank.org.

———. 2004a. "Making Deeper Trade Integration Work for Growth and Jobs." Republic of Tunisia, Development Policy Review. Report 29847-TN, World Bank, Social and Economic Development Group, Middle East and North Africa Region, Washington, DC.

———. 2004b. "Project Performance Assessment Report: Republic of Tunisia." Report 31017. http://www-ds.worldbank.org/servlet/WDSContentServer.

———. 2004c. "World Development Indicators." http://www.ddp-ext.worldbank.org.

———. 2003a. "Vers une meilleure gouvernance au Moyen-Orient et en Afrique du Nord: Améliorer l'inclusivité et la responsabilisation." Report on the development in the Middle East and North Africa. World Bank, Washington, DC.

———. 2003b. "Stratégie de développement touristique en Tunisie." World Bank, Washington DC.

———. 2000. "Poursuivre l'intégration à l'économie mondiale et pérenniser le progrès économique et sociale de la Tunisie." Sociale and structural review, World Bank, Washington, DC.

# 14

# Vietnam: "Good Practice" in Expanding Health Care Coverage—Lessons from Reform in Low- and Middle-Income Countries

*Björn Ekman and Sarah Bales*

## Background

*With a population of about 84 million and a GDP per capita of US$540, Vietnam is one of the larger low-income countries in the East Asia and Pacific Region of the World Bank. It is one of the world's most dynamic economies, with economic growth averaging between 6 and 8 percent a year over the past decade. Vietnam is predominantly rural: only 25 percent of the population lives in urban areas, but the ratio of the rural to urban population is rapidly falling. In 2003, Vietnam spent about 5.4 percent of its GDP on health—approximately US$26 per capita, which is about the average for its income level. Its health outcomes are excellent: in 2004, life expectancy was 70.3 years and the infant mortality rate was only 17.4 per 1,000 live births.*

*Vietnam's health care financing reforms have been motivated by three main considerations: its historic emphasis on good health, the important poverty-eradication component of health, and a desire to make health care affordable for the poor. Prior to the reforms, Vietnam's health system was geared toward provision of "health for all" via an extensive network of community health services and intercommunal policlinics for primary care and government hospitals for higher levels of care. Coverage was fairly widespread, but the quality of care was low primarily due to a lack of resources. The introduction of user fees in the late 1980s, however, posed barriers to access, and resulted in dissatisfaction among poor and nonpoor. In response, the government introduced targeted health financing support, initially as part of other broader poverty eradication policies and subsequently in the shape of stand-alone health financing programs for the poor and other target groups, including students and children.*

*The political-institutional framework of Vietnam—a one-party state—makes it difficult to assess the political economy of reforms, which take place within a less-open*

**439**

*system. For example, the lack of formal political opposition to the governing party and the absence of a free press in which political debate can be observed, complicates the study of the extent to which affordable health care is a central political-economic issue. Although the political economy dimensions of the health financing reforms have been little documented, some issues can be noted.*

*First, the political accountability of the Communist Party depends on an ability to provide the population with, among other services, affordable health care. Public dissatisfaction with user fees became an "embarrassment" for the party and led to reforms. More recently, with the National Assembly's expanding role in the country's general political debate, the minister of health has had to respond to questions and criticisms from the representatives about what the government is doing to help the poor obtain health care. Making the government accountable for the implementation of the program on Health Care Funds for the Poor (HCFP), for example, has contributed to some recent program adjustments.*

## Introduction

In the decade following the end of the armed conflict with the United States and the reunification of the country in 1975, Vietnam pursued a socialist economic policy, with the government controlling the production of most goods and services. Since then, liberalizations have been introduced that have affected the health sector.

### Economic Environment

In the immediate postwar period with an estimated gross domestic product per capita of US$130[1] a year, Vietnam was one of the world's poorest countries. Poor economic performance, stagnant school enrollments, and widespread malnutrition were endemic. By the mid-1980s, the Communist Party realized that a change was necessary to sustain food security and improve the welfare of the Vietnamese people.

Thus, the government adopted an economic reform program referred to as *Doi Moi* [renovation]. The program launched a series of policy changes continuing to this date. The most important changes involved extensive agricultural and trade liberalization. In the health sector, a far-reaching deregulation of the health care system was introduced in the early 1990s. Among other things, the changes meant that health professionals were allowed to operate private clinics and that private entrepreneurs could sell drugs in private outlets. User fees for health care were introduced to raise revenues. In addition, a social health insurance program was initiated and is now being expanded by further measures to broaden coverage and improve efficiency.

Table 14.1 shows the evolution of a set of key economic indicators since 1990. At the outset, economic growth in Vietnam lagged that of other geographically or economically comparable countries. Since then, as a direct result of the economic reform program, overall GDP growth has been comparable to that of other fast-growing countries in the region and well above that of other low-income countries

**Table 14.1   Vietnam: Economic Indicators, 1990–2004**

| Indicator | 1990 | 1995 | 2000 | 2001 | 2002 | 2003 | 2004 |
|---|---|---|---|---|---|---|---|
| GDP per capita (constant 2000 US$) | 226 | 305 | 397 | 419 | 444 | 471 | 502 |
| GDP per capita, PPP (current international US$) | 989 | 1,419 | 2,012 | 2,170 | 2,336 | 2,518 | 2,745 |
| GDP growth (annual %) | 5.10 | 9.54 | 6.79 | 6.89 | 7.08 | 7.34 | 7.69 |
| Poverty gap at US$1 a day (PPP) (%) | — | 181 | 92 | 0.53 | 0.5 | n.a. | n.a. |
| Poverty headcount ratio at national poverty line (% of population) | — | 581 | 372 | — | 28.90 | — | <20 |
| Revenue, excluding grants (% of GDP) | n.a. | n.a. | n.a. | n.a. | n.a. | n.a. | 22 |
| Tax revenue (% of GDP) | — | — | — | — | — | — | 17 |
| External debt (% of GDP) | — | — | 38.60 | 37.90 | 34.90 | 34.10 | 34 |
| Aid (% of GNI) | 3.12 | 4.08 | 5.47 | 4.50 | 3.70 | 4.52 | 4 |
| Unemployment, total (% of total labor force) | — | — | 2.30 | 2.80 | 2.10 | 2.30 | 2 |
| Inflation, consumer prices (annual %) | — | — | –1.71 | –0.43 | 3.83 | 3.10 | 7.80 |

*Sources:* WDI 2006; IMF Article IV Consultations, PRGF Reports; National Survey Data 1993, 1998, 2002.

*Note:* — = not available.

and some lower middle-income countries. Growth rates have been particularly strong in per capita terms due to Vietnam's reduction in fertility rates and subsequently limited population growth rates. The most recent estimate of gross national income (GNI) per capita is current US$540 (WDI 2006), thus placing Vietnam among the low-income countries that are rapidly moving into the group of lower-middle-income countries.

The changes in per capita income over this period suggest that the policies, in terms of economic stability, have provided Vietnam with a national income per capita of around US$2,700 a year in purchasing power terms. This is above the average for the low-income country group.

With its rapid economic growth Vietnam's income poverty rates have fallen steeply. Although estimates and definitions vary and are surrounded by some uncertainty, income poverty fell from around 58 percent in 1993 to 29 percent in 2002 (World Bank 2003a: i). The most recent estimates suggest that poverty has fallen even further, to a little more than 15 percent of the population in 2006 (GSO 2006).

Extreme poverty is relatively limited in Vietnam, and the remaining absolute poverty is concentrated mainly in some disfavored regions (flood-prone areas and mountainous regions) and among ethnic minorities (WHO 2003), who make up about 13 percent of the population. Income distribution remains an issue in Vietnam with the most well-off 20 percent receiving around 45 percent of available income compared with only around 7 percent for the poorest fifth of the population (WDI 2006).

In terms of government revenue, recent estimates suggest that Vietnam has a revenue-to-GDP ratio of around 22 percent, which is expected to increase slightly. The overall budget deficit is around 4.5 percent of GDP, suggesting that the overall fiscal situation is sustainable. Furthermore, national accounts data show that Vietnam has a tax revenue-to-GDP ratio of around 17 percent, mainly from income and profit taxes (IMF 2005).

Vietnam has managed to limit its external debt over this period. It is not a highly indebted poor country (HIPC) that can benefit from debt cancellation initiatives. Recent estimates put its total external debt at 33 percent of GDP, and debt servicing is less than 10 percent of total exports of goods and services (ibid.). An important issue for its external relations was accession to the World Trade Organization (WTO) on January 11, 2007, which is expected to affect the Vietnamese health sector in general and the pharmaceutical market in particular. Inasmuch as pharmaceuticals make up half of all health spending, drug prices are expected to fall significantly with possibly far-reaching consequences for both access to medicine and to health financing generally.

Vietnam has also limited its dependence on overseas development assistance (ODA). In the early reform period, former Soviet-bloc countries and Sweden provided assistance, a large part of it for the health sector. Since the late 1990s, when relations with the rest of the world were normalized, inflows of aid, including loans from development banks, have increased to 5 percent of GNI, much more than the regional average but substantially less than, for example, several countries in Sub-Saharan Africa.

## Demographic, Epidemiologic, and Social Environment

Vietnam covers 330,000 square kilometers (207,000 sq. miles) with a population of around 84 million resulting in some 255 inhabitants per square kilometer. The population consists of several different ethnic groups. The largest group, the Kinh, accounts for around 87 percent of the population. The remaining 13 percent consists of some 50 different ethnic minority groups with distinctive ethnolinguistic and cultural characteristics (WHO 2003). A quarter of the population lives in urban areas, although with migration from the countryside to the larger cities, the ratio of rural to urban population is falling.

Vietnam has pursued a relatively strict family and population policy over the past two decades that has resulted in a fertility rate barely above replacement level. Projections suggest that the population growth rate will be further reduced to less than 1 percent after 2025 (WDI 2006). Table 14.2 presents selected population, demographic, and social indicators for various years since 1990. Life expectancy at birth was much higher in Vietnam than in other countries at similar income levels well before the mid-1980s when the economic reform program was initiated.

One likely factor for Vietnam's good health outcomes is the comparatively high level of education, as reflected in the high literacy rates for both men and women. The Vietnamese literacy rates, for previous years not shown in the table, are also significantly higher than those of other low- and even some middle-income countries.

**Table 14.2  Vietnam: Selected Population and Social Indicators, 1990–2004**

| Indicator | 1990 | 1995 | 2000 | 2001 | 2002 | 2003 | 2004 |
|---|---|---|---|---|---|---|---|
| Population, total (millions) | 66.2 | 72.9 | 78.5 | 79.5 | 80.4 | 81.3 | 82.2 |
| Population ages 0–14 (% of total) | 38.92 | 37.02 | 33.46 | 32.67 | 31.87 | 31.08 | 30.30 |
| Population ages 15–64 (% of total) | 56.13 | 57.96 | 61.14 | 61.89 | 62.67 | 63.46 | 64.24 |
| Population ages 65 and above (% of total) | 4.95 | 5.03 | 5.40 | 5.44 | 5.46 | 5.46 | 5.45 |
| Median population age | 20.20 | 21.30 | 23.10 | — | — | — | — |
| Rural population (% of total population) | 79.74 | 77.79 | 75.68 | 75.20 | 74.72 | 74.24 | 73.76 |
| Population growth (annual %) | 2.18 | 1.80 | 1.29 | 1.23 | 1.16 | 1.10 | 1.04 |
| Age dependency ratio (dependents to working-age population) | 0.78 | 0.73 | 0.64 | 0.62 | 0.60 | 0.58 | 0.56 |
| Life expectancy at birth, female years) | 66.84 | 69.42 | 71.52 | — | 72.20 | 72.50 | 72.80 |
| Life expectancy at birth, male (years) | 62.82 | 64.96 | 66.70 | — | 67.30 | 67.60 | 67.90 |
| Life expectancy at birth, total (years) | 64.78 | 67.14 | 69.05 | — | 69.69 | 69.99 | 70.29 |
| Birth rate, crude (per 1,000 people) | 28.78 | 23.76 | 19.43 | — | 18.50 | 18.30 | 18.00 |
| Death rate, crude (per 1,000 people) | 7.26 | 6.68 | 5.80 | — | 6.20 | 6.10 | 6.10 |
| Fertility rate, total (births per woman) | 3.62 | 2.67 | 1.90 | — | 1.87 | 1.80 | 1.80 |
| Mortality rate, infant (per 1,000 live births) | 38.00 | 32.00 | 23.00 | — | — | 19.00 | 17.40 |
| Mortality rate, under-5 (per 1,000) | 53.00 | 44.00 | 30.00 | — | — | 23.00 | 23.20 |
| Mortality rate, adult, female (per 1,000 female adults) | 153.15 | — | — | — | 130.06 | — | — |
| Mortality rate, adult, male (per 1,000 male adults) | 215.02 | — | — | — | 181.67 | — | — |
| Maternal mortality ratio (modeled estimate, per 100,000 live births) | — | — | 130.00 | — | — | — | — |
| Literacy rate, adult female (% of females ages 15 and above) | — | — | — | — | — | — | 86.92 |
| Literacy rate, adult male (% of males ages 15 and above) | — | — | — | — | — | — | 93.92 |
| Literacy rate, adult total (% of people ages 15 and above) | — | — | — | — | — | — | 90.28 |

*Source:* WDI 2006.

*Note:* — = not available.

Figures 14.1 shows population pyramids for the years 1990, 2005, and 2020 (estimated), respectively. The figures reflect the effect of the government's family planning and population policy, one prominent feature of which is the active encouragement of a maximum of two children per family.

**Figure 14.1   Vietnam: Population Pyramids, 1990, 2005, and 2020**

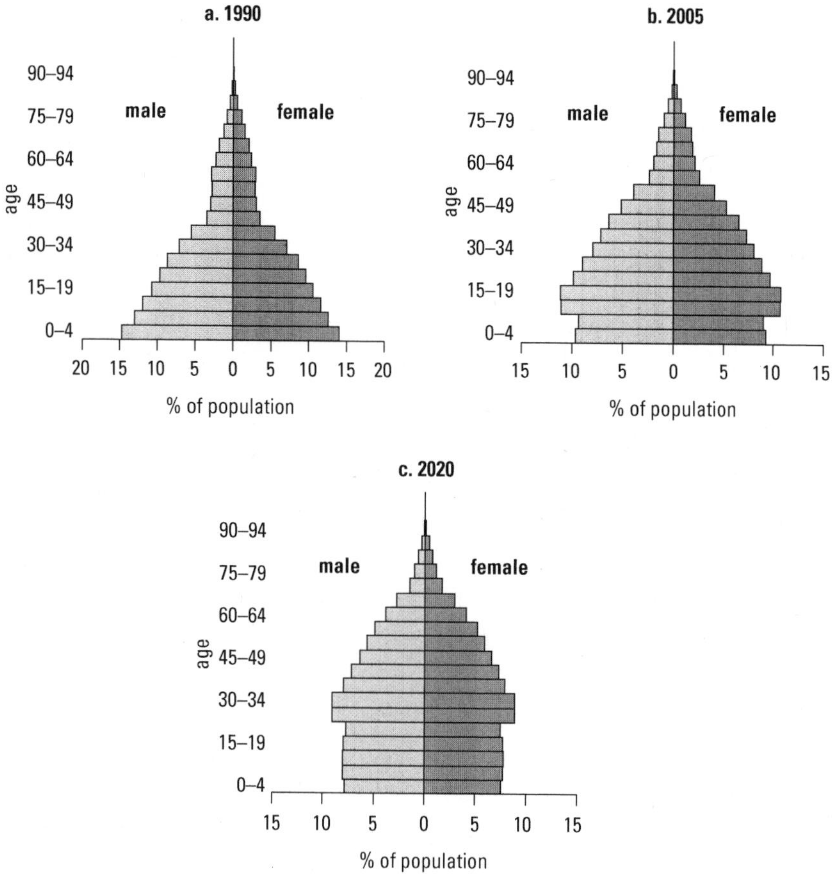

a. 1990

b. 2005

c. 2020

*Sources:* United Nations Population Division, World Population Prospects, the 2004 Revision Population Database (http://esa.un.org/unpp/index.asp).

Although the projections indicate that the total population will grow to around 125 million by 2025, it is plausible that Vietnam will be able to sustain its population with social services. The demographic transition of an aging population will, however, require continuous adaptation in the social service delivery system to the needs of elderly people.

Vietnam has made significant progress in its national health programs for targeting specific diseases. For example, it has dramatically reduced the incidence of and death from malaria. It has also reduced the incidence of polio, neonatal tetanus, and leprosy to the point where they are no longer regarded as threats to the health status of the population.

**Table 14.3  Vietnam: Estimated Burden of Disease, 2002**

**Top five diseases, by cause**

| Rank | GBD Cause | Estimated total deaths per 1,000 people |
|------|-----------|------------------------------------------|
| 1 | Cardiovascular diseases | 160.0 |
| 2 | Infectious and parasitic diseases | 74.6 |
| 3 | Malignant neoplasms | 64.1 |
| 4 | Respiratory diseases | 51.3 |
| 5 | Unintentional injuries | 36.1 |

**Burden of disease, by disease category**

| GBD rank / cause | Estimated total deaths per 1,000 | Share (%) |
|------------------|-----------------------------------|-----------|
| 1 Communicable, maternal, perinatal, and nutritional conditions | 126.2 | 24.5 |
| 2 Noncommunicable diseases | 341.1 | 66.1 |
| 3 Injuries | 48.5 | 9.4 |
| Total | 515.8 | 100.0 |

**Top five diseases, by cause**

| Rank | GBD cause | Estimated total DALYs, 1,000 |
|------|-----------|-------------------------------|
| 1 | Infectious and parasitic diseases | 2,337 |
| 2 | Neuropsychiatric conditions | 2,195 |
| 3 | Cardiovascular diseases | 1,389 |
| 4 | Unintentional injuries | 1,389 |
| 5 | Sense organ diseases | 809 |

**Burden of disease, by disease category**

| GBD rank/cause | Estimated total DALYs, 1,000 | Share (%) |
|----------------|-------------------------------|-----------|
| 1 Communicable, maternal, perinatal, and nutritional conditions | 4,305 | 32.2 |
| 2 Noncommunicable diseases | 7,334 | 54.9 |
| 3 Injuries | 1,721 | 12.9 |
| Total | 13,360 | 100.0 |

*Source:* World Health Organization, Department of Measurement and Health Information, December 2004 (http://www.who.int/healthinfo/bodestimates/en/index.html).

The estimated global burden of disease (GBD) for the main disease categories is shown in table 14.3. With respect to morbidity patterns, Vietnam has undergone an epidemiological transition along with the economic and social changes over the past two decades. In 1986, communicable diseases accounted for more than half of the entire estimated disease burden, with noncommunicable diseases making up almost the full balance (World Bank 2001). By the end of the 1990s, noncommunicable diseases accounted for 65 percent of the main causes of illness. Now communicable diseases make up around 27 percent, and accidents and injuries account for the rest. Accidents and injuries are expected to continue rising, not least as a result of road traffic incidents.

As table 14.3 indicates, Vietnam faces a dual burden of disease. Morbidity and mortality from noncommunicable diseases and injuries are rising, while the burden of disease from communicable diseases remains heavy.

As to specific causes of morbidity and mortality, it is estimated that the top 10 causes of hospital admissions were: pneumonia, acute pharyngitis and acute tonsillitis, acute bronchitis and acute bronchiolitis, influenza, transport accidents, diarrhea and gastroenteritis of presumed infectious origin, essential primary hypertension, gastritis and duodenitis, diseases of the appendix, and intracranial injuries (Ministry of Health [MOH] information system). Similarly, the main causes of hospital deaths were: intracranial injuries, HIV, pneumonia, intracerebral hemorrhage, transport accidents, acute myocardial infarction, stroke (not specified as hemorrhage or infarction), heart failure, respiratory tuberculosis, and intentional self harm (suicide). Information on causes of sickness and death is, however, very thin—deaths from the causes mentioned above explain only 5 percent of all deaths.

## Political and Governance Environment

Vietnam is a one-party socialist republic with a president as chief of state and a prime minister as head of government. The legislative branch, which elects the president from among its members, consists of a national assembly with representatives from the 64 provinces (comprising 611 districts/provincial towns and 10,600 communes/wards). The cabinet is appointed by the president and ratified by the national assembly. The national assembly is gradually assuming a more prominent role in policy debates and decisions, including in the social sectors. Given the country's relatively high decentralization, this is an important factor in terms of implementation of policies and possible adjustments. Formally, Vietnam is governed by People's Committees at various levels of the administration, including the commune. These committees have far-reaching authority over mobilization and allocation of resources at their respective level of administration. Furthermore, while it is fair to say that Vietnam is a centrally planned society, focused on production targets, attempts at active commune and village level participation in decision-making processes have been ongoing for many years.

In contrast with its administration, in terms of implementation Vietnam is highly decentralized, even in an international perspective (World Bank 2004, chap. 8). For example, spending at the subnational level has increased steadily since the early 1990s and now constitutes around 45 percent of state budget expenditures. An important factor in the decentralization process is the extent of interprovincial transfers, which are determined by the share of locally raised revenues that each province can retain and the grant received from the central government. Because resource availability varies considerably among provinces, some provinces are net contributors while most are net recipients of such grants. In general, the grants are directed toward a set of expenditure areas that include social and economic activities. A concern has been raised that the allocation formula is not sufficiently commensurate with local needs and resource mobilization abilities (World Bank 2003a). In particular, moving toward allocations based on development outcomes, including equity concerns, would most likely improve the incentive structure of the provincial and local authorities. This is a particular concern because the health sector is often given low priority when shortages of funds force cuts.

Another decentralization issue is the distribution of autonomy among administrative and service delivery units, including health care providers such as hospitals and clinics. The main point of conferring authority over resources is to improve operational efficiency. However, concern has been raised that the absence of transparency, accountability, and sound monitoring might lead to inappropriate use of resources and rent-seeking behavior among staff and managers of spending units (World Bank 2003a). This is a risk when decisions about investments in expensive equipment are made without any higher-level coordination and control. Continuity of care between different levels of the system is also threatened under the strong decentralization push underway.

As noted above, Vietnam has relied largely on a planning process that looks almost exclusively at the attainment of certain predefined production targets. Recently, the government has initiated a process that would give greater consideration to development goals (MPI 2005). Although this entails a much more analytically demanding planning process, it could be expected that the country would thereby manage to sustain or improve upon its recent record in economic development and poverty reduction.

## Overview of Health Financing

This section provides an overview of the Vietnamese health financing system. It starts by looking at the recent time trends in health financing followed by a description of the various health financing programs currently in existence in Vietnam and briefly reviews the main reimbursement systems. Finally, the section looks at some equity issues related to financing and utilization of care.

### Trends in Health Financing

Vietnam's health financing indicators show a continuing increase in per capita health expenditures but a relatively constant share of GDP spent on health (table 14.4). Private spending accounts for about three-fourths of all spending. Out-of-pocket spending accounts for the largest share, although it has seen a decline as

Table 14.4    Vietnam: Per Capita Total Expenditure on Health, 1999–2003

| Indicator | 1999 | 2000 | 2001 | 2002 | 2003 |
|---|---|---|---|---|---|
| Per capita total expenditure on health at (US$ at international dollar rate) | 111 | 129 | 145 | 143 | 164 |
| Total expenditure on health (US$ billion at international rate) | 8.6 | 10.1 | 11.5 | 11.5 | 13.3 |
| Total expenditure on health as share of GDP (%) | 4.9 | 5.3 | 5.5 | 5.1 | 5.4 |
| General government health expenditure as share of total government expenditure (%) | 6.7 | 6.0 | 6.7 | 5.1 | 5.6 |
| Out-of-pocket spending as share of total health expenditures (%) | 58.2 | 62.7 | 59.2 | 58.1 | 53.6 |
| Social insurance as share of general government expenditure on health (%) | 9.5 | 10.5 | 13.7 | 15.8 | 16.6 |
| Private health expenditures as share of total health expenditures (%) | 67.3 | 72.0 | 70.8 | 71.9 | 72.2 |
| Public health expenditures as share of total health expenditures (%) | 32.7 | 28.0 | 29.2 | 28.1 | 27.8 |
| External resources for health (% of total expenditure on health) | 3.4 | 2.7 | 2.8 | 3.5 | 2.6 |

*Source:* WHO 2006.

health insurance has increased its share. Starting in 2003 with the establishment of the Health Care Fund for the Poor (HCFP) and in 2005 with free health care for children under age six, the government has greatly increased its spending commitments on health care. These new entitlements to free health care constitute an impressive increase in government funding of health care not yet reflected in the figures in the following tables. Vietnam is not overly dependent on ODA for health care spending in general. Only 2.6 percent of total health spending comes from external sources, although the share of external funding for preventive care is somewhat higher (Vietnamese NHA).

Table 14.5 shows the share of health expenditures by type of service, and table 14.6 indicates the sources of funds by type of service. Most health spending goes for self-treatment—over-the-counter purchases of prescription and nonprescription drugs—not as part of a medical consultation, which accounted for a relatively stable high share of around 42 percent of all health spending from 2000 to 2003 (Vietnamese NHA). These purchases, mainly at private pharmacies, are not covered by health insurance or exemption programs. Self-treatment is the primary treatment choice of both poor and rich (Chang and Trivedi 2003).

Spending on inpatient care accounts for about 27 percent of all spending on health in Vietnam, mostly at state-run hospitals funded by user fees, government subsidies and health insurance reimbursements. Outpatient care accounts for about 14 percent of total health spending half of which comes from the state budget. Primary health care (PHC), funded largely by employers and school health programs, accounts for 7.5 percent of all spending.

**Table 14.5   Vietnam: Health Spending, by Type of Service (percentage)**

| Health care type | 1999 | 2000 | 2001 | 2002 | 2003 |
|---|---|---|---|---|---|
| Inpatient | 30.1 | 29.5 | 26.7 | 26.4 | 27.0 |
| Outpatient | 14.2 | 12.0 | 16.4 | 13.7 | 13.5 |
| Self-medication | 38.1 | 43.5 | 41.7 | 42.0 | 42.1 |
| PHC and school health | 4.8 | 4.9 | 6.3 | 7.7 | 7.5 |
| Preventive and public health | 10.5 | 7.9 | 6.6 | 7.7 | 7.4 |
| Other | 2.3 | 2.2 | 2.3 | 2.4 | 2.5 |
| Total | 100.0 | 100.0 | 100.0 | 100.0 | 100.0 |

*Source:* NHA 1998–2003; MOH, Statistical Publishing House 2006.

**Table 14.6   Vietnam: Sources of Funding, by Type of Service, 2003 (percentage)**

| Health care type | State budget | Health insurance | User fees | ODA | Other | Total |
|---|---|---|---|---|---|---|
| Inpatient | 27.2 | 15.2 | 37.5 | 1.4 | 18.8 | 100 |
| Outpatient | 49.6 | 19.8 | 10.1 | 1.3 | 19.3 | 100 |
| Self-medication | 0.0 | 0.0 | 100.0 | 0.0 | 0.0 | 100 |
| PHC and school health | 18.3 | 0.0 | 18.2 | 1.0 | 62.5 | 100 |
| Preventive and public health | 73.4 | 0.0 | 2.2 | 24.4 | 0.0 | 100 |
| Other | 67.3 | 10.8 | 0.0 | 6.1 | 15.8 | 100 |
| Total | 22.5 | 7.0 | 55.1 | 2.6 | 12.8 | 100 |

*Source:* MOH 2006.

Preventive health programs have declined in importance to 7.4 percent of total spending, three-fourths of it from the state budget and most the balance from external assistance. Government administration and regulation of the health sector, research, and training, account for a very small share of the total.

## Health Financing Programs

As Vietnam undergoes its transition to a market economy, the government continues to stress preventive care, maintaining state budgetary and ODA funding of national target programs and other preventive health measures. The government also continues to invest in the grassroots health network to implement these programs and to deliver primary and maternal and child health care. However, in recent years, financing of curative health care in Vietnam has increasingly relied on mobilizing resources from society (under the term *xa hoi hoa*, socialization), primarily through user fees at government facilities, expansion of the private sector, and a contributory social health insurance scheme. The share of expenditures of state-run health facilities covered by the government budget declined, from

**Table 14.7   Vietnam: Health Insurance Coverage, by Program Type, 1998–2004**

| Health insurance holders | 1998 | 1999 | 2000 | 2001 | 2002 | 2003 | 2004 |
|---|---|---|---|---|---|---|---|
| Percentage of population covered by health insurance | 12.7 | 13.4 | 13.4 | 15.8 | 16.5 | 20.3 | 27.7 |
| Of which: | | | | | | | |
| —poor (%) | — | 0.6 | 1.1 | 1.9 | 2.1 | 4.6 | 4.8 |
| —nonpoor (%) | 12.7 | 12.8 | 12.3 | 13.9 | 14.4 | 15.7 | 22.9 |

*Sources:* 1998–2002 Health Insurance Statistical Yearbooks. 2003–04 provisional figures from Vietnam Social Insurance Agency as presented in Lieu et al. 2005.

*Note:* — = not available.

62.7 percent in 1998 to 49.6 percent in 2003 (Lieu et al. 2005). User fees and, to a lesser extent, health insurance have taken up an increasing share, ensuring funding to maintain and improve the quality of health care facilities.

Social health insurance was introduced in 1992 as a solution to help mobilize resources and create a more appropriate mechanism for payment of user fees (table 14.7). The Vietnamese Communist Party and government have decided that health insurance should be the main health care financing mechanism and have set the challenging goal of reaching universal health insurance coverage in the near future. At the same time, social health insurance has gradually become the main mechanism for subsidizing users in an effort to increase government health spending to promote health equity goals and overcome the negative consequences of user fees. Figures from the Vietnam Social Insurance Agency (VSIA) indicate growing coverage of the population by health insurance, especially among the poor who receive government assistance to buy health insurance. Coverage by a prepayment mechanism is even higher if other government health financing programs are included.

The next section briefly describes the public and private health financing mechanisms for curative care currently available in Vietnam.

*Compulsory social health insurance.* As mentioned above, compulsory social health insurance was begun in 1992. There are two groups of beneficiaries, those who have made contributions to health insurance and those whose contributions were paid by governmental agencies.

The contributory compulsory social health insurance covers all Vietnamese employees with a contract of three or more months as well as pensioners and people on disability. Despite the compulsory nature of social health insurance for these groups, compliance is low for people in the private sector. Even among people making contributions for health insurance, there is some evidence of income underreporting so as to pay lower amounts into social insurance.

Many groups in the population are eligible for compulsory social health insurance paid through the government budget not covered through their employment. The first group is individuals who have served the government or provided meritorious service to the country, including elected officials, political beneficiaries who served in the revolution or wars protecting the nation, and family members of current military or police officers. The second group, the "vulnerable," for whom the government finances social insurance contributions, includes the elderly aged 90 and older, social assistance beneficiaries (such as the disabled, elderly without family to care for them, orphans), and foreign students on scholarships from the government of Vietnam.

In 2003, the government put in place the HCFP to ensure financing of health care services for the poor, ethnic minorities in disadvantaged provinces, and residents of remote communes (under Program 135). Provinces were allowed to choose whether to implement health care for the poor by purchasing health insurance or by reimbursing facilities directly for services used by the poor. When Decree 63 on health insurance was issued in 2005, the direct reimbursement option was discontinued, and the provinces were required to buy health insurance for these target groups with funding from the central budget.

*Voluntary health insurance.* Voluntary social health insurance, by law, covers individuals who need health insurance but are not covered under the compulsory scheme, such as the self-employed or the nonworking population, or individuals who have compulsory health insurance but want to contribute to voluntary health insurance to supplement their compulsory coverage. The voluntary part of the social health insurance program is intended for groups of people rather than individuals, so as to create a risk pool, reducing the risk of adverse selection. Most of the beneficiaries covered under voluntary health insurance are school pupils and students, a relatively easy group to enroll to meet the minimum coverage rate under the insurance regulations. Other options for risk pools include communes or various mass organizations and associations, but it has been more difficult to enroll enough members. Even then, the joiners tend to already have health problems and therefore pose a higher risk than healthy individuals to the insurance scheme.

In addition to social health insurance, several private and state insurance companies offer health insurance, usually as an add-on to life insurance products including policies for pupils and students as well as older working people to cover hospitalization, surgery, and emergency transport. In 2003, according to the latest National Health Accounts (NHA), private health insurance reimbursements to facilities constituted about one-third of all health insurance reimbursements (MOH 2006).

*Other government-sponsored programs.* There are two other government programs of note. One, by Decision 139 of October 2002 on the HCFP, covers health care costs for the poor and other target groups. It also provides—in theory—assistance to the nonpoor faced with unexpected and catastrophic health expenditures, but in practice implementation has been weak.

The other, under the Law on Protection and Care of Children, began in 2005. All Vietnamese children under 72 months of age are eligible for free health care at all government health facilities, with facility services reimbursed directly from the state budget. In 2006, the prime minister asked the MOH and Vietnam Social Security (VSS) to study how to convert this scheme into health insurance coverage for children under age six.

## Benefits Packages of Health Financing Programs

Compulsory and voluntary health insurance pay for outpatient and inpatient diagnosis and treatment at government and private facilities that have signed a contract with the social insurance agency agreeing to accept reimbursement at the rates set for public facilities. The package is generous, covering the costs of consultations, diagnosis, treatment, and rehabilitation during the time of treatment at the health facility; lab tests, diagnostic imaging, and other diagnostic techniques; medicines on the list drawn up by the MOH; blood and transfusions; medical procedures and surgery; use of materials, medical equipment, and treatment bed; and prenatal exams and assistance at delivery. Transportation costs for referrals from district- to higher-level hospitals are also covered by health insurance for the poor, political beneficiaries, and people living or working in mountainous and remote areas.

There are also some exclusions. For example, health insurance does not reimburse fees for certain health problems or treatments because of moral hazard issues, the elective nature of the intervention, or because those health problems are covered by other government programs.[2] Patients may also have to make copayments for any additional cost incurred beyond what basic services would have cost at an appropriate level of care in government facilities.[3]

For children under age six, the benefits include consultations, diagnosis, and treatment at all primary care public facilities (including commune health stations, district hospitals), and, if formally referred, treatment at provincial and central-level facilities. In an emergency, a family can seek treatment for the child at any level of facility without a referral. If the family of a child requests use of certain high-tech equipment, the family must pay additional fees. When this policy is converted to health insurance coverage for children under age six, the benefits will likely be the same as for other insured groups.

## Financing and Payment

This subsection discusses the main health financing and payment mechanism currently used in the Vietnamese health financing system, including contribution rates, sources of financing, and provider payment procedures. An important issue of health financing is the financial sustainability of the programs; this issue is discussed toward the end of the subsection.

*Contribution rates and financing sources.* Compulsory insurance contribution rates are set at a modest 3 percent of contractual salary and basic allowances, pension, social insurance payments, scholarship, or minimum wage, depending on the insured individual's entitlement group. Formally employed workers pay 1 percent of salary and their employers pay 2 percent. For retirees and people receiving social insurance benefits, the contributions are paid by the VSS. For the other groups, the government budget covers contributions. For the poor and the elderly aged 90 and older, the contribution is a fixed amount of US$3.10 per person per year with the contribution paid from the state budget. Voluntary social health insurance contributions range between US$1.90 and US$10.00, depending on the locality and the type of risk pool (e.g., school, association, commune) and are paid by individuals and their households.

For children under age six, the government has allocated US$4.70 per child per year, but if the total amount required exceeds this amount, funds from the reserve budget line of the national budget would be used to pay the excess. The HCFP requires provinces to allocate US$4.40 per eligible beneficiary, with 75 percent paid in from the state budget and most of that used to buy health insurance. The remaining amount, if it can be mobilized, can be used to pay for health care of ineligible groups confronted with catastrophic health care costs.

In the past, because of strict reimbursement ceilings imposed on hospitals, and despite low contributions, the health insurance fund has run a surplus. Since passage of Decree 63 on revised health insurance regulations in 2005, there has been some concern about the solvency of the social insurance fund because contributions remained low while the benefits package was expanded to include more than 200 additional medicines and many expensive high-tech services. In 2005, VSS estimated that health insurance reimbursements exceeded total contributions to health insurance by US$8.6 million, an amount equivalent to about 4.3 percent of total health insurance contributions. Currently this shortfall is being financed from accumulated reserves, but VSS has warned that these reserves may become exhausted in the coming years. Now, finding a solution for this issue is a top priority, by either increasing contribution rates or tightening cost controls.

To gauge their adequacy, contributions can be compared with per capita curative care spending. In 2003, according to NHA estimates, per capita annual spending amounted to US$7.10, counting only health spending at government hospitals and curative care facilities. Adding-in private curative care including self-treatment, annual per capita spending was US$20.30 (MOH 2006). There is some concern that with the generous package, coverage of a higher and higher share of people for whom low contributions have been paid (poor, elderly and soon children under age six), and with adverse selection among the voluntarily insured, major problems may arise in balancing the insurance fund. In addition, the cost of health care is fast increasing with the development of new technology and drugs, and contribution amounts will have to be raised periodically to keep up.

***Provider reimbursement procedures.*** Reimbursement of providers from health insurance and direct reimbursement of services for children under six and the poor not yet covered by health insurance is on a fee-for-service basis. The amount reimbursed to facilities is based on the partial schedule of user fees charged to uninsured patients, although in some cases the health insurance reimbursement is less than what facilities charge the uninsured.

Drugs and disposables are reimbursed at the facility's purchase price. The "major drugs list" of the MOH lists the drugs reimbursed by health insurance. It was updated in 2005 and now includes 646 modern and 91 traditional medicines. Regulations on certain drugs require committee approval before use, and the drug list also specifies which level of hospital (district, provincial, central) is allowed to dispense each type of medicine.

A list of procedures with prices reimbursed by health insurance was developed in 1995, and a price list covering new services was appended to it in 2006. Private facilities that sign contracts with the health insurance agency are reimbursed at the same rates as government facilities. Inherent in the fee-for-service payment mechanism are incentives to overprescribe certain health services and medications. Sepehri, Chernomas, and Akram-Lodhi (2005) found evidence that the inpatient admission rates and the average length of stay were higher for better-off individuals and for the insured.

To overcome this provider moral hazard problem (or provider-induced demand), Decree 63 called for alternative payment mechanisms, including capitation and case-mix options (such as diagnosis-related group, DRG). In 2004, WHO negotiated an experiment at selected districts in Hai Phong province. Initial results of the experiment were favorable both in terms of maintaining service quality, health insurance fund solvency, and provider and patient satisfaction. However, in 2005 when new health insurance regulations came into effect covering a wider range of services, especially high-tech services, the health insurance agency would not allow an increase in the capitation amount to cover the higher cost. Therefore, providers did not want to continue with the experiment. The MOH Department of Planning and Finance is doing a costing study as part of the process of developing a case-mix payment system to be pilot-tested in 2008. It is hoped that the case-mix system will improve the cost-effectiveness of health spending by reducing use of unnecessary services and drugs. This will contribute greatly to ensuring solvency of the health insurance fund.

*Measures to ensure solvency of the insurance fund.* At present, the health insurance scheme reimburses facilities only the partial user fees charged to patients paying out of pocket. The government continues to subsidize health facilities by paying salaries, buying equipment, and paying part of operating costs. If the government allows facilities to charge for the full cost of health care, the cost to patients and the insurance fund will increase substantially. Lieu, Long, and Bales (2007), studying the costs of treating five different medical conditions at provincial hospitals, found that the amount charged covers between 39 percent of full costs for pneumonia in children and 71 percent of full costs for intracranial injury.

Currently the MOH intends to continue subsidizing health care but would like to shift from direct payment to providers to payment through users, but it has not yet identified the appropriate mechanism for this purpose.

In the hospital costing study by Lieu, Long, and Bales (2007), drugs accounted for between 30 percent and 70 percent of the full cost of services. The cost of diagnostic procedures (depreciation, labor, and materials) was not found to be a high share of the total cost of care, but their share may increase with the development of high-tech services. The major drug list and list of user fees reimbursable by health insurance could theoretically be used to control costs. However, in establishing the lists of drugs and services, little attention was paid to the cost-effectiveness criterion. Thus, the benefits package is extremely generous—and ineffective as a tool for controlling costs.

Imposing ceilings on benefits is another way of ensuring solvency of the health insurance fund. Individual medical services costing less than VND 7 million are reimbursed by insurance, but any amount over VND 7 million is reimbursed in different amounts for different beneficiaries. Copayments are often instituted to discourage overuse of health services (moral hazard), but all copayments were eliminated in 2005 (Decree 63) in an effort to attract prospective health insurance subscribers. Neither ceilings on individuals nor copayments, however, gives practitioners any incentive to deliver cost-effective services. In health care, practitioners, not consumers, usually decide which services to provide and what to charge.

To avoid overspending the health insurance fund under the fee-for-service reimbursement mechanism, the VSS has capped the amount each first-contact facility will be reimbursed. In principle, the insurance fund available for reimbursements at each hospital is based on the number of people insured and the average contribution amount in the province. In practice, however, each facility subtracts an amount from the insurance fund as payment for referrals. The amount is calculated as 110 percent of the amount actually reimbursed to referral facilities in the previous year. Because no caps are imposed on services provided by referral hospitals, there are no incentives for cost-effective services at this level. Inherent in this payment mechanism is an incentive for first-contact hospitals to refer patients.

Although some expenditures in excess of the cap may be reimbursed by health insurance, there is a risk that they will not be or that reimbursement will be inordinately delayed. To avoid overspending, hospitals create their own controls on services to the insured, which often means that insured patients receive different services from those offered to patients paying user fees. Sometimes hospitals ask insured patients to "voluntarily" agree to pay the differential between the health insurance reimbursement and the amount the hospital would collect from fee-paying patients. This practice, though forbidden by the health insurance regulations, is not stopped because of sympathy with the difficulties of staying within the health insurance fund budget.

## *Equity: Health Indicators and Outcomes, and Their Distribution*

Several studies have reported inequitable utilization of health care services across living-standards groups, with the poor less likely to seek any care and, when they do, going to lower-level facilities. These studies have also shown differentials in the burden of health care expenditures with the heavier burden on the poor (Lieu, An, and Long 2005; Knowles et al. 2003; Minh, Khang, and Dung 2004; Chien 2005; Dong et al. 2002).

Earlier efforts by the Vietnamese government to improve health equity and access to health care for children under age six involved unfunded exemptions at government hospitals and provision of health insurance to a small share of the poor who were hard to target. The Vietnam National Health Survey (VNHS) of 2001/02 covered the period just before the approval of the HCFP policy (Decision 139). Low insurance coverage was found among the poor, ethnic minorities, and inhabitants of mountainous regions. In addition, fee waivers or health insurance reimbursements were obtained for only a third of inpatient visits by people eligible for Decision 139 benefits, compared with two-thirds of children under age six and nearly three-fourths of the people covered by health insurance (MOH 2003).

The negative consequences and inequities in access to curative health care and financial burdens for the poor have been documented in numerous studies (Knowles et al. 2003; Minh, Khang, and Dung 2004; Chien 2005; Dong et al. 2002; Wagstaff and van Doorslaer 2003). Wagstaff and van Doorslaer found that out-of-pocket expenditures for care contributed to increasing the number of absolute poor by 3.4 percentage points at the end of the 1990s.

The HCFP policy was developed because of the documented inequities in health outcomes, access to health care, and differential financial burden on the poor. Evidence of the strong impact of health insurance on access to health care helped to orient the policy toward subsidizing users through health insurance, although originally the policy also allowed direct government reimbursement to facilities for services used by the poor. Implementation of the HCFP policy began in 2003, and the results of the first impact evaluation only recently became available. Implementation of the policy on free health care for children under age six only began in 2005. During the implementation process, administrative reports from the provinces were compiled to identify shortcomings and implementation difficulties.

*Targeting specific populations.* The government's objective in targeting assistance to cover user fees is not based simply on need (that is, providing health care for the poor and the very old). It is also politically motivated (for example, covering people who have performed meritorious service to the country, nonpoor ethnic minorities) and anchored in concern about the health of future generations (health care for children younger than six).

One of the early complaints from the provinces about Decision 139 was prompted by perceived unfairness of providing assistance to some better-off people who happened to be part of the target group such as certain residents of disadvantaged communes or better-off ethnic minorities in mountainous provinces. In addition, it was felt that the many near-poor ethnic minorities residing outside of the 12 provinces targeted as disadvantaged also deserved assistance. In the first revision of the HCFP policy, in 2006, one of the main changes was to reduce leakages to better-off groups and undercoverage among near-poor ethnic minorities.

Its implementation has been hindered by a lack of clear-cut criteria for selecting the individuals who should receive assistance with catastrophic health expenditures from among the group of people who are ineligible for free health care cards or health insurance. The lack of well-defined criteria also makes it difficult to evaluate whether provinces are using these funds appropriately. According to administrative records of implementation, only about half the provinces have actually implemented this policy provision.

## Overview of the Health Delivery System in Vietnam

This section provides an overview of the Vietnamese health service delivery system, including the supply and organization of health care and the regulatory framework. Among other things, the data show that Vietnam is comparable with most other low-income countries in terms of service availability, albeit with large variation in quality across various parts of the country.

### Supply and Organization of the Health Care System

The health care system in Vietnam is organized in four tiers: the MOH, the Provincial health bureaus, the district health centers (DHCs), and the commune health stations (CHSs) (World Bank 2001). The MOH, together with the people's committees at the various administrative levels, is responsible for formulating and executing the country's health policy and programs. In addition to the MOH, several separate units and institutes function outside the ministry in areas such as training, research, and policy development in especially important areas, including family planning. In addition, 31 central-level hospitals provide mainly preventive care services together with training, research, and supervision of some targeted preventive care programs.

The second tier, the provincial health bureaus, is fairly influential, considering Vietnam's extensive decentralization. The provincial health bureaus, part of the provincial governments under the provincial people's committees, are charged with the overall planning of provincial health services and programs.

Immediately below the provincial health bureaus are the District Health Centers (DHCs). In 2006, as part of the decentralization process, the DHCs were split into three entities with distinct responsibilities: district health offices, district hospitals, and district preventive health centers. District hospitals and preventive health centers, for the most part, still supervised and managed by the provincial health bureaus, ensure curative and preventive care for district residents. The district health office, under the district people's committee, is responsible for government administration regarding overall management of the commune health stations, food safety and inspections, and disease prevention.

Finally, at the lowest level of the health care system are the CHSs, charged with delivering primary health care and executing the national health target programs. In addition to the CHSs, a system of village health workers (VHWs) provides residents of remote villages with basic health care, information-education communication (IEC), and first aid.

In terms of infrastructure, Vietnam has around 1101 hospitals with a total of 138,675 hospital beds. Fifty-five percent of the hospitals are district hospitals, 24 percent are provincial hospitals, and around 3 percent are central hospitals under the responsibility of the MOH. In addition, there are some 77 non-MOH hospitals that belong to other ministries and government units. In 2006, there were 62 private hospitals, a number that is expected to increase rapidly as a result of further deregulation and the government's intentions to further diversify health service provision.

As to the organization of health care and programs, most primary health care is delivered at the CHSs, although much is also provided higher up in the system in district, and even provincial, hospitals. The primary health care network in Vietnam has a long history. Until the mid-1980s, most care was provided by the local agricultural work brigades. This grassroots system formed the backbone of the service delivery system, but under the economic reforms at that time, these primary health care providers were largely dismantled. Recognizing the ensuing difficulties, in 1994 the government assumed the responsibility for paying the salaries of all health workers.

The national health programs, implemented from the top down, are an important feature of health care delivery in Vietnam. They are free or available at very low fees to the general public. The government has approved a revised list of national target programs in health to include: HIV/AIDS, community mental health (mainly schizophrenia and epilepsy), TB, leprosy, malaria, cancer, malnutrition, reproductive health, military-civilian medical collaboration, and an expanded program of immunization (EPI). In the CHS a large range of maternal and child health services are also provided, including prenatal care, deliveries, and health care for small children. Coverage of these primary health care and preventive programs is nationwide although evidence from a recent national health survey (MOH 2003 [VNHS 2001/02]) indicates that the programs are not being implemented uniformly across provinces and districts.

In addition to the public facilities, Vietnam's growing private health sector provides outpatient care and traditional medicine services and sells pharmaceuticals. As people's ability to pay for health care evolves and current policy reforms take hold, the size and scope of the private health care sector is expected to grow. Information is scant, however, about the size and scope of the private health care sector because private facilities come under the jurisdiction of the provincial health bureaus, and many private providers are not licensed. Distinguishing public from private facilities is also difficult, because many public doctors also operate private practices and many public hospitals are setting up semiprivate wings providing more "hotel-like" services to increase their revenues under the policy for promoting hospital autonomization. The most recent data on health care utilization suggest that private delivery of care may be as high as 30 percent of all care, with large variations across provinces and with a concentration in the urban areas (MOH 2003).

## Statistical Overview of the Health System

Using recent international health system statistics, this section presents a set of key health system indicators for Vietnam on human resources, service coverage, and some related health outcomes. In terms of nonfinancial health system inputs, table 14.8 shows human resources devoted to health care.

At around 1.3 government health workers per 1,000 inhabitants, Vietnam is on a par with other low-income countries. As professional training improves, the qualifications of health system personnel are also expected to improve. In addition to these formal health care providers, the many alternative (traditional) health care providers constitute a large and well-recognized part of the delivery system. Vietnam's ratio of 23 hospital beds to 10,000 inhabitants in 2003 compared with 39 for the region. The average numbers hide many details but seem to show that Vietnam has developed a relatively well-staffed delivery system with decent physical infrastructure, including hospitals and lower-level clinics.

Vietnam compares favorably in terms of per capita availability of health care facilities, but service quality, access, and utilization vary across regions. For example, although people in the most remote and mountainous areas have access to primary health care facilities, use is limited by poor quality, restrictions in physical access, financial obstacles, and possibly cultural factors. Furthermore, CHSs are perceived as implementing only target health programs, although their mandate extends to providing curative services as part of primary health care. There is some concern about low CHS utilization, estimated at an average of 12 consultations a day (World Bank 2001). Reasons for the low utilization rates at primary care level include the availability of alternative providers, staffing irregularities, and perceptions of low quality.

**Table 14.8  Vietnam: Human Resources for Health, Selected Indicators**

| Physicians | | Nurses | | Midwives | | Pharmacists | | Total |
|---|---|---|---|---|---|---|---|---|
| Number | Density/ 1,000 | Number | Density/ 1,000 | Number | Density/ 1,000 | Number | Density/ 1,000 | Density/ 1,000 (2003) |
| 42,327 | 0.53 | 44,539 | 0.56 | 14,662 | 0.19 | 5,977 | 0.08 | 1.3 |

*Sources:* WDI 2006; WHS 2006.

**Table 14.9   Vietnam: Selected Health Care Coverage and Health Outcome Indicators, 1990–2004**

| Indicator | 1990 | 1995 | 2000 | 2001 | 2002 | 2003 | 2004 |
|---|---|---|---|---|---|---|---|
| Births attended by skilled health staff (% of total) | — | — | 69.60 | — | 85.00 | — | 90.00 |
| Immunization, DPT (% of children ages 12–23 months) | 88.00 | 93.00 | 96.00 | 96.00 | 75.00 | 99.00 | 96.00 |
| Improved water source (% of population with access) | 72.00 | — | — | — | 73.00 | — | 80.00 |
| Improved water source, rural % of rural population with access) | 67.00 | — | — | — | 67.00 | — | — |
| Improved water source, urban (% of urban population with access) | 93.00 | — | — | — | 93.00 | — | — |
| Improved sanitation facilities (% of population with access) | 22.00 | — | — | — | 41.00 | — | 32.00 |
| Malnutrition prevalence, height for age (% of children under 5) | — | — | 36.50 | — | — | — | — |
| Malnutrition prevalence, weight for age (% of children under 5) | — | — | 33.80 | — | — | 28.40 | — |
| Diarrhea treatment (% of children under 5 receiving oral rehydration and continued feeding) | — | — | — | — | 39.00 | — | — |
| Prevalence of HIV, total (% of population ages 15–49) | — | — | — | 0.30 | — | 0.40 | — |
| Malaria prevention, use of insecticide-treated bed nets (% of under-5 population) | — | — | 15.80 | — | — | — | — |
| Incidence of TB (per 100,000 people) | 202.17 | — | — | — | — | — | 176.48 |
| Tuberculosis cases detected under DOTS (%) | — | 29.61 | 82.06 | 83.40 | 86.87 | 85.38 | 88.81 |
| ARI prevalence (% of children under 5) | — | — | 9.30 | — | — | — | — |
| ARI treatment (% of children under 5 taken to health provider) | — | — | 60.40 | — | 71.00 | — | — |
| Contraceptive prevalence (% of women ages 15–49) | — | — | — | — | 78.50 | — | — |

*Source:* WDI 2006.

*Note:* — = not available.

Table 14.9 presents a set of selected health service coverage indicators for Vietnam and some health outcome variables considered to be influenced by the health care system.

Among other things, the table indicates that immunization coverage in Vietnam is high. Since the mid-1980s, coverage has increased from less than 55 percent to more than 95 percent (World Bank 2001). Although immunization rates may be particularly high, other indicators of health service coverage also show similar increases. These improvements have contributed to the achievements in bringing down morbidity and mortality rates in Vietnam.

## Regulatory Framework

The MOH is the key regulator in the health sector. The ministry is responsible for developing national policies and monitoring and supervising the national public health programs. An important policy document is the Health Sector Master Plan to the Year 2010 and Vision to the Year 2020, recently developed by the MOH Department of Planning and Finance in collaboration with other sector departments. The government envisions a continued emphasis on care at grassroots while simultaneously developing more advanced medical technologies. The ministry is also responsible for developing and drafting central government health sector decisions and sending them to the provinces with specific implementation guidelines.

The private sector is regulated by the Ordinance on Private Practice of Medicine and Pharmacy, enacted in 1993 and updated in 2003, and by the decree detailing the implementation provisions. The ordinance stipulates the procedures and professional requirements for obtaining a private license to practice. The regulations specify 10 types of private health facilities, four types of private traditional medicine facilities, and four types of private pharmaceutical facilities. Licenses for private providers, including pharmacies, are issued by the provincial health bureaus after testing and screening the applicants.

The health insurance regulatory environment is changing fast. Currently, health insurance is regulated by Decree 63 of 2005, and VSS has overall responsibility for its implementation, including collecting contributions, managing the fund, and reimbursing providers. With technical assistance from the WHO, a law on health insurance is being developed (ILO 2006), and it is expected to be passed by the national assembly in 2008. As a reflection of the growing importance of health insurance as a financing instrument, a department for health insurance has been formed within the MOH. The new department is formally charged with developing legislation and strategies for attaining universal health insurance coverage and is expected to take an active part in the supervision and monitoring of current and new programs.

## Additional Components of the Health Delivery System

Together with the Ministry of Education, the MOH is responsible for educating and training all health care personnel at national and regional health training facilities. Vietnam has several medical universities that prepare health personnel and specialists in most medical areas. In line with its overall responsibility for the health sector, the MOH is also charged with generating most health statistics and information. The VSS is responsible for collecting and compiling health insurance data, a task expected to become more important as insurance coverage expands.

The government of Vietnam is planning technical advancements for the health sector so that it can also provide services and products for export purposes, including medical treatments for foreign visitors and pharmaceutical exportation. Central-level hospitals are becoming more technically sophisticated, and many demanding medical procedures can already be performed in Vietnam. Although improvements in medical technology will most likely play an important role in enhancing the quality of medical care, how much this process will help Vietnam achieve its major public health goals is not clear. For example, the main pediatrics hospital in the largest city can already deliver advanced neonatal care to save early preterm newborns. Such services are likely to be out of reach, however, for the many poor households on the fringes of society and the still large number of mothers giving birth at home.

The pharmaceutical sector has a prominent place in the Vietnamese health care system. Medicines, for example, absorbed half of all health spending in 2003 (MOH 2006). They were dispensed by a variety of providers only partly controlled and supervised systematically by the authorities. Despite existing laws and institutions to regulate the sale of pharmaceuticals, Vietnam is experiencing serious problems with antibiotic resistance, partly as a result of irrational use of drugs due to poor supervision and monitoring. Formally, responsibility for inspection and control of the pharmaceutical sector lies with the Drug Administration of Vietnam (DAV) and the MOH Department of Therapy. In practice, however, enforcing a policy for rational use of drugs is difficult, as indicated by the fact that 73 percent of all reported illnesses are treated by self-medication with over-the-counter drugs bought from public or private drug vendors (MOH 2003).

## The Health Coverage Reforms in Vietnam

The health system in 1986, prior to the Doi Moi series of socioeconomic reforms, was described in detail in a review of Vietnam's health sector (MOH 2001), on which this section strongly draws.

### *Rationale for Reforms in Vietnam*

The guiding principle of the Vietnamese health system prior to reform was "health for all." At grassroots, an extensive network of CHSs and intercommunal polyclinics provided the population with primary health care. Government hospitals treated people needing more intensive care. Despite the wide coverage, the quality of health care suffered from a lack of resources.

From a severe shortage of trained health workers at independence and very short-term basic training, the medical training of Vietnamese health workers improved as the system developed and medical schools expanded. Whereas in 1945 there were 180,000 persons per doctor, by 1985 the ratio had fallen to 3,137. Nevertheless, poor access to developments in medical science for training medical workers and low salaries were important causes of low-quality care. Materials and medicines, especially western drugs, were distributed through the health service but were generally insufficient, especially in CHSs. The health sector relied heavily on traditional medicine for treating common ailments, and distribution of the limited supply of modern drugs was tightly controlled. Supervision of health care services through inspections was infrequent due to limited availability of vehicles, fuel shortages, and absence of telephones in addition to limitations in clinical competence.

During the pre-reform period, only 3 to 4 percent of the state budget was allocated to health care, insufficient to cover the recurrent costs of government health facilities. Few funds were available to upgrade health facilities or provide medical equipment. Only some 8 percent of the perceived need for medical equipment was met. The basic operating costs of facilities above the commune level were covered solely through the government budget. The financing of CHSs depended on revenue from the agricultural cooperatives.

Foreign assistance from the former Soviet Union and other socialist countries dried up abruptly at the end of the 1980s. Because of the high dependency on foreign aid and the substantial government budget deficit at the time, health financing in Vietnam was severely constrained. Many health facilities did not even have enough money to maintain routine activities or pay salaries. Much of the medical equipment was obsolete or broken. The drug supply, already inadequate, worsened at every level. No longer could the government subsidize current expenditure for all health facilities, and alternative sources of finance had to be mobilized urgently to keep the health system afloat.

## Chronology of Reforms

The major economic and social reforms began with the Sixth Communist Party Congress, in 1986. The economy has gradually made the transition from a centrally planned to a socialist-oriented market economy. International trade and exchanges of information have increased. Dramatic economic growth and rapid improvements in living standards have been the result. However, gaps between rich and poor and between better-off and disadvantaged regions have widened in terms of both economic development and access to quality health care.

A series of health system financing reforms have been put in place at first to overcome resource constraints of the health system and more recently to narrow the gaps between rich and poor and advantaged and disadvantaged regions to ensure health for all. This section describes the main health financing reforms since Doi Moi began in 1986. A general overview of the chronology of the main reforms in Vietnam is provided in table 14.10.

The replacement of cooperative agriculture with family-based production in the Doi Moi reforms meant that the commune people's committees lost revenue from which to finance social services. The real income of CHS workers declined—their salary payments could be delayed by months—and their morale plummeted.

Starting in 1987 as part of the market-oriented reforms, private health and pharmaceutical sectors were officially sanctioned. As a result, Vietnam saw a rapid

**Table 14.10   Vietnam: Chronology of Health Reforms, 1989–2006**

| Year | Reform measure |
|------|----------------|
| 1989 | Fee for service<br>Private practice<br>Pharmaceutical sales |
| 1992 | Health insurance<br>Legal document on private practice |
| 1994 | Upgrading of the CHS system<br>Salary for the CHS staff<br>Health Policy Unit at MOH |
| 1996 | National drug policy<br>Policy for social mobilization (*Xa hoi hoa*) of health care<br>National target programs in health |
| 1997 | Provincial health system model |
| 1998 | Hunger Eradication, Poverty Reduction Program: Health Cards for the Poor |
| 1999 | Redefine goals of health sector reform |
| 2003 | Health Care Funds for the Poor (HCFP) |
| 2004 | Implement free health care for children under age 6 |
| 2005 | New health insurance regulations deepening coverage |
| 2006 | Drafting revision of HCFP and health care for the near-poor<br>Drafting health insurance law |

*Source:* Adapted from Adams 2005.

increase in private medical practice and retail pharmacies, but primarily in better-off areas and cities. Most private practices were small, and many of them were run by moonlighting government health workers. Greater freedom given to state pharmaceutical production and import companies and an increasing number of private pharmaceutical producers and distributors resulted in a rapid rise in the volume and diversity of pharmaceuticals on the market. As service at CHSs deteriorated, attendance at these facilities fell. People, including rural residents, resorted increasingly to more convenient and friendly over-the-counter drug purchases or private consultations for basic medical care despite its greater expense.

Also in 1987, in response to the dire state of many CHSs, the government decided that the provincial budget should subsidize salaries for a set number of CHS staff members per commune (typically three). However, by the early 1990s, only a third of CHSs were being subsidized in this way, and in 1994 the prime minister signed Decision 58/TTg, designating CHS staff members as government workers and allocating funds for their salaries to be paid from provincial budgets. This salary support has greatly improved income and morale among CHS workers, and it contributed to the strengthening of the Vietnam's public primary health care system.

Partial service fees and charges for drugs and diagnostics were officially introduced in public hospitals and other health facilities in 1989. The revenue was retained by the collecting facilities and was to be used to improve services. Certain population groups (such as children under age six, the poor, residents of remote or mountainous areas) were to be granted partial or total exemption from charges by the individual health facility, but this policy was inadequately funded and proved difficult to implement effectively or fairly. As a result, user charges have deterred people, especially the rural poor, from seeking public health care, and especially care at more expensive, higher-level hospitals. Although charging service fees has not been official policy for CHSs, many of them do levy a small fee. They may also earn substantial revenues from pharmaceutical sales.

Health insurance was introduced in Vietnam in 1992 to lighten the cost burden on the government health budget and increase people's access to health care. There was an initial surge in the number of people with compulsory, employment-related coverage and voluntary student insurance. Official documents have stated universal health insurance with equity of coverage and increased cost sharing of health service financing as a goal for 2010. However, attempts to extend voluntary health insurance to the general population have not met expectations and have led to serious problems of adverse selection. In 1998, and again in 2005, health insurance regulations were revised, gradually eliminating differences in the benefits packages between types of insurance and increasing the package of services and drugs reimbursable through health insurance. Cost-control measures put in place by the social security administration in charge of health insurance have forced some hospitals to underprovide health services to ensure that their costs do not exceed their annual allocation of health insurance funds.

Public health spending increased rapidly in real terms in the 1990s. In 1994, the MOH initiated a program to upgrade medical equipment in public hospitals. By 2000, central and provincial hospitals had most of the necessary equipment. Of district hospitals, 90 percent had X-ray machines; 70 percent, ultrasound machines; and 92 percent, ambulances. The Communist Party and the government issued guidelines for consolidating and strengthening the basic rural health network. External assistance helped finance the rehabilitation of CHSs and DHCs, focusing on disadvantaged areas. By 2002, 98 percent of the communes had a functioning CHS, and the goal is for every CHS to have a doctor by 2010.

Although the government is still increasing its contributions to the health sector, it is strongly pushing a policy of social mobilization (cost sharing) to mobilize additional funds for the health sector. An important component of this policy is the policy on semiautonomous public hospitals laid out in Decree 10 in 2002 and revised in 2006 by Decree 43. These facilities would move from state budget funding to a self-financing status with decentralized management powers. The purpose is to create incentives and conditions for public hospitals to operate more efficiently. There is some concern, however, that this policy will encourage commercialization of the Vietnamese hospital service, with perverse incentives to overuse investigations, drugs, and services to raise revenues and to concentrate on money-making activities to the detriment of other essential, but less lucrative, aspects of health care.

Household health care costs increased rapidly after the reforms and put a particularly heavy burden on poor rural households. Equitable access to, and utilization of, health care has always been a high priority of both the public health service and the Communist Party in Vietnam. Therefore in the mid-1990s, a policy of providing government-subsidized health insurance cards for the poor was put into effect to overcome the financial barriers to health care that resulted from the user-fee policy. Insufficient funds meant that not all the poor were covered, however, and the contribution per card was inadequate to cover the cost of services. To overcome these weaknesses, Decision 139/2002/QD-TTg provided for all provinces and cities to establish an HCFP with a major subsidy from the central state budget. The target beneficiaries include all poor people, as well as residents of disadvantaged communes and ethnic minorities in disadvantaged provinces. The amount allocated to the fund per poor person was increased substantially, and the provinces were allowed to use it either to purchase health insurance or to reimburse hospitals directly for health care services used by targeted beneficiaries.

In 2005, the Law on Protection and Care of Children came into effect, mandating free health care for children under six years of age. State budget funds were allocated, and the policy is being implemented as a direct reimbursement scheme from the state budget to state facilities providing health care to children under age six. Work is beginning on a health care policy for the elderly.

## Evaluation of Health Coverage Reforms

Vietnam's impressive achievements in reducing poverty and improving health and other outcomes among the population have attracted considerable interest from the international community, including health policy researchers and analysts. Quite a few studies have been published on several key outcomes, but only a handful of studies have applied rigorous quantitative analysis to gauge the causal effects of the policy interventions. The most important contributions to the impact are reviewed below.

Health insurance in Vietnam has been shown to have important impacts on health outcomes, access to health care, and out-of-pocket expenditures, especially for low-income individuals. Four recent studies have looked at the impact of the compulsory social health insurance program.

Wagstaff and Pradhan (2005) applied quantitative techniques, including double-difference and matching, to evaluate the impact of the government's social health insurance program on four outcomes: health, utilization, out-of-pocket spending, and poverty (nonmedical spending). Using panel data from the 1990s, they found that Vietnam's social health insurance has had a positive impact on height for age and weight for age of young school children and body mass index (BMI) of adults. This study also found that, for young children, health insurance increased use of primary care facilities and reduced self-medication. Among older children and adults, health insurance led to an increase in the use of hospital inpatient and outpatient care. Finally, the authors found that health insurance led to a reduction in annual out-of-pocket spending on health and an increase in nonmedical household consumption.

Using econometric modeling on the same data as the previous study, Sepehri, Sarma, and Simpson (2006) also found a positive effect of the compulsory social health insurance program on out-of-pocket spending. Controlling for unobserved heterogeneity, social health insurance reduced out-of-pocket expenditures between 16 and 18 percent with a more pronounced reduction for low-income individuals.

Wagstaff (2005) analyzed the effect of a negative health shock on income, medical spending, and household consumption. The author found that this type of health insurance does provide financial protection against the adverse effects of illness.

Finally, Chang and Trivedi (2003) also found a strong negative insurance effect on use of self-medication because the insured were much more likely than the uninsured to seek a medical consultation in case of illness. The application of these evaluation techniques to household survey data, including panel data, provides strong evidence of a positive and causal impact of this type of insurance on key policy outcomes.

With regard to the voluntary component of the Vietnamese health insurance program, Jowett, Contoyannis, and Vinh (2003) used a special survey to collect information from individuals on health care use and spending in three Vietnamese provinces in the late 1990s. Among other findings, the authors reported a 200 percent reduction in the average out-of-pocket spending for outpatient care. As to the effect of voluntary health insurance on utilization, Jowett, Deolalikar, and Martinsson (2004) found that, using the same data source and controlling for potential selection bias, voluntary health insurance in Vietnam led to higher use of outpatient facilities and public providers and less reliance on self-treatment and private providers, particularly strong effects at lower income levels. Although these studies are not national in scope, the finding that voluntary health insurance has had a positive impact is important for the government's policy development in the health sector.

Nguyen (2003) evaluated the impact of the health card initiatives introduced in the late 1990s as part of special programs to reach target groups. The author applies first-difference techniques coupled with propensity score matching on national household survey data from 2002 to analyze the impact on health care utilization and out-of-pocket spending. The results indicate only limited or no impact of the health care program on these outcomes. A recent report discusses several reasons for the apparent absence of an impact from these efforts to target the poor and other socially excluded groups, including incomplete implementation of the program, low levels of coverage, and finally, the need to improve the operation of the scheme so as to provide an effective protection mechanism (World Bank 2003a).

The policy of free health care to children under six has not yet been formally evaluated. However, a recent report discusses this policy, based on a case study of one central-level children's hospital in Hanoi (UNDP 2005). The report notes the hospital's increased patient load as a result of the policy. While it is too early to know for sure, the study discusses the possible effect on quality of care that the increase in utilization may have. In addition, future evaluations of this policy might usefully look at the benefit incidence of utilization of child care that may change to the advantage of the urban rich.

The impact of the program on Health Care Funds for the Poor has recently been evaluated using nonexperimental techniques, including propensity score matching (PSM) with national survey data. Among other things, the evaluation shows that the program has led to an increase in service utilization by the program beneficiaries (Axelson 2007). For example, those covered by the HCFP use services around 6 percent to 10 percent more than do the comparison persons. The program reduces out-of-pocket expenditure around 18 percent. The impact evaluation shows that catastrophic out-of-pocket payments are reduced by around 17 percent (personal communication). In addition, small studies designed to evaluate Decision 139 in particular provinces or regions have also shown promising results. Households interviewed in a WHO study in Bac Giang and Hai Duong provinces reported increased utilization of health services after implementation of the HCFP, especially for inpatient care (Axelson et al. 2005). The study also found a significant increase in health care seeking at the CHS as the first contact among HCFP beneficiaries.

Although these preliminary findings are encouraging, it is safe to say the implementation of this important program is not problem-free. The quality of primary health care, especially in remote areas, is still poor. Health insurance contributions are too low to cover the cost of the expanded package of services promised the insured, and dangerous deficits threaten the solvency of the health insurance fund. Incentives for both public and private health care facilities to overprescribe medicines or expensive diagnostic services have led to a rapid escalation in health expenditures and waste. The lack of adequate supervisory and quality control systems have exacerbated the overprovision of drugs and services and delayed further improvements in quality of care.

## Main Conditions for Success

During the implementation process of developing a policy for health financing in Vietnam, certain conditions for success have become evident. Providers need adequate funding to continue to provide health services. Although the state remains a primary financing source for government health services, user fees have helped fill the gap left by inadequate state financing so that provision, and the attempt to improve quality, can continue. Inadequate reimbursement of services by health insurance has led to underprovision of services or unofficial copayments by the insured. Finding out what full costs are is a precondition to ensuring their full coverage by existing financing sources. Only now, however, are studies being done to find out the full cost of services provided at state facilities.

Implementation of assistance programs for the poor or other target groups requires both clear targeting and adequate financing. The initial user-fee policy called for exemptions or reductions for the poor and children under age six. This policy failed because the facilities were not adequately reimbursed for the services provided, and targeting was unclear. A new policy to ensure health care for the poor promised a small amount of funding to buy health insurance for the very poorest. However, it did not provide clear criteria for targeting these people, and the contributions did not cover service costs. Since then, the policy for the poor and for children under age six has evolved so that more funding is available, and the targeting criteria are clear.

Monitoring and evaluating the impact of health financing policy has been important in orienting revisions or developing corrective policies for negative impacts. Findings from evaluations of the impact of user fees on access to care and the heavy burden of health expenditures on the poor was instrumental in convincing the government of the importance of a policy to assist the poor. Administrative monitoring of this policy, although it was not comprehensive and did not rely on a rigorous research process, was still adequate to show that earlier policies did not provide adequate coverage. This evidence impelled the development of the HCFP to ensure coverage for all poor and several near-poor groups.

### Assessment of Remaining Health System Strengths and Weaknesses

Compared with many other countries in a similar economic situation, Vietnam's health system is performing well, particularly at the primary health care level, despite some regional variations. Historically, the strong emphasis on the grassroots level with a wide organizational reach has likely contributed to the good health outcomes. The government continues to envision strong development of the health sector with an emphasis on developing medical technology in terms of both products and services. Moreover, its limited financial inputs compared with other countries and its favorable health outcomes suggest that Vietnam's health sector is relatively efficient.

Nonetheless, many difficulties persist in the performance of the health service delivery system. One problem that has been observed is high reliance on hospital care. Compared with other countries with similar national incomes, Vietnam ranks among the highest in terms of hospital beds per population, lower only than some of the countries of the former Soviet Union with its strong emphasis on hospital services (WHO 2006). Related to this is the inadequacy of the referral system, which leads to low utilization at lower levels and high use at upper levels of care, even for simple conditions. Moreover, the rational use of care is hampered by some weaknesses in the monitoring system where health information data are not systematically analyzed for use in planning and management.

A third issue is the observed differences in access to and utilization of health services in Vietnam. These differences have likely increased in the recent past and may continue to do so for some time. As discussed elsewhere in this chapter, however, the government has introduced measures to address these inequalities. The most important of these measures are Health Care Funds for the Poor and the policy of free health care for children under six years of age. Finally, the problem of irrational use of drugs and antibiotic resistance is an area in which the government will have to step up counteracting measures. Medical staff training, effective supervision, and the purposeful enforcement of existing regulations are important factors in this respect.

## Health Coverage Reforms: Enabling Factors and Lessons from Vietnam

The main health coverage reforms in Vietnam over the past two decades have been described in this chapter. During this period, the health sector has undergone many substantial transformations, including the introduction of cofinancing for health care, the private provision of services, and the gradual introduction of various types of prepayment mechanisms, including social health insurance and free health care for certain target groups. The discussion has also shown that coverage rates have increased steadily in terms of both services and health insurance. For example, today more than 90 percent of all children receive vaccinations compared with only around 55 percent in the mid-1980s. Over the same period, coverage by some type of health insurance has increased to almost 60 percent of the total population. Despite these successes, many problems remain, as illustrated by widespread child malnutrition, substantial inequalities in access to and utilization of health services, and the existence of catastrophic out-of-pocket payments for health care.

### Enabling Factors

The relative success of the Vietnamese government in extending health coverage to an increasingly larger share of the population, in terms of both services and health insurance, can be attributed to many different factors both inside and outside of the health sector. Among the most important such enabling factors outside of the health sector, three stand out. The first of these external factors is the rapid and sustained economic growth of the past 15 to 20 years that has enabled the government to embark on a series of ambitious health financing reforms and set the goal of universal health insurance by 2010. Although health spending as a share of GDP has remained largely constant over this period, per capita spending on health has increased from less than US$15 to over US$25. Moreover, the growth of national income has enabled the government to significantly increase its share of health spending. This has meant that substantial additional resources are now being channeled to the new entitlements of free health care for the poor and for children.

The importance of economic growth for sustainable financial support to government provision of health insurance is all the more evident, considering that Vietnam has received limited amounts of development assistance for health during this period. On average, less than 2 percent of total health spending has come from foreign assistance, compared with the much larger contributions seen in other low-income countries. Without economic growth of 6 to 7 percent a year, these reforms would still be wishes. Moreover, economic growth in Vietnam has been inclusive in that widespread poverty has been reduced. In light of the well-established importance of poverty reduction for improved health (and vice versa), this is a critical component of the Vietnamese experience.

One final result of sustained economic growth and limited dependence on development assistance for health is the fact that Vietnam has been able to develop and pursue policies that have been genuinely domestic in their scope and aims. This relative independence in policy making is not unique to the health sector. It can be seen in the country's overall development approach, which has meant that ownership of programs has been high and the incentive and ability to correct faulty implementation have been present.

The second enabling factor external to the health sector is the relatively well-structured and organized Vietnamese society. The political structure of the country, with at least nominally effective channels of communication from the central level down to the community level, has enabled the government to implement national policies fairly uniformly and in a timely fashion. As described above, the health care delivery system has a clear structure from village level up to the tertiary hospitals at the central level. This, combined with political stability in the postwar period, has most likely contributed to the government's ability to implement many of its policy programs.

Moreover, the relatively structured organization of Vietnamese society will probably be an important asset when the country computerizes its public management system, including the health information system, enabling the government to strengthen its monitoring and evaluation system. An effective information system will enable the authorities to implement even more effectively the special antipoverty programs targeting certain groups in difficult socioeconomic circumstances. Although recent reports have emphasized the limited leakage under these programs, the scope for further improvements should be evident from the broadened data bases after computerization of the health and other information systems.

One final enabling factor that can be seen as external to the health sector is the high esteem with which the Vietnamese people and the government have held health. For example, around a third of the population does some kind of regular exercise to stay healthy (MOH 2003). And the leadership has always emphasized public health as an important instrument for reducing widespread poverty. These sociocultural factors, combined with nutritional and healthy food consumption habits most likely also contribute to the good health outcomes in Vietnam compared with most other comparable countries. It can also be reasonably assumed that these factors have helped facilitate the uptake of the health coverage reforms, because the Vietnamese understand the importance of health for well-being.

In addition to these external factors, at least three elements within the health sector can help explain Vietnam's good performance in providing its people with health service and financial coverage over the past 20 years. The first of these is the inheritance of a wide network of primary health care services. The grassroots level of the system has long been seen as the most important part of an effective and equitable service delivery system. Over the course of reform, the government has built strategically on these past investments to further develop their efficiency in providing the population with needed services and interventions. Moreover, a clear policy goal of the government has long been able to provide the necessary interventions for disease prevention and eradication. The strategic approach of providing effective preventive care for specific infectious diseases has led to a decline in the burden of disease from those conditions and a relative increase in the disease burden due to conditions that cannot be easily prevented by traditional means.

The second important internal factor has been the timing, scope, and sequencing of the identified reform measures. In terms of service provision, the government identified a set of priority health problems and diseases on which to concentrate its attempts to diminish the burden of disease. Although other problems may have existed, setting priorities was seen as a necessary means for putting scarce resources to the best use. Furthermore, the priorities have been allowed to adapt to the gradually changing epidemiological pattern, for example, by the inclusion of HIV/AIDS prevention in the national disease priority program and the issuing of policies on tobacco control and prevention of accidents and injuries.

Finally, besides skilled health professionals and clinicians, effective and equitable health care requires extensive planning and management capacities, and the Vietnamese health sector is blessed with such skills. Within every level of the system, a formal structure delineates the management responsibilities of each type of provider. One result is the production of clear operational plans for the coming activity period. The weakness of the system is patchy monitoring. Related to the health planning and management skills of the health system is the capacity to develop useful health policies. A strategic effort on behalf of the central health authorities is to develop skills and capacities in health policy making, including analysis of the efficiency and distributional impact of policies and programs.

### Lessons from Health Coverage Reforms in Vietnam

Many of the health coverage reforms that Vietnam has introduced can be implemented in other countries, but some of the enabling factors might not be easy to replicate. For example, special funds to finance the health care needs of certain groups can theoretically be introduced in other contexts. The long-term sustainability of such programs, however, presumably requires relatively high economic growth for extended periods of time and rapid declines in the size of beneficiary groups.

With regard to political economy factors, an important dimension of the Vietnamese experience has been economic and political stability. The one-party structure of the Vietnamese governance system has enabled the country to develop policies that have been allowed to be implemented over a long period of time without interference from varying and sometimes competing political factions. The policy lesson from this factor points to the need to reach agreements on health policy reform measures that span the political divide in multiparty democracies. Otherwise, health reform measures may not be allowed to run their course over a sufficiently long time to take effect.

In terms of good value for money, the importance Vietnam has put on primary health care can serve as an important lesson to other low- and middle-income countries now introducing health coverage reforms. As noted, the grassroots level has been the backbone of the health care system. It has enabled the health sector to gradually introduce ever more advanced organizational and medical procedures, such as provider payment reforms and liberalizations of the health care production markets.

Low-income countries need to build a national capacity to develop, implement, and evaluate health coverage programs and other policies. Moreover, countries should attempt to use such capacities most effectively by pooling analytical resources, thereby creating a critical mass for effective health policy analysis. Lessons from Vietnam in this respect also include the strategic use of development assistance without allowing it to become too dominating. Generally, Vietnam has used its development assistance in health to develop health policy and other core competences and to implement the national disease priority programs.

In terms of health insurance coverage, the experiences of Vietnam with design and sequencing of implementation may be of interest to other countries. While universal coverage may be the long-term goal, countries should not attempt to reach it too quickly or by means of only one or two alternatives. Vietnam initiated its health financing coverage attempts by introducing social health insurance in the early 1990s. The eligible groups were well defined, and the benefits package of services was identified, although in the case of Vietnam it may be too broad. Gradually, more people were covered by prepayment as other programs were introduced, including voluntary health insurance and free health cards for the poor.

Importantly, the most recently implemented insurance benefits package was defined to dovetail with the initial program, thereby creating a certain level of transparency in the health insurance system. This pattern was repeated with introduction of the Health Care Funds for the Poor in 2003. Creating a uniform benefits package in this way limits the scope for overlap within the health insurance system, which reduces transaction costs. Should the government choose to liberalize the health insurance market by allowing private for-profit agents to enter, this last point may become even more important because private actors would then compete with existing insurance programs. From the client's perspective, a relatively uniform and generous benefits package would facilitate the choice between alternative programs and prevent private firms from skimming the market.

Inasmuch as every country attempting to achieve universal health coverage faces public resource limitations, one lesson from Vietnam concerns the importance of targeting those scarce resources to the people most in need. Recent analysis has shown that, compared with many other countries, Vietnam has been able to develop effective targeting mechanisms with limited leakage and undercoverage (World Bank 2003a). Because it has also been shown that these achievements are a result of a pragmatic approach by local authorities (Vietnam Dev Report 2004), another lesson from Vietnam would be that the successful implementation of target programs requires some operational decentralization. For administrative cost-effectiveness, it was also important that the health sector could latch on to the targeting being done by the Hunger Eradication and Poverty Reduction program, instead of having to fund the heavy administrative work of doing its own targeting.

Finally, the case of Vietnam also highlights the importance of introducing health coverage reforms gradually and incrementally. Vietnam introduced social health insurance for the formally employed first then made a concerted effort to cover the poor and the socially excluded. This approach gave the authorities important opportunities for learning by doing, lessons that will be valuable when tackling the persistent and most difficult challenges of increasing coverage rates for the rural poor. The importance cannot be sufficiently emphasized of having good information and knowledge about the health care–seeking behaviors of different target groups, such as children, the rural poor, and women.

## Endnotes

1. Unless otherwise noted, the October 24, 2006, exchange rate is used throughout this chapter: US$1 = Vietnamese Dong (VND) 16,080.

2. These exceptions are treatment of leprosy; medicines for treatment of TB, malaria, schizophrenia, epilepsy, and other diseases already covered by government-funded programs; diagnosis and treatment of HIV/AIDS, except when HIV tests are part of protocols for treatment of other diseases or if the individual was infected with HIV through work; syphilis and gonorrhea; immunizations, nursing care, early diagnosis of pregnancy, health checkups, family planning services, and infertility treatment; plastic surgery, prosthetics, false teeth, eyeglasses, and hearing aids; occupational diseases, labor accidents, and war-related accidents; treatment costs in suicide attempts, self-inflicted harm, drug addiction or health problems associated with illegal activities or behavior; health assessments for legal reasons; and consultations, treatments, rehabilitation, or home deliveries.

3. For example: special requests for services such as selecting their own practitioner, type of bed, or specific facility; bypassing a primary care facility without a referral; seeking treatment at a facility that does not have a contract with health insurance; seeking care at a private facility; or seeking treatment overseas.

## References

Adams, S. 2005. "Vietnam's Health Care System: A Macroeconomic Perspective." Paper prepared for the International Symposium on Health Care Systems in Asia at Hitotsubashi University, Tokyo, January 21–22.

Akal, A. 2004. "A Comprehensive Review of Health Insurance and Financing Regulations: FAQs." Background paper, WHO, Hanoi, September.

Axelson, H. 2007. "Impact of Decision 139 on Health Care Utilization: A Study Using Propensity Score Matching." Background Paper on Workshop on Impact Evaluation of Decision 139, Hanoi.

Axelson, H., D. V. Cuong, N. K. Phuong, T. T. M.Oanh, D. H. Luong, and K. A. Tuan. 2005. "The Impact of the Health Care Fund for the Poor on Poor Households in Two Provinces in Vietnam." Paper presented at Forum 9, Global Forum for Health Research, Mumbai, September 12–16. Health Strategy and Policy Institute and World Health Organization, Hanoi.

Baulch, B., Truong Thi Kim Chuyen, Dominique Hougton, and Jonathan Hougton. 2002. "Ethnic Minority Development in Vietnam: A Socioeconomic Perspective." WPS 2836, World Bank, Washington, DC.

Chang, F. R., and P. K. Trivedi. 2003. "Economics of Self-Medication: Theory and Evidence." *Health Economics* 12(9): 721–39.

Chien T. T. T., ed. 2005. *Health Care for the Poor in Vietnam.* Hanoi: Medical Publishing House.

———. 2003. *Vietnam Health Report 2002,* Hanoi: Medical Publishing House.

Dieleman, M., P. V. Cuong, L. V. Anh, and T. Martineau. 2003. "Identifying Factors for Job Motivation of Rural Health Workers in North Vietnam." *Human Resources for Health:* 10. http://www.human-resources-health.com/content/1/1/10.

Dong, Tham Tat, Pham Trong Thanh, Dam Viet Cuong, Duong Huy Lieu, and Nguyen Hoang Long, eds. 2002. *User Fee, Health Insurance and Utilization of Health Services.* Hanoi: Vietnam–Sweden Health Cooperation Programme.

Glewwe, P., Nisha Agrawal, and David Dollar, eds. 2004. *Economic Growth, Poverty, and Household Welfare in Vietnam.* Washington, DC: World Bank.

Government of Vietnam. 2003. "The Comprehensive Poverty Reduction and Growth Strategy (CPRGS)/Poverty Reduction Strategy Paper (PRSP)," Government of Vietnam/International Monetary Fund/World Bank, Hanoi.

Government of Vietnam and World Bank. 2005. *Vietnam—Management of Public Finances for Growth and Poverty Reduction: Public Expenditure Review.* Vols. 1 and 2. Hanoi: Finance Publishing House.

GSO (General Statistical Office). Various years. "Vietnam Household Living Standards Survey." GSO, Hanoi.

Gwatkin, D., Adam Wagstaff, and Abdo Yazbeck. 2005. *Reaching the Poor with Health, Nutrition, and Population Services: What Works, What Doesn't, and Why.* Washington, DC: World Bank.

Health Strategy and Policy Institute and World Health Organization. 2004. "Assessment of Decision 139 Implementation." Informal paper, Hanoi.

ILO (International Labour Office). 2006. "Enhancing Social Protection in Vietnam-Developing the New Social Security Law." Informal paper, Hanoi.

IMF (International Monetary Fund). 2005. "Vietnam: 2004 Article IV." Consultation–Staff Report, IMF, Washington, DC.

Jowett, Matthew, P. Contoyannis, and N. D. Vinh 2003. "The Impact of Public Voluntary Health Insurance on Private Health Expenditures in Vietnam." *Social Science and Medicine* 56: 333–42.

Jowett, M., A. Deolalikar, and Peter Martinsson. 2004. "Health Insurance and Treatment-Seeking Behaviour: Evidence from a Low-Income Country." *Health Economics* 13: 845–57.

Knowles, James C., Nguyen Thi Hong Ha, Dang Boi Huong, Nguyen Khang, Tran Thi Mai Oanh, Nguyen Khanh Phuong, Vu Ngoc Uyen. 2003. *Making Health Care More Affordable for the Poor: Health Financing in Vietnam*. Vol. 1: Main Report, MOH/ADB TA-3877-VIE. Hanoi.

———. 2003. *Making Health Care More Affordable for the Poor: Health Financing in Vietnam*. Vol. 2, Annexes, MOH/ADB TA-3877-VIE, Hanoi.

Lieu, D. H., N. H. Long, D. B. Huong, S. Bales, N. K. Phuong, C. Jiaying, M. Segall, and H. Lucas. 2005. "Alternative Approaches to Ensure Health Care for the Rural Poor: Lessons for Vietnam from the Chinese Experience." Draft Report, Ministry of Health, Hanoi.

Lieu, D. H., Nguyen H. Long, and Sarah Bales. 2007. *Study on Treatment Costs for Selected Disease Groups in Provincial General Hospitals*. Hanoi: Medical Publishing House.

Lieu, D. H., N. Q. An, and Nguyen H. Long. 2007. Study on Health Care Financing from a Household and User Perspective." Hanoi: Medical Publishing House.

Minh, H. V., N. Khang, and N. V. Dung. 2004. "Health Care Financing for the Poor in Vietnam," Working Paper No. 2004-8, World Bank, Washington, DC.

Ministry of Finance, Vietnam. 2005. "Medium-Term Expenditure Framework," Hanoi.

MOH (Ministry of Health, Vietnam). 2006. "National Health Accounts 1998–2003." Hanoi: Statistical Publishing House.

———. 2005. "Treatment Costs for Selected Disease Groups at Provincial General Hospitals." VSHC/HPC, Hanoi.

———. 2004a. "Assessment of 1-Year Implementation of Decision 139." MOH, Hanoi.

———. 2004b. *National Health Accounts: The Process of Implementation and Development in Vietnam*. Hanoi: Statistical Publishing House.

———. 2003. "Vietnam National Health Survey 2001/02." Main report, MOH, Hanoi.

———. 2001. *55 Years of Developing Vietnam's Revolutionary Health System* [55 nam phat trien su nghiep y te cach mang Vietnam] Hanoi: Medical Publishing House.

MPI (Ministry of Planning and Investment). 2005. *The Five-Year Socioeconomic Development Plan 2006–2010*. Hanoi: MPI.

Nguyen, V.C. 2003. "Assessing the Coverage and Impact of Vietnam's Programs for Targeted Transfers to the Poor Using the Vietnam Household Living Standard Survey 2002," World Bank, Hanoi.

Sepehri A., S. Sarma, and W. Simpson. 2006. "Does Nonprofit Health Insurance Reduce Financial Burden?—Evidence from the Vietnam Living Standards Survey Panel." *Health Economics* 15: 603–16.

Sepehri A., R. Chernomas, and H. Akram-Lodhi. 2005. "Penalizing Patients and Rewarding Providers: User Charges and Health Care Utilization in Vietnam." *Health Policy and Planning* 20(2): 90–99.

UNDP (United Nations Development Programme). 2005. "Preliminary Assessment of Free Health Care for Under-Six-Year-Old Children Policy at Central Pediatric Hospital." Report to UNDP workshop on Financial Policy Analysis, Hanoi.

Van de Walle, D. 2004. "Testing Vietnam's Public Safety Net." *Journal of Comparative Economics* 32: 661–79.

Van de Walle, D., and D. Gunewardena. 2000. "Sources of Ethnic Inequality in Vietnam." Policy Research Working Paper 2297, World Bank, Washington, DC.

Wagstaff, Adam. 2005. "The Economic Consequences of Health Shocks." World Bank Policy Research Paper 3655, Washington, DC.

Wagstaff, Adam, and Eddy van Doorslaer. 2003. "Catastrophe and Impoverishment in Paying for Health Care: With Applications to Vietnam 1993–1998." *Health Economics* 12: 921–34.

Wagstaff, Adam, and M. Pradhan 2005. "Health Insurance Impacts on Health and Nonmedical Consumption in a Developing Country," WPS 3563, World Bank, Washington, DC.

World Bank. 2006. World Development Indicators (WDI). World Bank. Washington, DC.

———. 2005. "Vietnam: Managing Public Expenditure for Poverty Reduction and Growth—PER and IFA." World Bank, Hanoi.

———. 2004. "Vietnam Development Report 2005: Governance." World Bank, Hanoi.

———. 2003a. "Vietnam Development Report 2004: Poverty." World Bank, Hanoi.

———. 2003b. "Ninh Thuan PPA, Poverty Task Force." World Bank, Hanoi.

———. 2001. "Growing Healthy: A Review of Vietnam's Health Sector." World Bank, Hanoi.

WHO (World Health Organization). 2006. *World Health Report 2006: Working Together for Health*. Geneva: WHO.

———. 2003. "Health and Ethnic Minorities in Vietnam." Technical Series No. 1, WHO, Hanoi.

# About the Coeditors and Contributors

## THE COEDITORS

*Pablo Gottret* is the lead economist of Health, Nutrition, and Population in the Human Development Network of the World Bank. Before joining the World Bank in 2002, he was viceminister of budgeting in his native Bolivia (1987–90) and chief executive of the Regulatory Body for Private Pensions, Private Insurance, and Securities (1998–2002). Gottret led the technical teams that developed Bolivia's Capital Markets Law, Insurance Law, and reforms to the Pension System Law approved by the Bolivian Congress between 1997 and 1998. He has worked in several countries in Latin America, Africa, and Eastern Europe. Gottret has a PhD in economics from Texas A&M University with specializations in econometrics, natural resource economics, and finance. He has published several books and articles in refereed journals.

*George J. Schieber* is a public finance economist with more than 30 years of domestic and international experience in health policy and economic issues, working in more than 40 countries. He has been an assistant professor of economics at the University of Pittsburgh, a staff member at the Urban Institute, and an economist at the OECD, Paris. He has held various positions in the U.S. government, including the director of the Office of Research and Demonstrations in the U.S. Health Care Financing Administration, and at the World Bank, including health and social protection manager in the Middle East and North Africa Region. He is currently a consultant to the World Bank and various governments. He has published more than 60 books and articles. Schieber holds a PhD in economics from Syracuse University.

*Hugh R. Waters* is a health economist and associate professor in the Department of Health Policy and Management at the Johns Hopkins Bloomberg School of Public Health. His areas of expertise are (1) health insurance and health financing reforms; (2) evaluation of the effects of health financing mechanisms on access, equity, and quality; and (3) economic evaluation of health care interventions. He has 19 years' experience working with public health programs and has worked extensively as a consultant with the World Bank, World Health Organization, and other international organizations. He currently teaches a course on comparative health financing systems at the Bloomberg School of Public Health. He holds a PhD in public health economics from the same institution and an MS in international economics from Georgetown University.

## THE AUTHORS

*Hédi Achouri, M.D.,* graduated from the Faculty of Medicine of Tunis (1980). He practiced general medicine and was regional director for public health until 1986. Since 1987, he has been director of public hospitals in the Tunisian Ministry of Public Health headquarters. He was a founding member and president of the Maghreb Economics and Health Systems Network, a nongovernmental organization working in the fields of health economics and health systems management in the Maghreb Region (Algeria, Morocco, and Tunisia). He is currently chairman of the Board of Habib Thameur Hospital (Tunis), a member of the Board of the National Health Insurance Fund, and general director of health public facilities in the Tunisian Ministry of Public Health headquarters. Among his recent publications is *Advances in Implementing Social Security: Lessons from Tunisia* (GTZ, Germany, 2007).

*Chokri Arfa* was a health economist at the National Institute of Public Health (1995-2002). He is currently assistant professor and head of the Research Department at the National Institute of Labor and Social Studies, University of Carthage. He is the coauthor of several health economics studies and a book on "Economie et Santé: Evaluation et stratégies de mise en œuvre". His research interests are national health accounts, health performance, and health surveys. He has worked as a short-term consultant for several national and international studies. His most recent expertise is Tunisian's health accounts and monography of health insurance. In 2007, he was awarded a prize at the European Workshop on Efficiency and Productivity Analysis X in Lille, France, for work on how to expand the use of production capacity in Tunisian's local hospitals.

*Sarah Bales,* a statistician, works as a health policy adviser to the Ministry of Health in Vietnam. She has extensive experience in health economic and policy analysis and has contributed statistical expertise to several national health and household surveys in Vietnam. Most recently, she was the principal statistical expert for the impact evaluation of the Vietnamese health financing program for the poor.

*Ricardo Bitrán D.,* an industrial engineer from the University of Chile, with an MBA in finance and PhD in economics from University of Boston, is a senior health economist with 25 years of experience in Chile, the United States, and more than 40 developing countries. At the University of Chile he is professor of public health in the School of Public Health, professor of health economics in the Master's in Public Policy Program, and adjunct assistant professor. His areas of expertise include economic evaluation of health investment and reform projects; study of health care markets; analysis of equity, efficiency, and financial sustainability; and delivery and financing of primary health care services. During his 10 years with Abt Associates Inc. of Cambridge, Massachusetts, first as a health economist and then as a senior scientist, he was also research director for the HFS Project, a US$18-million initiative funded by the U.S. Agency for International Development. Since 1994, he has been president and senior partner of Bitrán & Asociados. His 20 years of academic experience have encompassed teaching posts or assignments in Chile, China, France, Lebanon, Thailand, the United States, Zaire, and many other countries. He has been senior adviser to the GAVI Alliance and World Bank on health immunizations issues and academic director of the World Bank Institute Flagship Program in Health Sector Reform and Sustainable Financing in Latin American and the Caribbean Region. Bitrán is author of academic articles, books, and scientific papers.

*James Cercone* is an economist and president of Sanigest Internacional, a health care management and consulting company. He developed his interests in health economics and health reform through engagements with the World Bank (1990–94) and the government of Costa Rica (1994–97). He has more than 16 years' experience in the health sector, with particular emphasis on Latin America and transition countries. In the past five years, Cercone has been involved in the startup of several venture capital funds focusing on health sector investments, as well as provided investment and investment advice to clients around the world. His experience covers more than 40 countries, with emphasis on health policy reforms, private sector investment, impact of corruption in the health sector, hospital restructuring, health insurance reform and purchasing strategies, development of provider payment mechanisms, performance improvement, economic analysis of health projects, monitoring and evaluation, development of HIV/AIDS strategies, and management of health care services. Cercone has worked extensively on the design, implementation, and evaluation of projects for the World Bank, Inter-American Development Bank, ILO, and other development organizations.

*Björn Ekman* is an economist from Lund University in southern Sweden. He is currently assistant professor in the Health Economics Program (HEP) at Lund University. His research interests are health financing and health systems development in low- and middle-income countries and the economics of maternal and child health. He has worked as a consultant for WHO, Sida, and ADB in Asia and Africa.

**Lisa Fleisher** is a senior analyst with the Health Systems 20/20 Project, funded by USAID and implemented by Abt Associates Inc. She has worked in international health and development for the past six years. Her areas of expertise include health financing, health system strengthening, health policy analysis, and global public health. Currently, Fleisher's work is focused primarily on providing technical support to the HIV/AIDS and National Health Accounts components of Health Systems 20/20. Before that, Fleisher was a public health specialist at the World Bank, where she worked on health financing and health systems, issues related to the global health aid architecture, and the World Bank's new strategy for health, nutrition, and population. Other experience includes the implementation and administration of USAID-funded activities for youth reproductive health and HIV/AIDS prevention in Africa and Latin America, as well as grant making in health services research focused on domestic health care financing and organization. Fleisher received her master of public health in international health from the Johns Hopkins Bloomberg School of Public Health and her BA in human biology from Stanford University.

**Jarno Habicht, M.D.,** is head of the World Health Organization Country Office in Estonia, in the WHO Regional Office for Europe. Before joining WHO, he worked for the Ministry of Social Affairs in Estonia, the World Bank, and the Estonian Health Insurance Fund. He has previous experience in health services research and management of research programs. He is currently a PhD student in public health at the University of Tartu, Estonia.

**Triin Habicht** heads the Health Economics Department in the Estonian Health Insurance Fund. She has also been working for the Estonian Ministry of Social Affairs in the public health area. Habicht is currently doing her PhD in economics at the University of Tartu, Estonia.

**Melitta Jakab** is a WHO policy adviser in the Kyrgyz Republic, working mostly on health care financing issues and equity analysis. Previously, she worked at the World Bank in Washington, D.C., and in Hungary. Jakab has a PhD in health policy with concentration in economics from Harvard University.

**Adam Leive,** currently an economist with the Fiscal Affairs Department of the International Monetary Fund, worked in the Health, Nutrition, and Population Department of the World Bank during research for this volume. He has a master's degree in health economics from the University of York, United Kingdom, and a BA from Princeton University in the Woodrow Wilson School of Public and International Affairs.

**Elina Manjieva,** a WHO consultant, works in the Center for Health System Development under the Ministry of Health of the Kyrgyz Republic. Previously, she was a junior professional associate in the Human Development Unit of the World Bank Country Office in the Kyrgyz Republic. Elina has an MA in development economics and southwest Asian studies from the Fletcher School, Tufts University.

*José Pacheco Jiminez* holds an MA in development economics from the Institute of Social Studies in The Hague, the Netherlands. Between 2001 and 2003, he was a staff member of the Ministry of Finance of Costa Rica and worked as a consultant for the Congress, the National Bank, and the Telecommunications Company of Costa Rica. Since 2003, he has worked for Sanigest Internacional, where he is director of the Department of Social Economics and coordinator of R&D. Pacheco has participated in more than 25 projects in 17 countries around the world, particularly in Latin America, the Caribbean, Eastern Europe, and Central Asia, where he has focused on payment mechanisms, contracting, health insurance, financing, and poverty analysis.

*Diana Margarita Pinto Masís* received her MD and master in health administration from the Pontificia Universidad Javeriana, Bogotá, and her doctor of science from the International Health Policy and Economics program at the Harvard School of Public Health. She worked as a technical adviser at the Colombian Ministry of Social Protection, developing and executing projects to evaluate the design of the benefits packages and the financial sustainability of the health system. She is currently associate professor in health economics at the Department of Clinical Epidemiology of Pontificia Universidad Javeriana School of Medicine and an associate researcher at Fedesarrollo. Her research interests include impact evaluation of health policy and health interventions, technology assessment, and health system performance assessment.

*Ravi P. Rannan-Eliya* is a physician and economist who was graduated from the University of Cambridge with degrees in political science and medicine. After his internship in the United Kingdom, he specialized in international public health, earning a master's degree in public health and then his doctoral degree in health economics from Harvard University. From 1993 to 1997, he was a member of the research faculty at Harvard University, where he worked on a series of research projects in Latin America, Africa, and Asia. From 1997, he established and developed the leading health economics research group in Sri Lanka, at the Institute of Policy Studies, before transforming it in 2005 into a full-fledged, independent research center, the Institute for Health Policy, which he now heads. He has undertaken research and consulted in more than 30 countries, working with the World Bank, WHO, ADB, and other agencies and governments. His current research focuses on issues of health systems financing, aging, equity, and noncommunicable disease.

***Lankani Sikurajapathy*** was a research assistant at the Institute for Health Policy at the time of writing and now works for UNFPA in Sri Lanka. She was graduated with a degree in sociology with social policy from University of Warwick, before completing a master's degree in comparative social policy at the University of Oxford. While at IHP, she worked on a number of projects related to health systems financing and development of district health performance indicators.

***Ajay Tandon*** is a senior economist with the Health, Nutrition, Population hub at the World Bank in Washington, D.C. He has a PhD in economics from Virginia Tech. He has worked on a variety of issues related to health economics, including the measurement and evaluation of health system metrics. He worked previously with the Asian Development Bank in Manila, Philippines, as well as the World Health Organization in Geneva, Switzerland. He also held research appointments at the University of Oxford and Harvard University.

***Suriwan Thaiprayoon*** is a new health policy analyst. She earned her undergraduate degree in Nursing Science before she obtained her master's degree in international public health (Honors) from the University of Sydney, Australia. Her main interests are universal health care coverage, mechanisms of international cooperation and healthy public policy. Thaiprayoon served as a technical assistant to the Thai public health minister from October 2006 to February 2008. She currently works at the Bureau of International Health, Ministry of Public Health, Thailand.

***Gonzalo Urcullo C.,*** an economist from the Catholic University of Bolivia, holds a master's in management and public policy from the University of Chile. For more than a decade, he has worked in key posts in Bolivia's government, assessing the Council of Ministries in the areas of industry, tourism, telecommunications, mining, environment, and transport. He has worked in the fields of economic regulation, promotion of competition, public credit, and decentralization of planning. Urcullo also has experience in social areas. He has a diploma in labor economics from San Simon University in Cochabamba, Bolivia, and has worked in the Ministry of Education. He has also worked formulating public development strategies to reach the Millennium Development Goals. Urcullo has published in the areas of pension systems, regulation, economic development, and health financing. Since January 2006, he been an associate at Bitrán & Asociados, working on health projects in Bangladesh, Bolivia, Chile, El Salvador, Guatemala, and Peru.

***Suwit Wibulpolprasert, M.D.,*** is a general practitioner, a public health specialist, an administrator, and a policy advocate. He began his career as a director and a practitioner in four rural district hospitals in Thailand (1977–85). Later he was the director of the Northeastern Public Health College, the director of the Technical Division of the FDA, the director of the Bureau of Health Policy and Plan, and assistant permanent secretary and deputy permanent secretary of the Ministry of

Public Health. His main interests are in health policy and planning, and international health. He has been extensively involved in research and development in the areas of human resources for health, health economics and health care financing, international trade and health, health promotion, health information, and pharmaceuticals. He has published more than 100 papers, reports and books locally and internationally.

In Thailand, Dr. Suwit is the editor of a local journal for paramedical personnel and has produced radio and television programs on health and social issues for more than 15 years. He is currently president of the Folk Doctor Foundation; evaluation board member of the Thailand Research Fund; and board member of the Health Systems Research Institute, the National Health Security Board, the Thai Medical Research Council, the National Nanotechnology Centre, the Mahidol University Council, and the National Science and Technology Board.

As part of his international involvements, he represents Thailand in many international health forums and the World Health Assembly. He also represented Thailand and the Southeast Asia Region as a member and vice chair of the governing board of the Global Fund to Fight AIDS, TB, and Malaria from mid-2001 to March 2004. He was also president of the Intergovernmental Forum on Chemical Safety from November 2003 to September 2006 and a member and vice chair of the WHO executive board in 2004–07. At present, Dr. Suwit is a board member of the Health Metrics Network and the Mekong Basin Disease Surveillance Network. He chairs the steering committee of Asian Partnership on Avian Influenza Research and the steering committee of the Asia–Pacific Action Alliance on HRH. He is also a member and represents the chair of the Program Coordinating Board of the UNAIDS, and he is a member and chair of the Program and Policy Committee of the Interim Board of the Global Health Workforce Alliance. He served as a deputy permanent secretary at the Ministry of Public Health, Thailand, in 2000–03. Currently, he serves as a senior adviser in disease control and is also responsible for health policy and international health works of the ministry.

# Index